AF902255

HYDROCEPHALUS

Edited by **Sadip Pant** and **Iype Cherian**

Hydrocephalus
Edited by Sadip Pant and Iype Cherian

Published by InTech
Janeza Trdine 9, 51000 Rijeka, Croatia

Copyright © 2012 InTech
All chapters are distributed under the Creative Commons Attribution 3.0 license, which allows users to download, copy and build upon published articles even for commercial purposes, as long as the author and publisher are properly credited, which ensures maximum dissemination and a wider impact of our publications. After this work has been published by InTech, authors have the right to republish it, in whole or part, in any publication of which they are the author, and to make other personal use of the work. Any republication, referencing or personal use of the work must explicitly identify the original source.

As for readers, this license allows users to download, copy and build upon published chapters even for commercial purposes, as long as the author and publisher are properly credited, which ensures maximum dissemination and a wider impact of our publications.

Notice
Statements and opinions expressed in the chapters are these of the individual contributors and not necessarily those of the editors or publisher. No responsibility is accepted for the accuracy of information contained in the published chapters. The publisher assumes no responsibility for any damage or injury to persons or property arising out of the use of any materials, instructions, methods or ideas contained in the book.

Publishing Process Manager Anja Filipovic

Technical Editor Teodora Smiljanic

Cover Designer InTech Design Team

Additional hard copies can be obtained from orders@intechopen.com

Hydrocephalus, Edited by Sadip Pant and Iype Cherian
p. cm.
ISBN 978-953-51-0162-8

We are IntechOpen, the world's leading publisher of Open Access books

Built by scientists, for scientists

4,100+
Open access books available

116,000+
International authors and editors

120M+
Downloads

151
Countries delivered to

Our authors are among the
Top 1%
most cited scientists

12.2%
Contributors from top 500 universities

WEB OF SCIENCE™

Selection of our books indexed in the Book Citation Index
in Web of Science™ Core Collection (BKCI)

Interested in publishing with us?
Contact book.department@intechopen.com

Numbers displayed above are based on latest data collected.
For more information visit www.intechopen.com

For EU product safety concerns:
IN TECH d.o.o., Prolaz Marije Krucifikse Kozulić 3, 51000 Rijeka, Croatia,
info@intechopen.com or visit our website at intechopen.com.

Meet the editors

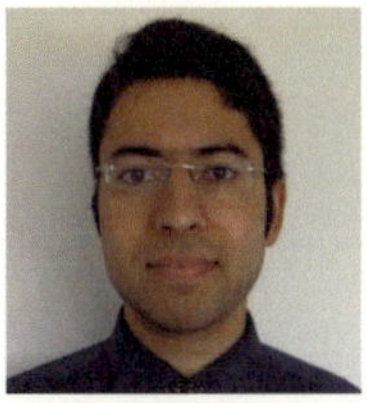

Dr Sadip Pant is currently affiliated to Department of Internal Medicine, University of Arkansas for Medical Sciences, USA. He graduated from Manipal College of Medical Sciences and has an outstanding clinical career. Besides being an excellent physician, he has a keen interest in translational research. He has published numerous papers in peer reviewed international journals, directed many book chapters and serves as a reviewer for McGill Journal of Medicine, Internet Journal of Medical Update, International Journal of Applied and Basic Medical Research, Calicut Medical Journal, Pan African Medical Journal and Journal of Bioengineering and Biomedical Research. Dr Pant is also a member of American Medical Association, American College of Physicians, Massachusetts Medical Society, Nepal Medical Association.

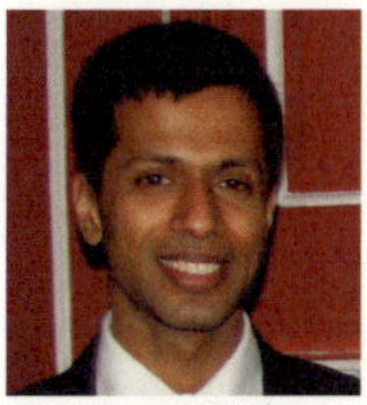

Dr Iype Cherian completed his MCh Neurosurgery from Christian Medical College, Vellore and Fellowship in Neurovascular Surgery from Fujita University, Japan. He has been credited for inventing the Mingwei technique which uses cisternostomy in head injuries. Dr Cherian has been teaching this technique to neurosurgeons in various countries and it is slowly getting popular. He is also a reviewer of the renowned Asian Journal of Neurosurgery and is a member of education committee of Asian Council of Neurosurgeons. Besides, he has authored various papers in peer reviewed international journals. He has delivered a talk in Cambridge as an invited speaker on the status of Neurosurgery in Nepal. He is currently the Chief of Neurosurgery and Program Director for MCh Neurosurgery program in College of Medical Sciences, Bharatpur, Nepal.

Contents

Preface

A child with a large head and a sick malnourished body was the epitome of poverty from the older days… But, the large head started getting noticed in children from well to do families as well. And then as the studies on Hydrocephalus progressed, simple ways of shunting the fluid away from the ventricles to any other cavity like the atrium, pleural cavity and peritoneal cavity evolved after considerable attempts to destroy the choroid plexus, but did not bear as much fruits.

The reasons for hydrocephalus (of course, the ones other than abject poverty) were looked into and the disease was classified to be either obstructive or non-obstructive (also termed communicative, a misnomer actually)… and then the logical ways of dealing with each appeared.

The shunt was a panacea for both, but then Endoscopy came along. The third ventriculostomy literally changed the scene with no implants, and thus abolishing the most feared complication of all, shunt infections.

Posterior third ventriculostomy, septostomy, stents across the aqueduct of sylvius and so on and so forth were treatments aimed at getting around the obstruction. And they proved to be successful as well, to an extent.

As is the usual cycle, time revealed the limitations of endoscopy. The shunts evolved into modern gadgets with programmability… and the evolution continues.

Lamina Terminalis was recognized as the anterior boundary of the third ventricle and fenestration of this thin membrane was thought to be helpful in resolution of hydrocephalus with subarachnoid hemorrhage. This was applied in very few cases in our center where Endoscopic third ventriculostomy could not be done due to a very thick and opalescent third ventricular floor. We did fenestration of Lamina terminalis through an eyebrow incision and a keyhole approach. We do think that in cases where an ETV is difficult or risky and the type of hydrocephalus is obstructive, this is something which could be an alternative to a shunt. Of course more work needs to be done to assess the feasibility.

However few things which were not considered earlier like the compliance of the brain and the fragile balance of the CSF system were studied later on and treatments started taking these factors into account as well. So evolved treatments for communicating hydrocephalus and normal pressure hydrocephalus where the compliance of the brain is important.

In the present scenario, surgeons have a lot to choose from. However, before doing anything it goes without saying that the surgeon weighs his options and goes ahead with the treatment, based on the familiarity and efficacy of a particular way of treating the hydrocephalus. After all, no surgeon would want a mismanaged case of hydrocephalus on his hands.

Dr. Sadip Pant
University of Arkansas for Medical Sciences, AR,
USA

Dr. Iype Cherian
College of Medical Sciences, Bharatpur,
Nepal

1

Hydrocephalus: An Overview

Milani Sivagnanam and Neilank K. Jha
Wayne State University
USA

1. Introduction

Hydrocephalus is a condition where an abnormal build-up of cerebrospinal fluid (CSF) fluid causes an increase in pressure in the ventricles or subarachnoid space of the brain. It can be caused by either the blockage of CSF flow (i.e. obstructive/non-communicating hydrocephalus) in the ventricular system or by inadequate re-absorption of CSF fluid (i.e. non-obstructive/communicating hydrocephalus). These features result in enlargement of the ventricles (i.e. ventriculomegaly) or subarachnoid space and increase intracranial pressure (ICP). The severity of ICP can compress surrounding brain parenchyma, manifesting into identifiable acute or chronic symptoms depending on the age of onset.

Major developments in the treatment of hydrocephalus have occurred since the 20th century, with the use of shunts and neurosurgical interventions being the most successful. Currently, no cure has been found for hydrocephalus.

2. Types and classification

Hydrocephalus can be grouped based on two broad criteria: 1) pathology and 2) etiology. Pathology can be grouped as either obstructive (non-communicating) or non-obstructive (communicating). Etiology can be grouped as congenital or acquired. Additionally, there is a form of hydrocephalus called normal pressure hydrocephalus (NPH), which primarily affects the elderly population.

Congenital hydrocephalus is present at birth, and can be caused by Dandy-Walker malformations, porenchphaly, spina bifida, Chairi I and II malformations, arachnoid cysts, and most commonly aquaductal stenosis. Very few cases of congenital hydrocephalus are inherited (X-linked hydrocephalus). Acquired hydrocephalus may be caused by subarachnoid haemorrhage, intraventricular hemorrage, trauma, infection (meningitis), tumour, surgical complications or severe head injury at any age.

Describing hydrocephalus based on type of CSF flow (i.e. communicating/non-obstructive or non-communicating/obstructive) is preferred because of the implications for treatment. Communicating hydrocephalus is often treated with shunt surgery while non-communicating hydrocephalus suggests treatment with endoscopic third ventriculostomy (ETV). Regardless of etiology, both groups present with ventriculomegaly and elevated intracranial pressure, which are responsible for the similar symptoms seen in both communicating and non-communicating forms of hydrocephalus.

2.1 Obstructive (Non-communicating) hydrocephalus

Obstructive hydrocephalus results from the blockage of CSF circulation, either in the ventricles or subarachnoid space. This can be caused by cysts, tumours, haemorrhages, infections, congenital malformations and most commonly, aqueductal stenosis or cerebral aqueduct blockage. An MRI or CT scan can be useful to identify the point of blockage. Patients can then be treated by removing the obstructive lesion or diverting the CSF using ETV or a shunt.

2.2 Non-obstructive (Communicating) hydrocephalus

Non-obstructive hydrocephalus may be caused by a disruption of CSF equilibrium. Rarely, hydrocephalus can be caused by an abundance of CSF production, as a result of a choroid plexus papilloma or carcinoma. Hydrocephalus is typically the underlying condition when CSF absorption is impaired, and can be caused by a complication after an infection or by hemorrhagic complications. Patients are often treated using a shunt.

2.3 Normal Pressure Hydrocephalus

Normal pressure hydrocephalus (NPH), which commonly occurs in the elderly, does not fit into either obstructive or non-obstructive hydrocephalus. NPH occurs in the sixth or seventh decade of life and is characterized with specific symptoms: gait disturbance, cognitive decline and urinary incontinence (i.e. Adam's or Hakim's triad). Ventricles appear enlarged, and there is an increase in intracranial pressure compared to baseline measurements. However, it is important to note that this increase in ICP is not as significant an increase as seen in obstructive or non-obstructive cases described previously. This is why this form of hydrocephalus is called 'normal' pressure hydrocephalus. Causes may include subarachnoid haemorrhage, trauma, infection (meningitis), encephalitis, tumour, subarachnoid inflammation, or surgical complications. Often, the cause of NPH is not clear and is referred to as idiopathic (INPH). Preferred treatment for NPH is often shunt surgery.

3. Pathological findings

CSF is the fluid which acts to serve as a cushion for the brain, and plays a role in haemostasis and metabolism of the brain. It is produced by the choroid plexus, found in the body and inferior horn of the lateral ventricle, the foramen of Monroe, roof of the third ventricle and inferior roof of the fourth ventricle. The flow of CSF through the ventricles is as follows: begins in the left and right lateral ventricles → interventricular foramen of Monroe → 3rd ventricle → cerebral aqueduct → 4th ventricle and out through the two lateral apertures of Lushka or the one medial aperture of Magendi into the cisternae magna. From there, CSF will flow into the cortico-subarachnoid space and the spinal subarachnoid space.

CSF is continuously being produced by the choroid plexus at a rate of 400-500ml/day and continuously reabsorbed by the arachnoids granulations into the dural sinuses, and eventually into the venous system. At any given time, there is approximately 140ml of CSF in the adult system, of which 25-40ml is in the ventricles. The rate of absorption is proportional to the difference in intracranial pressure and dural sinus pressure. An equilibrium between CSF production and CSF reabsorption maintains mean CSF pressure at 7-15mmHg in normal adults. In patients with communicating and non-communicating forms of hydrocephalus, the build up of extra CSF fluid within the ventricles will cause increased ICP. Clinicians can measure mean intracranial pressure either intracranially or by inserting a needle into the lumbar space. An abnormality in the mean ICP pressure or pattern of ICP changes can be indicative of hydrocephalus.

3.1 Normal Pressure Hydrocephalus (NPH)

Dr. Hakim first identified NPH over 4 decades ago, and a clear pathological model has not yet been proposed to explain the triad of clinical symptoms and the development of the paradoxical nature of near-normal intracranial pressure and ventricomegaly observed in NPH patients. Evidence suggests ventricomegaly is caused by impaired CSF absorption at the arachnoid granules or impaired CSF conductance through the subarachnoid space.

One theory suggests ICP increases due to accumulation of CSF as a result of reduced conductance and absorption. This causes an initial phase of ventricle enlargement, which then normalizes after the initial expansion. This theory has been supported by various experimental models of hydrocephalus.

Hakim hypothesized a transient increase in ICP was sufficient to initiate ventricular dilation. Using Pascal's law (force = pressure x area), if force were to remain constant, as ventricular area increased, the (intracranial) pressure could decrease and normalize, thereby explaining the paradoxical 'normal pressure' presenting in NPH patients. The transient increase in NPH patients is not detected in patients because they are examined in a clinical setting after ventricles have enlarged and ICP has normalized.

Other theories suggest ventriculomegaly develops as a combination of increased mean CSF pressure, and the increased frequency of CSF pressure waves. (Eide & Sorteberg, 2010; Madson et al., 2006)

4. Epidemiology

The true incidence of hydrocephalus in children and adults is unknown. It has been estimated that it affects 0.9 to 1.5 per 1000 births. When congenital abnormalities are included (e.g. spina bifida, myemeninocele), hydrocephalus can affect 1.3 to 2.9 per 1000 births. (Rizvi & Anjum, 2005) Due to the increased practice of pregnant females taking folic acid to reduce neural tube defects, it has been reported that the incidence of hydrocephalus in children has decreased over the recent decades. (Drake, 2008; Bullivant et al., 2008; Kestle, 2003) Without a central registry of hydrocephalus cases, however, it is difficult to accurately know the incidence of acquired cases of hydrocephalus.

Similarly, the incidence of NPH remains uncertain as well, mainly due to variability in diagnostic criteria between different centres. As well, many cases of NPH may be misdiagnosed as other common elderly diseases. Current reports estimate rates of 1.3 per million to 4 cases per 1000; variability due to different diagnostic criteria for NPH and sample populations. A recent study surveying 49 centers in Germany known to care for NPH patients estimated 1.8 cases per 100 000 people. (Krauss and Halve, 2004)

5. Clinical presentation of hydrocephalus

As noted earlier, irrespective of etiology, patient symptoms will present in a similar manner. However, depending on the type of hydrocephalus, age of onset, and severity, symptoms will vary greatly.

5.1 Infants (0-2 years)

In infants, the accumulation of CSF, enlargements of ventricles and increase in intracranial pressure (ICP) will manifest in an increase of head circumference (since the fontanelles have not yet fused), bulging fontanelles, and bulging scalp veins, which occurs especially when the infant cries. These are often the first presenting signs of hydroceaphlus in infants. The shape of the head may also indicate the location of an obstruction. For example, an occipital prominence is seen in Dandy Walker malformations and a larger forehead in comparison to the rest of the skull is seen in aqueductal stenosis. Other signs include an enlarged fontanelle and full anterior fontanelle. Also an infant will often present with signs of irritability, lethargy, fever, and vomiting.

As hydrocephalus worsens, the infant may suffer from 'sunsetting eyes'. This symptom is characterized by the child's inability to look upward, as the eyes are displaced downward due to the pressure on the cranial nerves controlling eye movement. As a result, the infant appears as though it is looking at the bottom lid of its eye. Vision may also be affected in advanced hydrocephalus due to compression of the optic chiasma as a result of a dilated 3rd ventricle. Stretching of periventricular structures can cause abducent nerve paresis, presenting in nystagmus and random eye movement.

Infants with advanced hydrocephalus may also present with increased deep tendon reflexes and muscle tone in lower extremities, growth failure, delayed neurological development, and limited control in the head and trunk regions. Left untreated, this can progress and can result in seizures and/or coma.

5.2 Children and adults

Children presenting with hydrocephalus, may have had a pre-existing and unrecognized hydrocephalus and may have normal or delayed neurological development. These children have slightly enlarged heads, optic atrophy or papilloedma caused by increased ICP. These children also have abnormal hypothalamic function (i.e. short stature, gigantism, obesity, precocious puberty, diabetes insipidus, amonerrea), spastic lower limbs and hyperreflexia. In school, they may present with learning difficulties, and often have lower performance IQ than verbal IQ.

When hydrocephalus occurs in children and adults (after fontanelles have fused), hydrocephalus will manifest with different symptoms. Affected individuals will have normal head size and present with headache, vomiting, irritability, alerted consciousness, lethargy and ventriculomegaly. Papilloedema, absucens nerve pareis, and lower limb hyper reflexia are also seen. The stretching of cranial nerves that are responsible for eye function may lead to impaired or dysfunctional eye movement and/or tunnel vision.

Toddlers may present with loss of previously gained cognitive and motor abilities, delays in reaching milestones (e.g. walking, talking, etc.), poor coordination and decreased bladder control. Older children often complain of headaches as their primary symptom (due to increased ICP), feel sleepy and lethargic, and also show a decline in school performance. Adult symptoms may vary from weakness to spasticity, difficulties with balance, poor motor control, headaches and nausea.

If an individual with suspected hydrocephalus is left untreated or poorly managed, the chronic increase in intracranial pressure may lead to convulsions, mental retardation, gait disturbances, dementia and personality changes in adults. In young girls, it may also lead to early onset puberty.

5.3 Adult normal pressure hydrocephalus

Normal pressure hydrocephalus results from a decrease in CSF absorption, and ICP may range from normal to high depending on the time of day. It is often characterized by Hakim's triad of symptoms: incontinence, dementia and gait disturbance. Symptoms start off mild, often beginning with gait impairment, and eventually progress in severity. Patients present with varying degrees of symptom severity, and not all symptoms may be present.

5.3.1 Gait

Gait dysfunction is the most common symptom present in adults with NPH and develops over many months or years. Enlarged lateral ventricles compress corticospinal tract fibers in the corona radiata, which are responsible for voluntary skilled movements of the legs.

Patients present with a slower, wide based gait, small shuffling steps, poor balance and a tendency to take many small steps during a turn, as well as a tendency to fall (positive Romberg test). Steps are of reduced height and small clearance, characteristic of a 'magnetic gait'. However, there is no significant motor weakness in limbs. A patient's clinical history may reveal that the patient originally presented with difficulty walking on uneven surfaces, which later developed into an increasing number of falls, needing the use of a walking stick, walker or wheelchair. The Tinetti Assessment Tool is a quick way to assess gait and balance.

Causes for gait disturbances in the elderly population can be multifactorial. As a result, it is important for physicians to rule out other possibilities or co-morbidities before a patient's diagnosis or treatment for NPH is confirmed by taking a detailed clinical history and clinical exam. A history of significant back pain, lower extremity weakness and radicular pain can be due to cervical or lumbar canal stenosis, and can be assessed with MRI. Steppage gait suggests peripheral neuropathy. Differentiation between Parkinson's disease and NPH can be challenging due to similarities in gait dysfunction: hypokinetic, smaller steps, and freezing. However, NPH is specifically associated with a wider base, outward rotated feet, an erect trunk, preserved arm swing, smaller step height, no response to levadopa treatment, and the absence of a resting tremor.

5.3.2 Urinary incontinence

Compression of sacral fibers along the corona radiata by enlarged lateral ventricles impairs inhibitory fibers to the bladder. Patients can present with a variation of urinary symptoms, ranging from urgency or increased frequency to (near) incontinence.

Since urinary incontinence is also extremely common in the elderly population, a detailed history and examination must be taken to rule out other causes of similar symptoms, such as urethral stricture (prostate hypertrophy), diuretic use, detruster instability or pelvic floor weakness leading to stress incontinence. The type of incontinence (stress, urge, etc.) and use of cystoscopy and urodynamic testing can be helpful in diagnosing patients.

5.3.3 Cognitive dementia

Patients with NPH suffer subcortical dementia, characterized by forgetfulness, disrupted visuospatial perception, psychomotor slowness, decreased attention, and preserved memory storage. A patient history may reveal the patient is incapable of daily tasks, such as shopping, or managing bank accounts. Physicians may use the Montreal Cognitive Assessment test or HIV Dementia Scale as a quick screening tool to identify subcortical cognitive dysfunction.

Cognitive decline in NPH can be similar to other common dementias seen in the elderly population, including Alzheimer's, vascular dementia, and Lewy body disease. An onset of symptoms over a few months, rather than a few years, and lack of apraxia, agnosia, aphasia and complete memory loss can differentiate subcortical dementia found in NPH from Alzheimer's. However, other types of dementia may be more difficult to differentiate from dementia due to NPH.

6. Diagnostic evaluation

6.1 Infants

Head circumference should be routinely measured in infants. Any excessive growth in serial measurements is a risk factor for hydrocephalus and should be followed up with a physician. Additionally, failure of sutures to close in a child may indicate the development of hydrocephalus, as progressive growth of ventricles in a young infant can prevent the fusion of sutures. This may also lead to a larger than normal head circumference. If hydrocephalus is suspected, x-rays of a child's head may provide further evidence such as an enlarged head, craniofacial disproportion, or elongated interdigitations of suture lines, indicating increased ICP in older children.

Hydrocephalus can be diagnosed before birth with the use of ultrasound. Also, in premature infants and very young infants with open fontanelles, ultrasound can be used to image the size of ventricles. If possible, a CT or MRI scan can be performed on the infant to assess the cause of hydrocephalus (e.g. aquductal stenosis, loculated ventricles, tumour, etc.) and to choose appropriate follow up interventions. However, due to the invasive nature of these diagnostic procedures, it is difficult to monitor ICP in a very young infant to detect an increase ICP.

6.2 Children and adults

Children and adults presenting with symptoms of hydrocephalus need to confirm the presence of enlarged ventricles with CT or MRI. Using an MRI, Evan's ratio is defined as the ratio of the maximum width of the anterior ventricular horns to the maximum width of the calvarium at the level of the intraventricular foramen of Monroe. A ratio of 0.3 or greater defines ventriculomegaly. CT or MRI may also reveal the presence of infection or tumours causing an obstruction and enlarged ventricles. Gating MRI to the cardiac cycle can track CSF flow and monitor movement through the ventricles to identify any blockages. Lumbar puncture can also be used to assess intracranial pressure, and screen for the presence and/or type and severity of infection.

Signs indicating non-communicating hydrocephalus include: lack of indication of obstruction on an MRI, increased CSF flow velocity in the aquaduct, rounding of lateral ventricles, and thinning and elevation of the corpus collosum on sagittal MRI images.

7. Predictive tests for shunt surgery for NPH

Although the use of neuroimaging to identify ventriculomegaly and assessment of clinical symptoms (i.e. the presence of one or more features of Hakim's triad for INPH), can be used to diagnose NPH, additional testing must be conducted to identify patients who qualify for shunt surgery. The use of supplementary tests can help improve diagnostic accuracy and stratify patient populations into those who would be considered good candidates for surgery and those who would not.

7.1 Cisternography

In cisternography, a radioactive isotope is injected via lumbar puncture into the CSF and is allowed to distribute within the ventricular and subarachnoid system over a 1-2 day period. Flow and speed are assessed using a gamma camera. In a normal patient, the material can be seen accumulating over the cortical space. Any accumulation or reflux of the isotope in the ventricles indicates NPH. Although this method was used heavily in the past, a review in the early 1990s (Vanneste et al., 1992) concluded that this method did not improve diagnostic accuracy, and this method has been abandoned since.

7.2 Infusion methods

To examine CSF dynamics, two needles are used: one to infuse artificial CSF into the lumbar subarachnoid space, and another needle at a second side in the spine to record intracranial pressure and resistance of CSF absorption pathways in the subarachnoid space. Patients with an ICP >18mmHg/mL/min would have a good outcomes after shunt surgery (high specificity). However, certain patients still benefit from surgery, despite failure to meet the >18mmHg/mL/min cutoff, indicating low sensitivity of this test. Though this test can be quite useful to physicians recommending patients for surgery, it requires technical skill, and is currently only available at very few centers in the US.

7.3 Intracranial pressure measurement

Measuring intracranial pressure (ICP) can be done using an intraventricular or lumbar catheter. From recordings, mean pressure and systolic and diastolic pulsations of CSF can be calculated. Measurements >50mmHg for 15-20 minutes time segments on ICP recordings indicate A-waves (plateau waves). B-waves are often low amplitude waves (1-5mmHg) lasting a short period of time and have been recently explored as a possible indicator of shunt surgery outcomes. However, other studies have shown low correlation between the incidence of B-waves and good surgical outcome. (Stephensen et al., 2004) ICP monitoring is only available at a few centers in the world, and studies have found varying results on the use B waves as a positive indicator for shunt surgery. This is likely due to the different interpretation of recordings at different centers.

7.4 CSF tap test

A CSF tap test removes 40-50ml of CSF and involves assessment of gait performance and cognitive ability before and after the procedure. The act of removing CSF simulates what would happen if the patient were to undergo placement of a shunt. The test may be done in an outpatient setting, and has low risk, low costs associated, and is a popular test to use for stratifying good surgical candidates. Although the specificity of this test is high, the sensitivity is low. Physicians should keep in mind a patient who does not respond well to this test, should not be excluded from surgical consideration. Rather the patient should be followed up with other supplementary tests, such as continuous CSF drainage before treatment is finalized. Currently, there is an ongoing European multicentre study to investigate the reliability of this test. (Malm & Eklund, 2006)

7.5 Continuous CSF drainage

Removal of large amounts of CSF over a 2-3 day period through a spinal catheter and comparison of symptoms (e.g. gait and cognitive ability) before and after this procedure has proven to be useful in consideration of shunt surgery. Factora & Luciano (2006) found at their institution, that clinical symptomatic improvement after this test was performed on patients with ideal NPH presentation (ventriculomegaly and clinical symptoms), was indicative of a high success rate after surgery.

Although this test is valuable, it is a high risk procedure. Patients may suffer from headaches, meningitis, infection, nerve root irritation, catheter blockage, as well as the associated cost of hospital stay. Additionally, the sensitivity and specificity of this test in multiple studies has been variable and only certain centers in the US specialize in this technique, suggesting continuous CSF drainage may not be best suited for widespread clinical use.

7.6 CSF flow using MRI

MRI can be used to assess CSF flow in the brain. Studies have shown increased CSF volume through the aqueduct during systole to be associated with positive outcome to shunt surgery. This technique is advantageous due to its non-invasive nature, yet further research is needed to assess reliability in a clinical setting.

7.7 Conclusion

In addition to the supplementary tests, it is important to keep in mind the likelihood of patient recovery following shunt surgery decreases the longer the NPH patients has presented with clinical symptoms.

The various ancillary tests have varied risks and benefits as well. Many studies have demonstrated that these tests also vary in terms of sensitivity and specificity. Currently, in the absence of a true gold standard for the diagnosis of NPH, studies have highlighted CSF drainage as the best available test to indicate successful surgical outcome.

8. Treatment

Treatment of hydrocephalus is dependent on a number of factors, mainly etiology, severity, age of patient, and response to previous treatments or supplementary tests. After careful consideration and review of a patient's neuroimaging, clinical symptoms, contraindications and response to alternative treatments/tests, a physician may offer to treat a patient conservatively with pharmacotherapy or surgically with implantation of a shunt or endoscopic third ventriculostomy (ETV).

8.1 Pharmacotherapy

CSF production in choroid plexus cells is based on movement of ions on the basolateral and apical side of the cells. Carbonic anhydrase is responsible for catalyzing the following reaction: $H_2O + CO_2 \rightarrow H_2CO_3 \rightarrow HCO_3 + H^+$. The bicarbonate and hydrogen ion are exchanged on the basolateral side for Na^+ and Cl^- while on the apical side, NaCl, $NaHCO_3$ and H_2O are secreted to form CSF.

In the past, in an attempt to reduce CSF production, acetazolamide, a carbonic anhydrase inhibitor was prescribed. Although this treatment has been shown to reduce CSF production slightly and mediate milder forms of hydrocephalus, it cannot be used as a long-term treatment modality. Patients who progress to more severe forms will have to either undergo a shunt placement or ETV.

8.2 Shunt surgery

Patients with communicating hydrocephalus, including adult NPH, are primarily treated with shunt surgery. As described earlier, patients offered shunt surgery as an option have typically undergone ancillary testing to determine their response to placement of a shunt.

The purpose of a shunt in a hydrocephalic patient is to divert CSF flow to another area of the body, where it can be absorbed. This allows intracranial pressure to return to normal levels and improves clinical symptoms. The procedure involves placing a proximal catheter in a ventricle through the brain or in the lumbar subarachnoid space, to drain CSF. This catheter is connected to a one-way resistance valve which controls CSF drainage and is usually placed against the skull, under the skin. The fluid then drains through a distal catheter which collects the excess fluid and drains into the peritoneal cavity (ventriculoperitoneal shunt), right atrium (ventriculoatrial shunt), or pleural space.

In addition to considering the risk to benefit ratio of the surgery, surgeons must carefully evaluate patients for specific sites of distal and proximal catheter placements, type of valve to be used, and possible co-morbidities, making shunt surgery highly individualized. Placement of proximal catheter is often in the ventricles, but in patients with specific concerns of brain injury from insertion of a catheter (e.g. patient already has left hemisphere injury, and placement of catheter in right hemisphere could result in bilateral lesions), the physician may opt to place it in the lumbar subarachnoid space. Studies have also shown that placement of the proximal catheter within the ventricles has best outcomes when placed away from the choroid plexus. This will help to avoid catheter occlusion that would normally lead to shunt failure. The preferred location for the placement of the distal catheter is the peritoneal cavity because of ease of access and because there are typically fewer complications. If a patient has previously had an abdominal surgery or peritonitis, their ability to absorb CSF may be decreased and a surgeon may opt for a ventriculoatrial shunt. Placement of distal catheter in the heart or lung increases the risk of complications, such as: risk of emboli, pleural effusion, pneumothorax, respiratory distress, and endocarditis. Ventriculoatrial shunts also have increased and more serious risks in the long term (e.g. renal failure, great vein thrombosis).

8.2.1 Valves

There are two types of shunts used today: 1) single valve setting (fixed-resistance valves/differential pressure valves) and 2) programmable/adjustable shunts (variable resistance).

8.2.1.1 Fixed resistance valves

These valves are designed to open if the intracranial pressure is greater than the opening pressure of the valve and abdominal pressure (in VP shunt) or outlet area. This allows CSF to flow through the shunt pathway along with regular CSF pathways in the ventricles and subarachnoid spaces.

These shunts cannot be adjusted (i.e. opening pressure altered) after they are implanted and are not susceptible to alteration of function when in proximity to a magnetic field. If patient does not seem to improve symptomatically following surgery, it may become necessary to repeat the surgery and replace the shunt with a shunt that has lower opening pressure. Shunts are typically available in low, medium or high pressure.

When a patient sits upright, the hydrostatic pressure gradient may be greater than the opening pressure of the valve, and cause over drainage of the ventricles. The siphoning effect can create postural headaches (headaches which cease when patient lies down) and increases the risk of subdural hygromas and/or hematomas. Current fixed-resistance valves now have anti-siphon features to minimize disturbances when patients sit upright.

8.2.1.2 Variable Resistance Valves

The mechanism of these valves is the same as fixed-resistance valves, but they have opening pressures ranging from 20-200mmH_2O and can be adjusted after implantation using a magnetic device. Thus, after surgery, the valve can be adjusted to optimize benefit to the patient (i.e. as seen by best relief of clinical symptoms) and/or to avoid over drainage, and manage subdural hygromas/hemotomas.

Variable resistance valves are advantageous in comparison to fixed-pressure valves because they can be adjusted non-invasively. However they are susceptible to external magnetic fields. If a patient undergoes an MRI or comes in close contact with small kitchen magnets, the patient risks unintentionally changing the valve settings and causing unexpected changes in CSF flow. Patients are forewarned, and should visit a physician after an MRI scan to re-evaluate shunt settings.

A study looking at outcome with patients with fixed resistance vs. variable resistance valves showed no significant benefit of one valve over the other. (Pollack et al., 1999)

Selection of type of valve is dependent on the surgeon as well as the patients' etiology of hydrocephalus.

8.2.2 Complications

Implantation of a shunt can have complications that arise from the surgery itself, complications related to the shunt system or complications reflected in overall suboptimal shunt function.

The INPH guidelines list several complications, including shunt malfunction (20%), subdural hematoma (2-17%), seizure (3-11%), shunt infection (3-6%) and intracerebral hematoma (3%). (Bergsneider et al, 2005) McGirt et al. (2005) sampled 132 INPH patients, and found 7% developed an infection, 2% developed a subdural hematoma, and 1% developed an intracerebral hematoma.

8.2.2.1 Infection

Infection is a common complication resulting from the implantation of a shunt and has been reported to appear in ~8-10% of cases, most arising within the first year after shunt surgery. Evidence of infection should be taken seriously and treated immediately. The most common infection is caused by *Staphyloccoccus aureus* adhering to the shunt system, causing shunt occlusion and/or poor wound healing, and creating the risk of under drainage of CSF through the shunt. Patients experiencing an infection can present with a variety of symptoms, including fever, nausea, vomiting, lethargy and irritability. Upon presentation of these non-specific symptoms, physicians should examine patients for skin tenderness around the surgical incision and catheter and abdominal tenderness. If the entire system is infected, it must be removed surgically and replaced. As well, the patient must undergo antibiotic treatment. Current shunt catheters are impregnated with antibiotics, and have lower shunt infection rates as a result.

8.2.2.2 Shunt dysfunction

Shunt systems have a risk of the individual parts disconnecting or migrating, and tubing segments breaking apart. In growing children, there is a risk of the distal catheter being pulled out of the peritoneal cavity or causing 'inguinal hernias in male infants'. If there is a mechanical issue suspected with the shunt system, a series of plain X-rays should be taken to identify a break down in the system. Any shunt dysfunction can lead to excessive CSF in the ventricles, which may lead to a recurrence of original hydrocephalus symptoms.

8.2.2.3 Shunt occlusion

The most common complication with shunt surgery is occlusion of the proximal or distal catheter leading to shunt dysfunction. Occlusion may be suspected if a patient initially had a period of improvement, then a slow deterioration back to their original condition, or if there was no improvement after surgery at all.

Possible occlusion of the proximal catheter could be due to choroid plexus, and can be minimized if the catheter tip is positioned away from this region. If the distal catheter is positioned in the peritoneal cavity, occlusion and immobilization of the tip are caused by omentum or adhesions. Certain cases have reported catheter tip migration in the cavity, causing bladder or bowel perforations. Poor absorption of drained CSF flow may result in peritoneal cysts. If this is suspected, an X-ray can be taken on separate days, and degree of mobilization of the distal tip can be assessed.

If an occlusion is suspected, a physician may conduct a patency test to check for shunt flow-through by injecting a 'radioisotope into the shunt reservoir' and noting the movement through the system. Obstruction(s) will be evident if there is a delay or restriction of the radioisotope to a certain area or no flow at all.

8.2.2.4 Over drainage

Over drainage of the ventricles may occur due to a siphoning effect, and requires the opening pressure of the shunt valve to be set higher if an adjustable valve was used, or replacement of the valve if a non-adjustable valve was used. Patients often complain of headaches when they are sitting up, which resolve when they lie down.

Excessive over drainage may result in a subdural hematoma and occurs in children and adults with completed sutures. The rapid drainage causes a compression of the ventricles, and the accompanying brain shift into space previously occupied by ventricles tears bridging veins. Prolonged overdrainage may result in slit ventricle syndrome, in which patients present with intermittent headaches and small slit-like ventricles on imaging.

8.2.3 Outcome

8.2.3.1 Children

With appropriate identification of surgery candidates, patients will often see improvement of their symptoms. Patient response to shunt surgery is variable, and there are still no tests to predict how quickly a patient will respond or to what extent symptoms will be reversed. As well, there are no tests to predict how long the improvements will last. Patients treated for infantile hydrocephalus may have complications in the long run. Often, many children will lead full, active lives, while others may still suffer from vision and motor difficulties, and learning disabilities. The majority of children are able to graduate from normal school. Routine follow-ups and management are required to ensure proper maintenance and optimal use of the shunt.

8.2.3.2 Adult NPH

Patients suffering from NPH, and who have undergone shunt surgery often show improvement, at least in one symptom, especially if shown to respond positively to pre-surgical tests. The degree of improvement and recovery time can range from immediate recovery to many months after surgery. Improvement in balance and gait are seen in the majority of patients and this symptom improves to a greater degree than other symptoms.

Marmarou et al. (2005) found improvement in at least one symptom in 90% of patients who had been selected as surgical candidates based on positive response to CSF drainage tests. Wilson and Williams (2006) selected shunt surgery candidates based on selecting surgical candidates including ICP monitoring and CSF drainage tests, and found improvement of at least one symptom in 75% of their 132 patients 18 months following surgery. Improvement in cognitive function or slowing decline in cognitive function occurs to a lesser extent in patients and can be assessed using a Mini-Mental State Exam. An international study in 2005 developed INPH guidelines, and reported "improvement rates of 30-60%"(Klinge et al,.

2005). The results of such studies indicate the variability in patient improvement, which is often due to differing criteria of patient selection, differences in postoperative assessment and variation of follow up time from surgery in various studies.

Patients may be followed up with imaging and periodic revisions to shunts. Careful follow-ups with physicians must be done to identify infection and prevent any loss in improvements of symptoms made with surgery. Patients who show no improvement in any symptoms up to 6 months after surgery should be re-evaluated for possible misdiagnosis, or shunt function.

8.2.4 Follow Up

During routine follow up visits, blood and CSF samples should be drawn for signs on infection, which is a common complication of shunt surgery. Additionally, physicians should perform routine assessments on patients to evaluate any improvement or decline in symptoms. A lack of clinical improvement after surgery may indicate a non-functional CSF shunt system (which should be evaluated for repair), a misdiagnosis, or symptoms of another developing disease. In patients with INPH, the state of disease may have reached a point in which symptoms are irreversible, thus placement of a shunt will not benefit the patient.

A patient who had previously shown improvement, but then deteriorates symptomatically may indicate improper shunt function. A patient may present with features of hydrocephalus, but not to the degree they presented prior to surgery. Thus, a follow up should include an extensive examination of the shunt system itself. If the reservoir does not refill after mechanically pumping the valve, there might be an obstruction in the proximal catheter. A proximal catheter obstruction may be due to a change in position and/or of the tip, which should be in the right frontal horn, as not to be obstructed by choroid plexus. Ultrasound can be used to examine the distal catheter position, to identify a cyst or abscess of distal tip catheter occlusion. A series of plain x-rays (i.e. shunt series) may be useful in visualizing the entire shunt system, to identify position, disconnection of components, or mechanical damage in the shunt system. Any identification of a displaced catheter would have to be fixed surgically. Shunt disconnection is usually not a problem in adults, but may present more often in children, due to increased activity, and growth.

Shunt placement comes with the risk of over drainage and the possibility of developing subdural hematomas and slit ventricle syndrome. If a shunt was placed in a very young child, as they grow up and spend more time upright, there may be excessive drainage of CSF into the distal catheter because of the siphoning effect. Children with fixed sutures and large ventricles have a high risk of developing a subdural hematoma. (Kestle 2003) Children must have frequent follow-ups and monitoring after shunt surgery and may need contrast CT/MRI scans to visualize a hematoma. For minor subdural hematomas, a physician may choose to manage with monitoring and adjustment of valve opening pressure. However, in many cases, it is necessary to surgically remove the shunt and drain the subdural hematoma.

Slit ventricle syndrome (SVS) is a rare condition, seen in patients who have had a shunt for many years. They present with symptoms of a shunt malfunction, and with periods of recurrent headaches, and show small ventricles on imaging. Current theories suggest long term over drainage results in smaller ventricles, and the brain to filling in any excess intracranial space. Any subsequent increases in intracranial volume presents as symptoms of high ICP. Small ventricles can also cause the proximal catheter to be obstructed. SVS occurs in a very small population of patients.

8.3 Endoscopic Third Ventriculostomy (ETV)

Endoscopic third ventriculostomy (ETV) is an alternative to treating hydrocephalus with a shunt. ETV was first attempted in the early 1920s, but the practice was abandoned in the 1950s when shunt surgery gained popularity. Increasing evidence of potential shunt complications (e.g. shunt failure, infection rates, etc.) and effectiveness in identifying patients with obstructive hydrocephalus due to modern imaging has led to an increasing popularity of ETV surgery. ETV is now considered the primary form of intervention for patients with aquaductal stenosis or tumours obstructing flow between the 3rd and 4th ventricle but also have adequate CSF reabsorption capacity in the patent subarachnoid space. Patients with minimal CSF reabsorption capacity (i.e. previous case of IVH, meningitis, myelomeningocele) may not be considered suitable for this procedure, and in studies have shown a lower success rate with ETV. (Rezaee et al, 2007)

A neuroendoscope enters through a precoronal burr to visualize the anatomy of the ventricles and the floor of the 3rd ventricle. It is guided through the cerebral mantle, through the lateral ventricle and the foramen of Monro into the 3rd ventricle. Forceps and a balloon are used to perforate a hole downward and widen a stoma in the floor of the 3rd ventricle, anterior to the mammillary bodies and bifurcation of the basilar artery, creating a passage to divert excessive CSF into the prepontine space. This diverted fluid will be absorbed through normal pathways (i.e. subarachnoid space). A pathway for excess CSF to leave the ventricles will result in normalizing the ICP, and decreasing the excessive pressure and damage of chronic systolic CSF pulsations on brain parenchyma. Cerebral blood flow and perfusion to these areas are restored, and normal CSF dynamics are restored, resulting in a reversal of symptoms.

It is important to visualize the proximity of nearby structures, namely the basilar artery, mammillary bodies, hypothalamus and thalamus prior to surgery, to avoid injury prior to surgery. However the fenestration may close in the future, resulting in a rise in ICP and a recurrence of symptoms, and the possibility of another surgery.

The lack of foreign objects in this procedure makes it a viable and suitable surgical alternative to shunt placement and current studies are examining the effectiveness of using ETV for non-communicating forms of hydrocephalus. Hadar et al. (2008) assessed the outcome of obstructive hydrocephalus patients undergoing ETV as a primary surgery or as a secondary surgery for patients who originally had shunt surgery. Results showed that those who had ETV as their second surgery had the worst outcomes overall. A similar study by Woodworth et al. (2007) showed patients who were initially treated with a CSF shunt and subsequently underwent ETV were 2.5 times more likely to suffer from treatment failure in comparison to patients who had ETV as their primary surgical treatment. Results from such studies indicate physicians should carefully select the primary surgery offered to a patient as initial treatment to avoid excessive complications later.

Treatment of NPH with ETV has been explored as well. Gangemi et al. (2004) looked at 25 patients with NPH to be treated with ETV. ETV provided symptom relief that was comparable to shunt treatment in patients who had a short duration of symptoms and suffered primarily from gait disturbance. This suggests that a particular subgroup of NPH patients may benefit from ETV and thereby avoid shunt insertion.

8.3.1 Complications

Drake (2008) reports the overall surgical complication rate for ETV surgeries to be 10-15%.

Risks associated with ETV include hemorrage, CSF leak, and perforation of nearby structures during the procedure, including the basilar artery, hypothalamus, and cranial nerves.

If the floor of the 3rd ventricle cannot be clearly visualized, or is thin enough to see the basilar artery, a surgeon may choose to place a VP shunt to avoid risking basilar artery rupture. Injuries to the hypothalamus have been reported in the literature to manifest as hormonal disorders, such as diabetes insipidus and weight gain. Possible injury to the occulomotor nerve may result in gaze palsy as well. Bouras & Sgouros (2011) examined reports of ETV complications in multiple sites, including their home institution, and found a low percentage of complications relating to injuries to periventricular structures. These injuries were caused by an abrupt insertion of the endoscope into the lateral ventricle or through the foramen of Monroe. Other extremely rare complications included decreased consciousness, memory disorders, and hemiparesis.

A rare, but fatal risk after ETV is late rapid deterioration. Patients will respond well after the procedure, but will then complain of headache, and rapidly deteriorate. If not given immediate care by a neurosurgeon, this condition may be fatal. A recent study collected autopsy results from patients who had late rapid deterioration, and reported the stoma of the 3rd ventricle had been closed. (Drake, 2008) Further studies in this area need to be conducted to determine if closure of the stoma precipitates the risk of late rapid deterioration.

8.3.2 Outcome

Generally, outcome after surgery in adults is good. Reports on ETV trials have claimed success rates greater than 75% (50-94%) for carefully selected patients. (Rezaee et al., 2007)

ETV offers an opportunity for children suffering from hydrocephalus to avoid a lifetime of shunt dependency. A large multicenter study (Drake 2008) showed complication rates are higher in children less than one year old, and include symptoms such as uncontrolled intraoperative bleeding. This suggests it is best to treat an infant with a shunt surgery early on, and then revaluate the patient for ETV later in life. Thus age is a critical factor in determining whether a patient would be a good candidate for ETV, and is currently under further investigation. (Bouras & Sgouros, 2011)

8.3.3 Follow Up

Patients should be tested for improvement of their specific symptoms, and possible recurrence of original symptoms, which may indicate a potential closure of the stoma. After surgery, the size of ventricles may decrease with clinical improvement, but it has been shown that the degree of volume shrinking is not a good indicator of surgical outcome. CSF flow void via MRI can determine whether ETV function is optimal.

9. Conclusion and controversy

Current research on hydrocephalus patient populations is limited in that many cases are lumped together, irrespective of etiology and prognosis, and is likely the cause of the variable results in similar studies from different centres. Much of the issue, especially in NPH studies, is the lack of a universal set of diagnostic criteria to create homogenous control groups and patient populations, as well as standards of pre and post operative assessments. Additionally, most of the research to date has been focused on reporting any improvement or lack of improvement after surgery, instead of the degree of improvement. Specifically, there is little work looking at whether surgery on a patient with very mild symptoms would be beneficial for reversing the disease process. Focus is now aimed at identifying a set of diagnostic criteria that can be evaluated in studies to determine which set of criteria yield the highest success after shunt implantation.

Identifying a universal set of diagnostic criteria can determine the best candidates for surgery and yield the highest success rate is of key importance in this field. McGirt et al. (2005) reported having one of the highest long-term response rates (75% at 18 month follow up) for NPH patients undergoing shunt surgery. Their criteria for choosing surgical candidates included: 1) ventriculomegaly identified using imaging, 2) two or more clinical features of NPH, 3) no risk factor for secondary NPH, 4) A or B waves present during ICP monitoring and 5) improvement of clinical symptoms following a 3 day trail of CSF drainage. 93% of patients had improvement in gait, and patients who classified gait disturbance as their primary debilitating symptom, instead of incontinence or dementia, saw twice the improvement.

Much interest has been shown in using A or B CSF waves on ICP readings as a predictor of shunt surgery outcome in NPH. Increasing studies of successful surgery outcomes by incorporating pulsatile waves abnormalities in the criteria of selecting successful candidates for shunt surgery suggests possible modification of the hydrocephalus model. Incorporation of the rapid pulsations of CSF into the current bulk-flow CSF model may provide clues to the pathophysiology of NPH and may improve predictions and better cater treatment options for patients.

As previously mentioned, ETV is not routinely performed on children under a year old due to the poor outcome. Instead, infants with hydrocephalus are treated with shunts, and at a later date, may be successfully treated with ETV. One of the reasons that allow this to occur is that CSF absorption ability may be restored at an older age, after a period of shunt drainage during infancy. (Beni-Adani et al, 2006) Thus, studies are now aimed at redefining how long one should wait before offering ETV treatment (i.e. could ETV be offered before 12 months?)Although there is insufficient evidence in the literature to effectively answer this question, it is important to explore, since it could help infants avoid being dependant on shunts.

10. References

Beni-Adani, L., Biani, N., Ben-Sirah, L., & Constantini, S. (2006). The occurrence of obstructive vs. absorptive hydrocephalus in newborns and infants: relevance to treatment choices. Child's Nervous System, Vol.22, No.12, (December 2006), pp. 1542-1563.

Bergsneider, M., Black, P.M., Klinge, .P, Marmarou, A., & Relkin, N. (2005). Surgical management of idiopathic normal-pressure hydrocephalus. Neurosurgery. Vol 57, No. 3 Suppl (September 2005), pp. S2939.

Bouras, T., & Sgouros, S. (2011). Complications of endoscopic third ventriculostomy. Journal of Neurosurgery: Pediatrics. Vol.7, No.6, (June 2011), pp. 643-649.

Bullivant, K..J., Hader, W., & Hamilton, M. (2009). A pediatric experience with endoscopic third ventriculostomy for hydrocephalus. Canadian Journal of Neuroscience Nursing. Vol.31, No. 2, (March 2009), pp. 16-19, ISSN: 1913-7176

Chiafery, M. (2006). Care and management of the child with shunted hydrocephalus. Pediatric Nursing. Vol. 32, No. 3, (May-June2006), pp.222-225.

Cinalli, G., Salazar, C., Mallucci, C., Yada, J.Z., Zerah, M., & Sainte-Rose, C. (1998). The role of endoscopic third ventriculostomy in the management of shunt malfunction. Neurosurgery. Vol. 43, No. 6, (December 1998), pp.1323-1329.

Czosnyka, M., & Whitfield P. (2006). Hydrocephalus: a practical guide to CSF dynamics and ventriculoperitoneal shunt. *Advances in Clinical Neurosciences and Rehabilitation.* Vol. 6, No. 3, (July/August 2006), pp. 14-17, ISSN 1473-9348.

Drake, J.M. (2008). The surgical management of pediatric hydrocephalus. Neurosurgery. Vol.62, No. 2, (February 2008 supplement), pp 633-642.

Eide., P.K., & Sorteberg, W. (2010). Diagnostic intracranial pressure monitoring and surgical management in idiopathic normal pressure hydrocephalus: a 6-year review of 214 patients. Neurosurgery. Vol. 66, No. 1, (January 2010), pp. 80-91.

Factora, R., & Luciano, M. (2006). Normal pressure hydrocephalus: diagnosis and new approaches to treatment. Clinics in Geriatric Medicine. Vol. 22, No. 3, (August 2006), pp.645-657.

Feng, H., Huang, G., Liao, X., Fu, K., Tan, H., Pu, H., Cheng, Y., Liu, W., & Zhao, D. (2004). Endoscopic third ventriculostomy in the management of obstructive hydrocephalus: an outcome analysis. *Journal of Neurosurgery.* Vol.100, No.4 , (April 2004), pp.626-633.

Gallia, G.L., Rigamonti, D., & Williams, M.A.The diagnosis and treatment of idiopathic normal pressure hydrocephalus. Nature clinical practice: neurology. Vol.2, No.7, (July 2006), pp.375-381.

Gangemi, M., Maiuri, F., Buonamassa, S., Colella, G., & de Divitiis, E. (2004). Endoscopic third ventriculostomy in idiopathic normal pressure hydrocephalus. *Neurosurgery.* Vol. 55, No.1 (July 2004), pp. 129-134.

Hader, W.J., Walker, R.L., Myles, S.T., & Hamilton, M. (2008). Complications of endoscopic third ventriculostomy in previously shunted patients. *Neurosurgery.* Vol 63, No. 1 Suppl 1, (July 2008), pp. 168-174.

Jenkinson, M.D., Hayhurst, C., Al-Jumaily, M., Kandasamy, J., Clark, S., & Mallucci, C.L. (2009). The role of endoscopic third ventriculostomy in adult patients with hydrocephalus. *Journal of Neurosurgery.* Vol. 110, No. 5, (May 2009), pp. 861-866.

Kestle, J.R. (2003).Pediatric hydrocephalus: current management. *Neurologic Clinics*. Vol. 23, No. 4, (November 2003), pp. 883-895.

Klinge, P. Marmarou, A., Bergsneider, M., Relkin, N., & Black, P.M. (2005). Outcome of shunting in idiopathic normal-pressure hydrocephalus and the value of outcome assessment in shunted patients. *Neurosurgery*. Vol. 57, No. 3 Suppl (September 2005), pp. S40-52.

Krauss, K.J. & Halve, B. Normal pressure hydrocephalus: survey on contemporary diagnostic algorithms and therapeutic decisions-making in clinical practice. *Acta Neurochirurigca (Wein)*. Vol. 146, No. 4, (April 2004), pp. 379 - 388.

Koch-Wiewrodt, D., & Wagner, W. (2006). Success and failure of endoscopic third ventriculostomy in young infants: are there different age distributions? *Child's Nervous System*. Vol 22, No. 12, (December 2006), pp. 1537-1541.

Madson, J.R., Egnor, M., & Zuo, R. (2006). Cerebral fluid pulsatility and hydrocephalus: the fourth circulation. *Clinical Neurosurgery*. Vol. 53, No. (2006), pp. 48-52.

Malm, J., & Eklund, A. (2006). Idiopathic normal pressure hydrocephalus. *Practical Neurology*. Vol.6, No. 1, (January 2006), pp. 14-27.

Marmarou, A., Young, H.F., Aygok, G.A., Sawauchi, S., Tsuji, O., Yamamoto, T., & Dunbar, J. (2005). Diagnosis and management of idiopathic normal-pressure hydrocephalus: a prospective study in 151 patients. *Journal of Neurosurgery*. Vol. 102, No.6 (June 2005), pp. 987-997.

McGirt, M.J.,Woodworth, G.,Coon, A.L.,Thomas, G.,Williams, M.A., & Rigamonti, D. (2005). Diagnosis, treatment, and analysis of long-term outcomes in idiopathic normal-pressure hydrocephalus. *Neurosurgery*. Vol. 57, No. 4, (October 2005), pp. 699-705.

Pollack, I., Albright, A., Adelson, P., Group H-MI. (1999). A randomized, controlled study of a programmable shunt valve versus a conventional valve for patients with hydrocephalus. *Neurosurgery*. Vol. 45, No.6, (December 1999), pp 1399-1411.

Rezaee, O.,Sharifi, G,Samadian, M.,Haddadian, K,Ali-Asgari, A, &Yazdani, M. (2007). Endoscopic third ventriculostomy for treatment of obstructive hydrocephalus. *Archives of Iranian Medicine*. Vol 10, No. 4, (October 2007), pp.498-503.

Rizvi, R., & Anjum, Q. (2005). Hydrocephalus in children. *The Journal of Pakistan Medical Association*. Vol. 55, No. 11, (November 2005), pp. 502-507.

Stephensen, H., Anderrson, N., Eklund, A., Malm, J., Tisell, M., & Wikkelso, C. (2004). Objective B wave analysis in 55 patients with non-communicating and communicating hydrocephalus. *Journal of Neurology, Neurosurgery and Psychiatry*. Vol. 76, No. 7, (July 2004), pp.965-970.

Vanneste, J., Augustijn, P., Davies, G.A., Dirven, C., & Tan, W.F. (1992). Normal-pressure hydrocephalus. Is cisternography still useful in selecting patients for a shunt? *Archives of Neurology*. Vol. 49, No. 4, (April 1992), pp. 366-370.

Wilson, R.K. & Williams, M.A. (2006). Normal pressure hydrocephalus. *Clinics in Geriatric Medicine*. Vol. 22, No. 4, (November 2006), pp. 935-951.

Woodworth, G.,McGirt, M.J.,Thomas, G.,Williams, M.A., & Rigamonti, D. (2007). Prior CSF shunting increases the risk of endoscopic third ventriculostomy failure in the treatment of obstructive hydrocephalus in adults. *Neurological Research*. Vol. 29, No. 1, (January 2007), pp. 27-31.

2

Intraventricular Cerebrovascular Pathologies of Hydrocephalus and Managements

Ahmet Metin Şanlı, Hayri Kertmen and Bora Gürer
Ministery of Health Diskapi Yildirim Beyazit
Education and Research Hospital
Turkey

1. Introduction

Hydrocephalus, "water in the brain", had been amazed and challenged clinicians throughout the history of medicine till Galen. Vascular causes of hydrocephalus had been a mystery until the discovery of modern neuroradiological techniques such as digital subtraction angiography and magnetic resonance imaging.

Vascular lesions of the ventricular system are rare. Despite the rarity, they may cause symptomatic hydrocephalus. These kinds of lesions cause hydrocephalus in the CSF pathways by either obstruction or hemorrhage. Because of the rarity of this entity, there is no conciliation for the treatment. Four types of intraventricular vascular lesions causing hydrocephalus were categorized as follows:

1. Cavernomas
2. Aneurysms
3. Arteriovenous malformations
4. Venous malformations

2. Intraventricular Cavernomas (IVCs)

Cavernous malformations (CM), also called cavernous angiomas and cavernomas, are low-flow vascular malformations that constitute 5-13% of all central nervous system vascular malformations (Moriarity et al., 1999; Raychaudhuri et al., 2005). On the other hand, IVC are rare pathological entities, constituting 2,5-10.8% of cerebral CM (Kivelev et al., 2010). The first report of an IVC was published in 1905 by Finkelnburg. As to our knowledge, so far 102 IVCs have been summarized published cases in the literature (Table-1).

2.1 Embryogenesis

The exact pathogenesis of the CM is still unknown; but they are thought to arise from early stages of embryogenesis and may be due to aberrant vasculogenesis (Sure et al., 2005). The CMs are known to exhibit an unpredictable dynamic behavior and may increase in size

(Moriarity et al., 1999). The growth most likely occurs by a process of cavern proliferation in the setting of repetitive hemorrhages (Shenkar et al., 2007).

2.2 Pathology

CMs are histologically benign, hamartomatous vascular malformations, consisting of lobulated sinusoidal vascular channels which are lined with thin endotelia. CMs are classified along with capillary telangiectasia, venous angiomas and arteriovenous malformations (AVM) as vascular malformations (Raychaudhuri et al., 2005). CMs are typically lacking interventing neural parenchyma, large feeding arteries or large draining veins; but may have surrounding gliosis. Hemorrhages at all stages of evolution are present within the lesion and cause occlusion and thrombosis of the vascular channels. Organization of the hematoma results in hyaline-degenerative changes, chronic granulation and scar formation; and includes pseudotumorous evolution of the mass (Voigt & Yaşargil, 1976). Further bleeding may occur in the immediate vicinity of CM leading to hemosiderin deposits and gliosis (Chen et al., 2006).

2.3 Location and symptoms of the intraventricular Cavernomas (IVCs)

The most frequent symptoms for all intracranial CM are seizures (60%), progressive neurological deficits (50%) and hemorrhages (20%) (Coin et al, 1977). IVCs are more likely to present with increased intracranial pressure.

The most common location of the IVC is lateral ventricles followed by the third and the fourth ventricles. CM can be asymptomatic; when symptoms are present they depend on the size and the location of the lesion.

Third ventricular CMs have different symptomatology due to its location. The most common presentation of third ventricle CM is hydrocephalus followed by hemorrhage. Some patients presented with memory loss, diabetes insipidus, seizures, visual field deficits and intermittent postural headaches (Fagundes-Pereyra et al., 2000; Katayama et al., 1994; Mizutani et al., 1981; Milenkovic, 2005; Reyns et al., 1999).

On the other hand, symptoms of IVCs are most likely to present late, since the ventricular cavity allows for tumor growth to large sizes (Kumar et al., 2006). This could be explained by the fact that the surrounding cerebrospinal fluid (CSF) allows the increase in size of the lesion without restrictions from parenchyma. Surprisingly, in spite of being intraventricular lesions, hydrocephalus is seldom reported unlike choroids plexus papillomas in the same location (Nieto et al., 2003). For CM of the third and the fourth ventricles, the presence of acute obstructive hydrocephalus is anticipated and can easily explain the patients' symptoms of intracranial hypertension. For CM of the lateral ventricles intracranial hypertension is not so readily explained. Although CSF outflow obstruction from hemorrhagic elements present within the ventricle or on the arachnoid villi from previous microhemorrhages cannot be excluded as the reason for the raised intracranial pressure. A focal non-communicating hydrocephalus due to entrapment of a horn (most commonly temporal horn) may be the cause (Stavrinou et al., 2009). The temporal horn contains the choroids plexus where CSF is produced continuously, so focal obstructive hydrocephalus will result from the CSF production-absorption imbalance. Moreover temporal horn dilatation and the subsequent stretching of the ventricular wall vessels results in disturbance of the venous blood flow and contributes significantly to the development of periventricular edema and intracranial hypertension (Tsugane et al., 1992).

Authors & Year	Age (y),Sex	Presentation	Hydrocephalus	Location	Treatment	Outcome
Finkelburg, 1905	2, M	mass effect	NR	4V	PR	died
Dandy, 1928	31, M	mass effect	yes	4V	TR	improved
Meritt, 1940	16, F	mass effect	none	LV	TR	comatose
Arnstein et al., 1951	2 days, M	mass effect	none	LV	no op	died
Latterman, 1952	68, F	mass effect	NR	3V	no op	died
McGuire et al., 1954	3 mos, M	mass effect	yes	LV	NR	NR
Schneider & Liss, 1958	33, F	mass effect	NR	LV	TR	HH
Jain, 1966	15, M	mass effect	yes	LV	TR	improved
McConnel & Leonard, 1967	31, F	IVH	none	LV	no op	death
Coin et al., 1977	36, F	seizure	none	LV	TR	hemianopia
Numaguchi et al., 1977	43, M	mass effect	none	LV	TR	hemiplegia & hemianopia
Giombini & Morello, 1978	27, M	mass effect	yes	4V	PR	died
Terao et al., 1979	29, F	IVH	yes	4V	TR	improved
Pau & Orunesu, 1979	56, NA	IVH	NR	LV	no op	died
Namba et al., 1979	45, F	IVH	NR	LV	PR	improved
Vaquero et al., 1980	18, F	mass effect	none	3V	TR	improved
Britt et al., 1980	11, F	mass effect	none	LV	TR	improved
Pozzati et al., 1981	31, F	mass effect	yes	3V	TR	improved
Iwasa et al., 1983	8 days, F	mass effect	yes	LV	TR	improved
Kendall et al., 1983	60, F	mass effect	yes	4V	PR	symptom recurrence
Lavyne & Patterson, 1983	48,F	mass effect	yes	3V	PR	hydrocephalus, bleeding
Amagasa et al., 1984	40, M	mass effect	none	3V	TR	improved
Harbaugh et al., 1984	44, F	IVH	yes	3V	TR	improved
Chadduck et al. 1985	21, F	seizure	none	LV	TR	hemianopia
	29, F	mass effect	none	LV	TR	improved
	4 mos, F	seizure	none	LV	TR	improved
Simard et al., 1986	22, M	mass effect	NR	LV	NR	NR
	13, F	mass effect	NR	LV	NR	NR
Yamasaki et al., 1986	73, M	mass effect	NR	LV	TR	improved
	9, M	mass effect	NR	3V	PR	improved
	36, M	mass effect	yes	3V	TR	improved
	47, M	mass effect	NR	4V	TR	improved
	15, F	mass effect	yes	3V	NR	NR

Authors & Year	Age (y),Sex	Presentation	Hydrocephalus	Location	Treatment	Outcome
Suzuki, 1988	40, M	mass effect	none	LV	TR	improved
Sabatier et al., 1989	9 mos, M	IVH	NR	LV	no op	cerebellar dysfunction
Voci et al., 1989	19, F	IVH	NR	3V	TR	improved
Ogawa et al., 1990	16, M	mass effect	yes	3V	TR, shunt	improved
	40, M	mass effect	none	3V	TR	transient DI, HH
Andoh et al., 1990	62, F	mass effect	none	LV	TR	HH
Tatagiba et al., 1991	33, M	IVH	none	LV	TR	improved
	35, M	seizure	none	LV	TR	died
	24, F	mass effect	yes	LV	TR	improved
Itoh & Usui, 1991	44, F	IVH	yes	4V	TR	improved
Miyagi et al., 1993	3, F	IVH	none	LV	TR	mild hemiparesis
Lynch et al., 1994	39, F	seizure	none	LV	TR	improved
	5, M	seizure	none	LV	TR	improved
	10, F	mass effect	none	LV	TR	improved
Katayama et al., 1994	9, F	seizure	yes	3V	PR, shunt	died
	50, F	mass effect	yes	3V	NR	NR
	45, F	IVH	NR	3V	NR	NR
	49, M	mass effect	NR	3V	NR	NR
	47, F	mass effect	NR	3V	TR	transient DI
Sinson et al., 1995	43, F	mass effect	yes	3V	TR	died
	36, F	mass effect	yes	3V	TR	hemiparesis, hydrocephalus
	52, F	mass effect	yes	3V	TR	improved
	32, F	mass effect	yes	3V	TR, shunt	improved
Hashimoto et al., 1997	2 days, M	mass effect	yes	LV	TR, shunt	mild MR
Kaim et al., 1997	64, M	mass effect	yes	3V	TR	NR
Gaab & Shroeder, 1999	44, F	mass effect	yes	LV	TR	permanent memory loss
Reyns et al., 1999	16, F	mass effect	none	LV	TR	improved
	36, M	seizure	none	LV	TR	hemihypertonia
	42, M	asymptomatic	none	3V	PR	improved
Fagundes-Pereyra et al., 2000	15, F	mass effect	none	LV	TR	improved
Attar et al., 2001	30, M	mass effect	none	LV	NR	improved
	30, M	mass effect	none	LV	NR	improved
	18, M	mass effect	none	LV	NR	improved
	30, M	mass effect	none	LV	NR	improved
Suess et al., 2002	36, F	mass effect	yes	3V	TR	improved
Crivelli et al., 2002	38, M	mass effect	yes	3V	TR	improved

Authors & Year	Age (y),Sex	Presentation	Hydrocephalus	Location	Treatment	Outcome
Nieto et al., 2003	11, F	seizure	none	LV	TR	HH
Tatsui et al., 2003	17, F	seizure	none	LV	TR	improved
	52, M	IVH	none	LV	TR	improved
Wang et al., 2003	62, F	mass effect	yes	3V	TR	improved
Anderson et al., 2003	45, F	mass effect	none	LV	TR	improved
Michaelson et al., 2004	22, F	mass effect	none	LV	TR	improved
Darwish et al., 2005	47, F	asymptomatic	none	3V	TR, shunt	improved
Milenkovic et al., 2005	56, M	mass effect	yes	3V	TR	improved
Chen et al., 2006	51, F	mass effect	yes	3V	TR	improved
Kumar et al., 2006	8, M	mass effect	none	LV	TR	improved
	19, F	seizure	none	LV	TR	seizure remained
	20, M	mass effect	none	LV	TR	improved
Longatti et al., 2006	35, M	mass effect	yes	3V	TR	improved
Zakaria et al., 2006	8, M	mass effect	yes	3V	TR	improved
Sato et al., 2006	47, F	mass effect	yes	3V	TR	improved
Gonzalez-Darder et al., 2007	25, M	mass effect	none	LV	TR	improved
Prat & Galeano, 2008	56, NA	mass effect	yes	3V	TR	improved
Stravrinou et al., 2009	52, F	mass effect	yes	LV	TR	improved
Carrasco et al., 2009	60, F	mass effect	none	LV	TR	hemiparesis
	70, M	mass effect	yes	LV	PR, shunt	improved
	66, M	seizure	none	LV	TR	seizure remained
Kivelev et al., 2010	66, M	mass effect	yes	LV	shunt only	improved
	43, F	mass effect	none	4V	TR	improved
	65, M	IVH	yes	LV	TR	improved
	58, F	IVH	none	4V	TR	mild deficit
	20, M	IVH	none	LV	PR	improved
	15, M	IVH	none	4V	TR	mild deficit
	52, M	mass effect	none	3V	TR	improved
	49, F	mass effect	none	4V	TR	mild deficit
	35, M	IVH	none	LV	no op	improved
	49, F	IVH	yes	4V	TR	improved
	65, M	IVH	yes	LV	no op	improved
	53, M	IVH	none	LV	TR	improved

IVH=intraventicular hemorrhage, LV=lateral ventricle, 3V=third ventricle, 4V=fourth ventricle, PR=partial resection, TR=total resection, NR=not registered, HH=homonymous hemianopia, MR=mental retardation, DI=diabetes insipidus

Table 1. Presented cases of IVC in the literature.

2.4 Natural History of the IVCs

According to the review of the literature, the natural history of IVCs may be different from intraparenchymatous lesions. In IVCs, most common symptoms occurred due to mass effect (65%) followed by hemorrhage (20%) and seizure (15%). In children, clinical presentation does not differ significantly from adults. The annual risk of hemorrhage from supratentorial CM is about 0.25-0.7% (Moriarity et al., 1999; Raychaudhuri et al., 2005). The natural history of the IVC cannot be determined due to small number of cases.

2.5 Diagnosis

2.5.1 CT scan

Typical computed tomography (CT) findings associated with CM consist of a well circumscribed high density nodular lesion with minimal or no mass effect, absence of perifocal edema and mild or no contrast enhancement (Chen et al., 2006; Iwasa et al., 1983; Stavrinou et al., 2009). Sometimes calcification of the lesion and intraventricular bleeding may be demonstrated (Tatagiba et al., 1991). Calcifications may appear on conventional x-rays. Several authors have described atypical images, such as hypodense areas within the lesion caused by cystic components (Khosla et al., 1984; Ogawa et al., 1990; Ramina et al., 1980). Nonetheless, these CT findings can be mimicked by AVM, venous angioma, low grade glioma, craniopharyngioma, meningioma, teratoma, neurocytoma, ischemia enhancing infarct and inflammatory lesions (Chadduck et al., 1985).

2.5.2 MRI

The major diagnostic tool of choice in the detection of the IVC is magnetic resonance imaging (MRI). MRI is both highly sensitive and specific. The introduction of MRI has led to diagnosis of an increasing number of CM that had been clinically silent, angiographically occult and undetected by CT. The common MRI features include a heterogeneous core with multiple foci of high signal on short and long TR/TE images, which correspond to hemorrhages of different ages. Interspersed fibrosis shows low signal intensity. The lesions are well delineated by a pseudocapsulate and typically show a low signal hemosiderin rim on T2-weighed images (T2WI). Edema surrounding the CM is unusual and, if present, always mild. Contrast enhancement ranges from strong to moderate or none (Gomori et al., 1986; Kaim et al., 1997; Lemme-Plaghos et al., 1986; Sigal et al., 1990). The radiological appearance of IVC differs from the parenchymatous CM. The typical hypointese perilesional rim on T2WI is absent, probably because no gliotic reaction towards the hemosiderin is established. Another differential aspect is the intense gadolinium enhancement similar to that of neoplastic lesions (Nieto et al., 2003).

2.5.3 DSA

Since CMs are lack of well-formed vessels supplying or draining them, they are often angiographically occult (Simard et al., 1986). Despite CMs have been classically considered as angiographically occult or cryptic vascular malformations, a tumoral blush (supplied by an enlarged choroidal artery) or a feeding artery can be identified on cerebral angiography (Chadduck et al., 1985). Numaguchi et al., have described the presence of tiny strands of the contrast medium in the avascular mass in the capillary and venous phase, without large draining veins or early venous filling being observed. But digital subtraction angiography (DSA) is also indicated to exclude AVM.

2.5.4 Differential diagnosis

The differential diagnosis on MRI includes primary and secondary hemorrhagic neoplasms that can be seen at the ventricle. Anaplastic astrocytomas, glioblastomas and oligodendrogliomas are usually heterogeneous because of intratumoral necrosis, hemorrhage or calcification and may mimic CM. However anaplastik tumor tissue showing nonhemorrhagic, abnormal signal intensity with contrast enhancement and surrounded by prominent high signal edema on long TR/TE images should permit distinction from CM (Sze et al., 1987). In young adults rare but important differential diagnosis include central neurocytoma and subependymal giant cell astrocytoma (Kaim et al., 1997). One should also consider cystic and hemorrhagic metastases which may occur together with metastatic melanoma, adenocarcinoma or bronchogenic carcinoma (Atlas et al., 1987). Most of these malignancies, however have multiple lesions and present with known systemic metastases. Furthermore, ventricles are very uncommon site for solitary metastasis. Colloid cysts and germinomas may occur at foramen of Monro, but can be excluded by their different appearance on CT and MRI (Kaim et al., 1997). IVCs are frequently misdiagnosed as tumors and this can lead the use of invasive diagnostic procedures such as steriotactic biopsy which can cause iatrogenic bleeding (Carrasco et al., 2009). On the other hand, several authors have reported that steriotactic biopsies have been performed safely in patients with CM despite the apparent danger of hemorrhage (Sedan et al., 1989).

2.6 Managements

Still, little is known about natural history of the IVC. The lack of through prospective series and long-term follow-up make decision making the treatment of the IVC difficult. Surgery is advocated when rebleedings are frequent and the mass effect causes hydrocephalus and progressive neurological deficits.

2.6.1 Conservative treatment

A conservative approach to an asymptomatic supratentorial CM is appropriate. However, the tendency for rapid growth and extralesional hemorrhage of IVC may suggest the need to treat these lesions more aggressively (Katayama et al., 1994; Reyns et al., 1999; Sinson et al., 1995). In addition, the radiological diagnosis of IVC may be difficult as these lesions may mimic neoplasms. Incorrect preoperative diagnosis has sometimes resulted in inappropriate treatment, such as radiotherapy (Reyns et al., 1999).

2.6.2 Surgical treatment

The management of hydrocephalus associated with IVC has not been well established. An early resection of the mass might solve the CSF obstruction. In fact, the presence of ventricular dilatation may help during surgery. However insertion of a ventriculoperitoneal shunt or external ventricular drainage before removing the lesion represents a safe choice, because it allows an early relief of the symptoms of high intracranial pressure while studying the mass. The avascular nature of the CM minimizes the risk of shunt device obstruction caused by intraoperative bleeding during lesion removal (Carrasco et al., 2009). On the other hand, shunting CSF may contribute to lesion's rapid growth by altering the hydrodynamic equilibrium between malformation and the ventricular system (Sinson et al., 1995).

The preferable routes for the resection of CM located within the frontal horn are either the transcortical, transventricular or the interhemispheric transcallosal approaches. Transtemporal and superior parietal approaches have been used for the excision of trigonal and temporal horn lesions. The transsylvian transventricular approach is a good alternative for the resection of trigonal lesions with the benefit of a minimal disruption of the visual pathways (Carrasco et al., 2009).

Surgical approaches used to reach foramen of Monro and the third ventricle are transcallosal, transfrontal transventricular and translamina terminalis approaches.

Surgery for an IVC in the lateral or third ventricles is safer than in the fourth ventricle. Patients with CM close to the brainstem frequently present preoperatively with cranial nerve deficits as a sign of brainstem damage. Thus surgery in this already affected region can worsen neurological status and cause new deficits; even after minimal manipulation (Kivelev et al., 2010).

Endoscopic ventriculoscopy may be very useful in establishing the diagnosis or narrowing the differential diagnosis. Despite the increasing role of neuroendoscopy in the treatment of intraventricular lesions, in the cause of IVC the use of endoscopy has been used to confirm the diagnosis under direct vision of the lesion (Sato et al., 2006). Complete endoscopic resection of an IVC has been reported to be performed successfully only in two cases (Gaab & Schroeder, 1999; Prat & Galeano, 2008).

3. Intraventricular Aneurysms (IVAs)

Intraventricular localization of an aneurysm is a very rare entity. To our knowledge, 59 cases were presented in the literature (Table-2).These aneurysms are either true intraventricular or its dome extending into the ventricle cavity(Sanli et al.,2011)For the former aneurysms, most common location is lateral ventricle followed by the third ventricle. Only few cases were located in the fourth ventricle. Most aneurysms in the lateral ventricle are originated from anterior choroidal artery. More specifically, aneurysms in the third ventricle arise from a major branch of the circle of Willis and aneurysms in the fourth ventricle arise from a distal branch of posteroinferior cerebellar artery. Most IVAs are idiopathic, but the most common association is with Moyamoya disease. IVAs can also be found in association with AVM, atherosclerosis and trauma (Lévêque et al., 2011).

Main clinical presentation of IVA is hydrocephalus with either mass effect or hemorrhage.

3.1 Diagnosis

3.1.1 CT scan

CT shows pure intraventricular hematoma (IVH) in most ruptured IVA and IVH with slight subarachnoid hemorrhage (SAH) in some. In some cases, the site of the IVA can be

Author, year	Age, sex	Presentation	Location	Origin	Treatment	Outcome	Associated disease
Lemmen et al., 1953	8mo, ND	HCP	3V	PostChoA	Conservative	dead	none
Strully, 1955	27, F	HCP	LV	AntChoA	Trapping	poor	none
Cressman & Hayes, 1966	34, M	SAH	LV	AntChoA	Conservative	died	trauma
Schürmann et al., 1968	23, F	IVH	LV	MCA	resection	good	none
Butler et al., 1972	15, F	SAH	LV	AntChoA	Trapping	fair	AVM
Papo et al., 1973	57, F	SAH + HCP	LV	AntChoA	Trapping	poor	Atherosclerosis
Kodoma & Suzuki, 1978	16, F	SAH	LV	PostChoA	Conservative	good	Moyamoya
	39, M	SAH	LV	PostChoA	Conservative	good	Moyamoya
	48, F	SAH	LV	PostChoA	Conservative	good	Moyamoya
Babu & Eisen, 1979*	52, M	HCP	3V	AComA	VPS + Ligation	died	none
Tanaka et al., 1980	57, F	IVH	LV	AntChoA	Conservative	died	Moyamoya
Tyson et al., 1980*	75, F	IVH	3V	Basilar tip	External ventriclostomy	died	none
Pasqualin et al., 1981*	32, M	SAH	4V	PICA	clipping	good	none
Bose et al., 1983*	55, F	HCP	3V	Basilar tip	VPS + Clipping	died	none
Koga et al., 1983*	65, F	HCP	3V	Basilar tip	VPS	good	none
Piek et al., 1983*	60, F	HCP	3V	Basilar tip	V-A shunt	good	not registered
Kasamo et al., 1984	55, F	SAH + HCP	LV	AntChoA	clipping	died	Moyamoya
Nehls et al., 1985	18, F	ICH	LV	PostChoA	resection	good	AVM
Konishi et al., 1985	13, M	IVH	LV	AntChoA	Conservative	fair	Moyamoya
	57, F	IVH	LV	AntChoA	Conservative	died	Moyamoya
	34, F	IVH	LV	AntChoA	Conservative	died	Moyamoya
Borrie et al., 1985*	72, F	HCP	3V	Basilar tip	VPS	good	none
	70, M	HCP	LV	MCA	V-A shunt	good	none
Ungersböck & Perneczky, 1986	18, F	NR	LV	PostChoA	clipping	good	none
Knuckey et al., 1988	46, F	SAH	LV	AntChoA	Ligation	good	Atherosclerosis
Morota et al., 1988*	69, F	HCP	3V	ICA bif	VPS	good	none
Inagawa et al., 1990	75, F	SAH + HCP	LV	AntChoA	Conservative	died	none
Nishihara et al., 1993	34, F	SAH + IVH	LV	AntChoA	Excision	good	none
Hamada et al.,	48, F	IVH	LV	AntChoA	Trapping	good	Moyamoya

Author, year	Age, sex	Presentation	Location	Origin	Treatment	Outcome	Associated disease
1994							
Smith et al., 1994*	60, F	HCP	3V	PComA	clipping	good	none
Uranishi et al., 1994	65, F	IVH	4V	PICA	resection	moderate	none
Bergsneider et al., 1994	65, M	IVH	3V	PComA	resection	moderate	none
Urbach et al., 1995*	55, M	IVH	4V	PICA	clipping	good	not registered
Morgenstren et al., 1996	33, M	Ischemia	LV	AntChoA	Conservative	good	none
Koyama et al., 1996*	52, F	HCP	3V	Basilar tip	VPS	died	none
Kawai et al., 1997	19, M	IVH	LV	AntChoA	Conservative	fair	Moyamoya
Watanabe et al., 1999*	60. M	HCP	3V	Basilar tip	Coil embolization	good	none
Yanaka et al., 2000	8, F	IVH	LV	AntChoA	Trapping	good	AVM
Miyake et al., 2000	30, F	IVH + HCP	4V	SCA	resection	good	Moyamoya
	47, M	IVH	LV	PostChoA	resection	good	Moyamoya
	11, F	IVH	LV	PostChoA	Conservative	good	Moyamoya
Lee et al., 2001	48, M	ICH + IVH	LV	AntChoA	Trapping	good	Moyamoya
Hongo et al., 2001*	70, F	HCP	3V	Basilar tip	Endovascular occlusion	died	none
Gelal et al., 2002*	58, M	HCP	3V	Basilar tip	VPS	good	none
Kwok-chu Wong, 2003	62, F	ICH + IVH	LV	AntChoA	clipping	good	Moyamoya
Horie et al., 2003	77, F	IVH + HCP	4V	PICA	resection	died	none
Ali et al., 2004	26, M	IVH	LV	PostChoA	trapping + resection	good	Moyamoya
Liu et al., 2005*	55, M	HCP	3V	Basilar tip	ETV	good	none
Inci et al., 2007	19, F	ICH + IVH	LV	AntChoA	Trapping	good	none
	37, F	ICH + SAH	LV	AntChoA	Trapping	died	none
Koç & Ceylan, 2008*	58, F	SAH	3V	AComA	clipping	good	AVM
Tsutsumi et al., 2008*	58, M	HCP	3V	Basilar tip	VPS + Embolization	good	none
Oertel et al., 2009*	80, M	HCP	3V	Basilar trunk	ETV	good	none
	55, M	HCP	3V	Basilar tip	ETV + Coil embolization	died	none
	32, F	HCP	3V	Basilar trunk	ETV + Endovascular occlusion	died	none
Yurt et al., 2009	70, M	IVH	LV	AntChoA	clipping	good	none

Author, year	Age, sex	Presentation	Location	Origin	Treatment	Outcome	Associated disease
Leveque et al., 2011	50, F	IVH	LV	AntChoA	Endoscopic resection	good	Moyamoya
Sanli et al., 2011*	41, M	Mass effect	LV	Distal ACA	Coil embolization	good	none

ND= not determined, HCP= hydrocephalus, NR=not registered, LV=lateral ventricle, 3V=third ventricle, 4V=fourth ventricle, IVH=intraventricular hematoma, SAH=subarachnoid hemorrhage, ETV=endoscopic third ventriculostomy, VPS=ventriculoperitoneal shunt, PostChoA=posterior choroidal artery, AntChoA=anterior choroidal artery, MCA=middle cerebral artery, PComA=posterior communicating artery, ACA=anterior cerebral artery, PICA=posteroinferior cerebellar artery, SCA=superior cerebellar artery, asterics(*)=aneurysm's dome extending into the ventricle cavity.

Table 2. Presented cases of IVA in the literature.

estimated on the basis either as the IVH defect or as the prolonged presence of a hyperdense area on the ventricle wall (Hamada et al., 1994). In the course of a giant aneurysm, the appearance on CT is characteristic, consisting of a well-circumscribed round an oval mass (Artmann et al., 1984). The presence of thrombus determines the central attenuation characteristics, which may range from iso- to hyperdense. A peripheral zone of increased attenuation is frequently seen due to mural thrombus (Schubiger et al., 1987). After administration of the contrast media, CT scans show intense enhancement of the residual aneurysm lumen, and this rapidly declines after cessation of contrast media injection (Artmann et al., 1984).

3.1.2 MRI

MRI taken after resolution of IVH usually shows the site of the aneurysm clearly, precise location within the ventricle and the relation of the lesion to the parent vessel (Smith et al., 1994). The aneurysm usually appeared as flow void signs with marked gadolinium enhancement (Fig.1). Old blood clots often surround the aneurysm, with signal intensity depending on clot age.

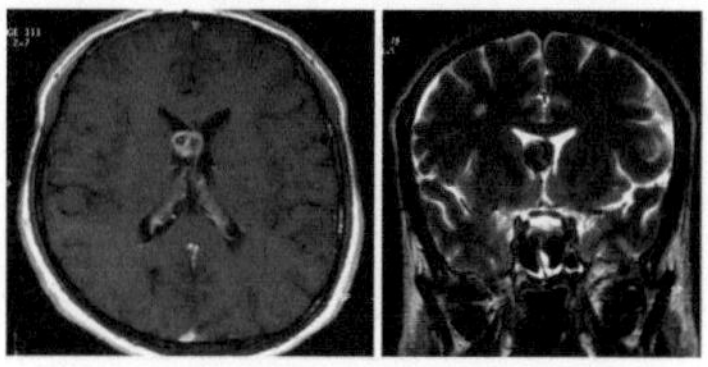

Fig. 1. MRI view of intraventricular aneurysm. Left, T1W image with gadolinium shows a nodular lesion in the lateral ventricle; right, T2W image shows a heterogenous lesion hypointense to brain tissue.

3.1.3 DSA

DSA is the method of choice in diagnosing aneurysms and provides reliable delineation of the aneurysmal lumen and its relationship to the parent vessel and adjacent arteries (Fig.2). But it has limitations; first it is invasive. Especially in the posterior fossa, where invasive surgical treatment is less often considered, less invasive diagnostic methods may be preferred. Second, in DSA only the patent lumen is visualized, thus the thrombosed lumen and the aneurysm may be missed. However MRI-angiography and/or CT-angiography may provide complementary information in cases of thrombosed aneurysm, where the mass of the aneurysm is much larger than what is seen on angiographic filling. Although, IVA often cannot be found during the acute stage after hemorrhage, since the aneurysm or its parent artery is easily compressed by a packed IVH (Miyake et al., 2000). Therefore neuroradiological examination shall be repeated to confirm the diagnosis.

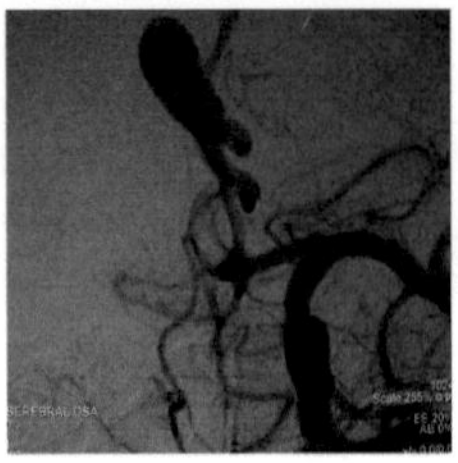

Fig. 2. Left carotid angiogram shows a saccular aneurysm of the distal anterior cerebral artery in the right lateral ventricle.

3.1.4 Differential diagnosis

Sometimes aneurysms in a ventricle cavity can cause difficulties in the differential diagnosis with mass lesions including AVM, CM, and tumors (colloid cysts and non-enhancing meningiomas) (Inci et al., 2007). Cross-sectional imaging modalities can usually be used to distinguish aneurysms from other mass lesions (Smith et al., 1994). Initially, a correct preoperative diagnosis is vital, and the wrong diagnosis of an aneurysm in an unusual location may encourage surgical removal of these lesions (Bose et al., 1983; Liu et al., 2005).

3.2 Managements

3.2.1 Conservative treatment

Conservative treatment can be effective for IVA, which may disappear spontaneously (Kodama & Suzuki, 1978; Konishi et al., 1985; Miyake et al., 2000). Rebleeding during observation may also occur (Hamada et al., 1984; Konishi et al., 1985). So, neuroradiogical examinations should be repeated; DSA is essential for this purpose.

3.2.2 Surgical treatment

Direct surgery should be seriously considered for most of the IVAs, especially for persistent IVAs, enlarged or reruptured aneurysms. Cerebral revascularization should be performed when the parent artery needs an important collateral route or in the case of misery cerebral perfusion.

Aneurysmal clipping and resection are the treatments of choice for IVAs depending on the size of the parent artery. For very small arteries, aneurysmal resection rather than clipping is preferred to prevent postoperative distortion and tears of the parent artery.Neuronavigation is helpful to minimize surgical damage when treating small and deeply situated lesions.

Direct aneurysmal coil embolization is difficult because the lesion is usually situated on a deep small branch and the aneurysm wall is fragile (Watanabe et al.,1999; Sanli et al., 2011). Endovascular occlusion of the parent artery is a choice when the parent artery can be sacrifided.

After aneurysmal SAH, ventriculoperitoneal shunt dependence due to hydrocephalus is a frequent observation with an incidence up to almost 20% (de Oliveira et al., 2007). Most patients require shunt treatment for malabsorbtive hydrocephalus, although some patients with aneurysms suffer from hydrocephalus due to CSF pathway obstruction rather than malresorption. CSF shunting is the most frequently performed procedure for treating obstructive hydrocephalus induced by a non-ruptured IVA (Hongo et al., 2001). For a ruptured aneurysm, experimental and clinical evidence suggests an increased risk of rebleeding when the pressure gradient across the aneurysm wall is increased (Nornes, 1973; Rosenørn et al., 1983). Several reports explain that ventricular drainage is not conclusively associated with an increased incidence of repeated aneurysmal rerupture (Hasan et al., 1989; Voldby & Enevoldsen, 1982). On the other hand, Pare et al., demonstrated an increased risk of aneurismal rebleeding in patients undergoing ventricular drainage, particularly in the presence of hydrocephalus. Obstructive hydrocephalus due to IVA was also treated with microsurgical ventriculostomy via transcallosal approach (Liu et al., 2005). Also, Oertel et al., reported 3 cases with obstructive hydrocephalus due to basilar artery aneurysm that were treated by endoscopic third ventriculostomy.

4. Intraventricular Arteriovenous Malformations (AVMs)

AVM located entirely in the ventricular system are uncommon and account for 4% of AVM in child (Humphreys, 1986) and 1.3% of AVM in adults (Jomin et al., 1985). Less than 40 intraventricular AVM have been reported. The most common locations are lateral ventricle and foramen of Monro. Only two well documented cases have been reported in the third ventricle in the literature (Heafner et al.,1985; Sanli et al., 2007).

Most intraventricular AVM have been manifested with spontaneous hemorrhage into the ventricle, and this causes posthemorrhagic hydrocephalus via blockage CSF absorption or mechanical blockage of CSF pathways. There were only two cases with an aqueductal lesion causing hydrocephalus have been reported (Song et al., 2008).

4.1 Diagnosis

4.1.1 CT scan

CT may be better than angiography in detecting angiographically occult intraventricular AVM (Song et al., 2008). AVM characteristically have high signal attenuation on CT scans and can be enhanced intensely (Fig.3). Miyasaka et al., considered that CT is more useful for;

- precise determination of the anatomical location of the lesion
- detection of angiographycally occult vascular malformations including CM or venous agiomas.
- recognition of the extent of the hemorrhage or the degree of hydrocephalus accompanying the small vascular malformation

Therefore, when angiography fails to reveal the responsible lesion, CT is very helpful for detection of the intraventricular vascular lesion. But it may give very little information about the type of the vascular lesion.

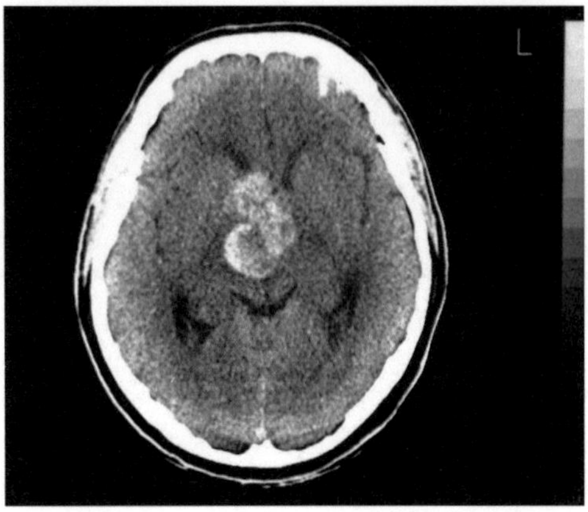

Fig. 3. CT scan shows an irregular hyperdense lesion in the third ventricle and mild hydrocephalus due to mass effect.

4.1.2 MRI

At this point MRI offers more detailed information about the primary lesion and its differential diagnosis. In MRI the nidus is hypointense on T1 weighed images (T1WI) and hyperintense on T2WI. This high signal intensity on T2WI is due to vascular stasis. The signal void linear straits belonging to drainage vessels seen on angiography give a clue to AVM (Fig.4). Therefore, MRI can be helpful in differential diagnosis of granulomatous or highly vascular neoplastic lesions such as choroids plexus papilloma and carcinoma (Gürcan et al., 1998).

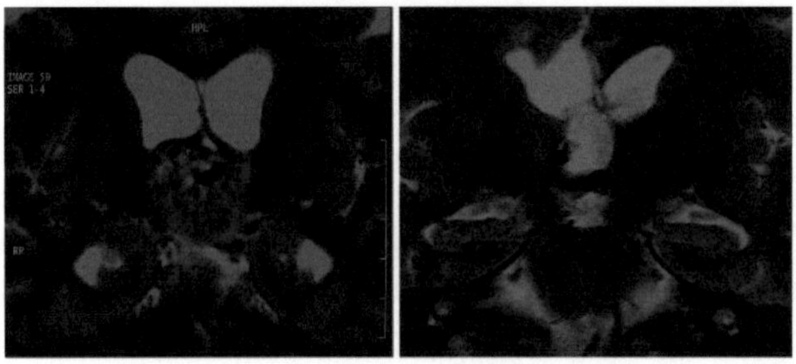

Fig. 4. left, coronal T2W image shows a mass with heterogeneous signal intensity in the third ventricle and dilated temporal horns of the lateral ventricles. The lesion includes tubular signal void areas. Right, early postoperative MRI after right transcallosal approach.

4.1.3 DSA

Cerebral DSA is the most reliable radiological examination for the diagnosis of AVM (Fig.5). Intraventricular AVMs are commonly angiographycally occult, because these lesions are often too small to be detected by angiography or because hemorrhage or thrombosis of the involved vessels may destroy them (Roda et al., 1981; Sanli et al., 2007). Angiography showed no evidence of AVM in about 20% of intraventricular AVM (Tamaki et al., 1994).

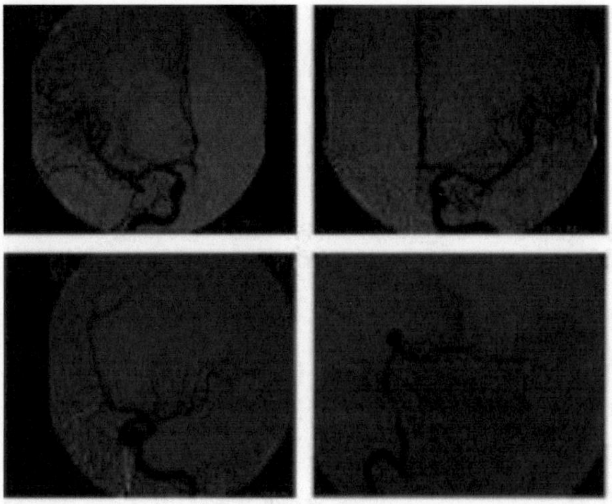

Fig. 5. Both carotid arteries and left vertebral artery angiographies show no any vascular pathologies.

4.1.4 Differential diagnosis

Intraventricular AVM with a typical images are not rare. Misdiagnosis is common because the characteristic signal void may be absent or angiographic results may be negative. Moreover, some intraventricular AVM may radiologically mimic tumors (Britt et al., 1980).

Transfontanel ultrasonography is helpful for finding hydrocephalus, IVH and intracerebral hemorrhage secondary to AVM. Transfontanel ultrasonography is safetly used for diagnosing intraventricular AVM in neonates (Ceylan et al., 1993; Heck et al., 2002). Correct preoperative diagnosis of intraventicular AVM is important for appropriate treatment planning.

4.2 Managements

Overall, 2-4% of brain AVM bleed, and the hemorrhage rates are higher in children than adults (Song et al., 2008). Bleeding rates of the intraventricular AVM are 81% in children and 95%in adults, and incidences of rebleeding and resultant are also high (Tamaki et al., 1994).

4.2.1 Conservative treatment

Despite the fact that intraventicular AVMs are often seemed inoperable because of their deep location and sometimes intimidating vascular patterns, there is evidence to suggest that their natural history is unfavorable with a high incidence of hemorrhagic complications, so that intraventricular AVMs must be treated (Batjer & Samson, 1987). But the treatment of these lesions remains a challenging matter. Surgical excision, endovascular embolization, radiosurgery or a multimodality approach have been used to treat this condition, however studies are not conclusive yet (Ogilvy et al., 2001).

4.2.2 Surgical treatment

The ideal treatment for a cerebral AVM is total surgical resection. AVM of the ventricles are generally small enough to be removed safely by microsurgical techniques (Tamaki et al., 1994). Preoperative embolization may be helpful, although embolization is rarely curative.

Fahim et al., reported that the transtubular microendoscopic approach may be advantageous for resecting intraventricular lesions by avoiding unnecessary retraction; therefore, it may reduce the risk of injury to the surrounding brain tissue.

Yamada et al., reported the endoscopic resection of the intraventricular AVM.

Total surgical excision is very important for intraventricular AVM because any mass left after surgery, radiosurgery or embolization can result in hemorrhage or hydrocephalus.

Regarding the craniotomy microsurgery and neuroendoscopy; former is safer for managing bleedings during surgery (Moftakhar et al., 2006). Surgery for pediatric cases may be delayed because procedures become less difficult as child grows (Heck et al., 2002).

5. Intraventricular venous malformations

Developmental venous anomalies (DVA) and venous loops or varices may cause hydrocephalus by blocking CSF pathways at the Sylvian aqueduct. Also they may cause unilateral dilatation of a ventricle due to blockage at the foramen of Monro. DVA, also known as venous agiomas, represent nonpathological variations in venous drainage. DVA represent the most common intracranial vascular malformations, composing of 63% of such lesions in autopsy series (Garner et al., 1991). To our knowledge, there were only 12 reported cases of intraventricular venous anomalies causing hydrocephalus (Table-3).

DVA and venous varices have similar wall characteristics; where the walls of both are composed of intima and adventitia without presence of media (Kelly et al., 1995). DVA consist of multiple dilated anomalous veins with interposed neural tissue and ≥1 dilated draining vein, typically presenting pathologically as a conical or wedge-shaped lesion with its base at the meninges and its apex toward the ventricle (Fierstien et al., 1979). The intervening parenchyma is normal. Venous varices, on the other hand, are characterized as a focal dilatation of a single vein without neural tissue (Kelly et al., 1995). Although intraventricular DVA may not have the characteristic interposition of neural tissue, they are characterized by dilatation of multiple anomalous veins (Leonardo & Grand, 2009).

The most popular theories for the etiology of these benign lesions include primary dysplasia of capillaries and small transcerebral veins (Ostertun & Solymosi, 1993) or a compensatory mechanism when normal venous pathways are by-passed due to accidental thrombosis in the intrauterine period (Saito & Kobayashi, 1981).

Most common location of the CSF pathway obstruction causing hydrocephalus is Sylvian aqueduct. There are only two reports of unilateral hydrocephalus caused by venous malformation due to obstruction of the foramen of Monro (Leonardo & Grand, 2009; Tien et al., 1990).

Author, Year	Age, Sex	Symptom	Imaging	Treatment	Outcome
Rosenheck, 1937	58, F	Mental deterioration	Postmortem	none	dead
Avman & Dinçer, 1980	35, F	Headache	Ventriculography + CT + angiography	ventriculostomy	good
Tien et al., 1990	37, F	Headache, gait instability	MRI + CT	septum pellucidum fenestration	good
Watanabe at al., 1991	39, M	Headache	CT + MRI + angiography	shunt	good
Oka et al., 1993	43, F	Seizure	CT + MRI (cine) + angiography	ETV	good
Blackmore & Mamourian, 1996	16, F	Headache, behavior abnormalities	MRI (cine)	none	good
Bannur et al., 2002	11, M	Headache	CT + MRI (cine)	shunt	good
Sato et al., 2004	28, F	Headache	CT + MRI + angiography	ETV	good
Yagmurlu et al., 2005	7, F	Headache	MRI	none	good
Giannetti et al., 2008	42, M	Headache, behavior abnormalities	MRI + CT	ETV	good
	18, M	Headache	MRI + CT	ETV	good
Leonarda & Grand, 2009	28, M	Headache	MRI + CT + MR angiography	Endoscopic septum pellucidum fenestration	good

CT=computed tomography, MRI= magnetic resonance imaging, ETV=endoscopic third ventriculostomy

Table 3. Presented cases of intraventricular venous lesions in the literature.

5.1 Diagnosis

CT may not be helpful in the diagnosis, and MRI has proven to be the most sensitive diagnostic tool (Oka et al., 1993). In general, the lesions are hypointense in T1WI and enhance intensely after the contrast media administration. On T2WI they have high or low signal intensity depending on the flow velocity, the orientation and the pulse sequence. Cine

MRI has also used to confirm the location of hydrocephalus in some cases (Blackmore & Mamourian, 1996). The role of DSA is limited and can, at least, document the anomaly of the associated anomalous venous drainage (Bannur et al., 2002).

5.2 Managements

DVA and venous varices are benign lesions that do not need any treatment because there is no risk of rupture or bleeding. Also, they present normal blood outflow pathways, and any attempt in removing them surgically, can cause venous infarction or edema (Bannur et al., 2002; Blackmore & Mamourian, 1996; Yagmurlu et al., 2005).

Hydrocephalus caused by venous anomalies can easily be treated by shunts or endoscopic third ventriculostomy. As listed in the table 3, the outcome is almost always good.

6. Conclusion

The cerebrovascular pathologies cause hydrocephalus by obstruction of CSF pathways due to the slow growing of the vascular lesion or hemorrhage. Since the cerebrovascular lesions are complex pathologies, there is not an agreement among neurosurgeons on treatment. The lack of more clinical and surgical experiences makes a decision with difficulty in the treatment of the intraventricular cerebrovascular lesions.

7. References

Atlas, SW.; Grossman, RI.; Gomori, JM.; Hackney, DB.; Goldberg, HI.; Zimmerman, RA. & Bilaniuk, LT. (1987). Hemorrhagic intracranial malignant neoplasms: spin-echo MR imaging. *Radiology*, vol.164, No.1, pp. 71-77

Artmann, H.; Vonofakos, D.; Müller, H. & Grau, H. (1984). Neuroradiologic and neuropathologic findings with growing giant intracranial aneurysm. Review of the literature. *Surgical Neurology*, Vol.21, No.4, pp. 391-401

Bannur, U.; Korah, I. & Chandy, MJ. (2002). Midbrain venous angioma with obstructive hydrocephalus. *Neurology India*, Vol.50, No.2, pp. 207-209

Batjer, H. & Samson, D. (1987). Surgical approaches to trigonal arteriovenous malformations. *Journal of Neurosurgery*, Vol.67, No.4, pp. 511-517

Blackmore, CC. & Mamourian, AC. (1996). Aqueduct compression from venous angioma: MR findings. *American Journal of Neuroradiology*, Vol.17, No.3, pp. 458-460

Bose, B.; Northrup, B. & Osterholm, J. (1983). Giant basilar artery aneurysm presenting as a third ventricular tumor. *Neurosurgery*, Vol.13, No.6, pp. 699-702

Britt, RH.; Silverberg, GD.; Enzmann, DR. & Hanbery, JW. (1980). Third ventricular choroid plexus arteriovenous malformation simulating a colloid cyst. Case report. *Journal of Neurosurgery*, Vol.52, No.2, pp. 246-250

Carrasco, R.; Pedrosa, M.; Pascual, JM.; Navas, M.; Liberal, R. & Sola, RG. (2009). Cavernous angiomas of the lateral ventricles. *Acta Neurochirurgica (Wien)*, Vol.151, No.2, pp.149-154

Ceylan, S.; Kuzeyli, K.; Kalelioğlu, M.; Aktürk, F. & Ozoran, Y. (1993). Choroid plexus arteriovenous malformation (AVM) in a newborn. Case report. *Neurosurgical Review,* Vol.16, No.3, pp. 241-243

Chadduck, WM.; Binet, EF.; Farrell, FW.; Araoz, CA. & Reding, DL. (1985) Intraventricular cavernous hemangioma: report of three cases and review of the literature. *Neurosurgery,* Vol.16, No.2, pp.189-197

Chen, CL.; Leu, CH.; Jan, YJ. & Shen, CC. (2006). Intraventricular cavernous hemangioma at the foramen of Monro: Case report and literature review. *Clinical Neurology and Neurosurgery,* Vol.108, No.6, pp. 604-609

Coin, CG.; Coin, JW. & Glover, MB. (1977). Vascular tumors of the choroid plexus: diagnosis by computed tomography. *Journal of Computer Assisted Tomography,* Vol.1, No.1, pp. 146-148

de Oliveira, JG.; Beck, J.; Setzer, M.; Gerlach, R.; Vatter, H.; Seifert, V. & Raabe, A. (2007). Risk of shunt-dependent hydrocephalus after occlusion of ruptured intracranial aneurysms by surgical clipping or endovascular coiling: a single-institution series and meta-analysis. *Neurosurgery,* Vol.61,No.5,pp. 924-933

Fagundes-Pereyra, WJ.; Marques, JA.; Sousa, LD.; Carvalho, GT. & Sousa, AA. (2000). Cavernoma of the lateral ventricle: case report. *Arquivos de Neuro-psiquiatria,* Vol.58, No.3B, pp. 958-964

Fahim, DK.; Relyea, K.; Nayar, VV.; Fox, BD.; Whitehead, WE.; Curry, DJ.; Luerssen, TG. & Jea, A. (2009). Transtubular microendoscopic approach for resection of a choroidal arteriovenous malformation. *Journal of Neurosurgery: Pediatrics,* Vol.3, No.2, pp. 101-104

Fierstien, SB.; Pribram, HW. & Hieshima, G. (1979). Angiography and computed tomography in the evaluation of cerebral venous malformations. *Neuroradiology,* Vol.17, No.3, pp. 137-148

Finkelburg, R. (1905). Zur DifferentialDiagnose zwischen Hirntumoren und chronischem Hydrocephalus. (Zugleich ein Beitrag zar Kenntnis der Angiome des zentralnervensystems). *Deutsche Zeitschrift für* Nervenheilkunde, Vol.29, pp. 135-151

Gaab, MR. & Schroeder, HW. (1999). Neuroendoscopic approach to intraventricular lesions. *Neurosurgical Focus,* Vol.15, No.6, pp. e5

Garner, TB.; Del Curling, O.; Kelly, DL. & Laster, DW. (1991). The natural history of intracranial venous angiomas. *Journal of Neurosurgery,* Vol.75, No.5, pp. 715-722

Gomori, JM.; Grossman, RI.; Goldberg, HI.; Hackney, DB.; Zimmerman, RA. & Bilaniuk, LT. (1986). Occult cerebral vascular malformations: high-field MR imaging. *Radiology,* Vol.158, No.3, pp. 707-713

Gürcan, F.; Aribal, ME.; Baltacioğlu, F. & Aslan B. (1998). Arteriovenous malformation of the choroid plexus. *Australasian Radiology,* Vol.42, No.1, pp. 69-71

Hamada, J.; Hashimoto, N. & Tsukahara T. (1994). Moyamoya disease with repeated intraventricular hemorrhage due to aneurysm rupture. Report of two cases. *Journal of Neurosurgery,* Vol.80, No.2, pp. 328-331

Hasan, D.; Vermeulen, M.; Wijdicks, EF.; Hijdra, A. & van Gijn, J. (1989). Management problems in acute hydrocephalus after subarachnoid hemorrhage. *Stroke,* Vol.20, No.6, pp. 747-753

Heafner, MD.;Duncan, CC.; Kier L.;Ment, LR.; Scott, DT.; Kolaski, R. & Sorgen, C.(1985). Intraventricular hemorrhage in a term neonate secondary to a third ventricular AVM. Case report. *Journal of Neurosurgery,* Vol.63,pp.640-643

Heck, DV.; Gailloud, P.; Cohen, HL.; Clatterbuck, RE.; Tamargo, R.; Avellino, AM. & Murphy, KP. (2002). Choroid plexus arteriovenous malformation presenting with intraventricular hemorrhage. *Journal of Pediatrics,* Vol.141, No.5, pp. 710-711

Hongo, K.; Morota, N.; Watabe, T.; Isobe, M. & Nakagawa, H. (2001). Giant basilar bifurcation aneurysm presenting as a third ventricular mass with unilateral obstructive hydrocephalus: case report. *Journal of Clinical Neuroscience,* Vol.8, No.1, pp. 51-54

Humphreys, RP. (1986). Hemorrhagic stroke in childhood. *Journal of Pediatric Neuroscience,* Vol.2, pp.1-10

Inci, S.; Arat, A. & Ozgen, T. (2007). Distal anterior choroidal artery aneurysms. *Surgical Neurology,* Vol.67, No.1, pp. 46-52

Iwasa, H.; Indei, I. & Sato F. (1983). Intraventricular cavernous hemangioma. Case report. *Journal of Neurosurgery,* Vol.59, No.1, pp. 153-157

Jomin, M.; Lesoin, F. & Lozes, G. (1985). Prognosis for arteriovenous malformations of the brain in adults based on 150 cases. *Surgical Neurology,* Vol.23, No.4, pp. 362-366

Kaim, A.; Kirsch, E.; Tolnay, M.; Steinbrich, W. & Radü, EW. (1997). Foramen of Monro mass: MRI appearances permit diagnosis of cavernous haemangioma. *Neuroradiology,* Vol.39, No.4, pp. 265-269

Katayama, Y.; Tsubokawa, T.; Maeda, T. & Yamamoto, T. (1994). Surgical management of cavernous malformations of the third ventricle. *Journal of Neurosurgery,* Vol.80, No.1, pp. 64-72

Kelly, KJ.; Rockwell, BH.; Raji, MR.; Altschuler, EM. & Martinez AJ. (1995). Isolated cerebral intraaxial varix. *American Journal of Neuroradiology,* Vol.16, No.8, pp. 1633-1635

Khosla, VK.; Banerjee, AK.; Mathuriya, SN. & Mehta, S. (1984). Giant cystic cavernoma in a child. Case report. *Journal of Neurosurgery,*Vol.60, No.6, pp. 1297-1299

Kivelev, J.; Niemelä, M.; Kivisaari, R. & Hernesniemi J. (2010). Intraventricular cerebral cavernomas: a series of 12 patients and review of the literature. *Journal of Neurosurgery,* Vol.112, No.1, pp. 140-9

Kodama, N. & Suzuki, J. (1978) Moyamoya disease associated with aneurysm. *Journal of Neurosurgery,* Vol.48, No.4, pp. 565-569

Konishi, Y.; Kadowaki, C.; Hara, M. & Takeuchi, K. (1985). Aneurysms associated with moyamoya disease. *Neurosurgery,* Vol.16, No.4, pp. 484-491

Kumar, GS.; Poonnoose, SI; Chacko, AG. & Rajshekhar, V. (2006). Trigonal cavernous angiomas: report of three cases and review of literature. *Surgical Neurology,* Vol.65, No.4, pp. 367-371

Leonardo, J. & Grand, W. (2009). Enlarged thalamostriate vein causing unilateral Monro foramen obstruction. Case report. *Journal of Neurosurgery: Pediatrics,* Vol.3, No.6, pp. 507-510

Lemme-Plaghos, L.; Kucharczyk, W.; Brant-Zawadzki, M.; Uske, A.; Edwards, M.; Norman, D. & Newton, TH. (1986). MRI of angiographically occult vascular malformations. *American Journal of Roentgenology,* Vol.146, No.6, pp.1223-1228

Lévêque, M.; McLaughlin, N.; Laroche, M. & Bojanowski, MW. (2011). Endoscopic treatment of distal choroidal artery aneurysm. *Journal of Neurosurgery,* Vol.114, No.1, pp. 116-119

Liu, JK.; Gottfried, ON. & Couldwell, WT. (2005). Thrombosed basilar apex aneurysm presenting as a third ventricular mass and hydrocephalus. *Acta Neurochirurgica,* Vol.147, No.4, pp. 413-416

Milenkovic, Z. (2005). Postural intermittent headaches as the initial symptom of a cavernoma in the third ventricle. *Acta Neurochirurgica,* Vol.147, No.1, pp. 105-106

Miyake, H.; Ohta, T.; Kajimoto, Y.; Ogawa, R. & Deguchi, J. (2000). Intraventricular aneurysms--three case reports. *Neurologia Medico-Chirurgica,* Vol.40, No.1, pp. 55-60

Miyasaka, Y.; Kitahara, T.; Saito, T.; Ohwada, T. & Yada, K. (1982). Small vascular malformation of choroid plexus in lateral ventricle. Diagnostic problems of the lesion. *Neurologia Medico-Chirurgica,* Vol.22, No.2, pp. 159-166

Mizutani, T.; Goldberg, HI.; Kerson, LA. & Murtagh, F. (1981). Cavernous hemangioma in the diencephalon. *Archives of Neurology,* Vol.38, No.6, pp. 379-82

Moftakhar, R.; Salamat, MS.; Sahin, S. & Iskandar, BJ. (2006). Endoscopically-assisted resection of a choroid plexus vascular malformation traversing the cerebral aqueduct: technical case report. *Neurosurgery,* Vol. 59, No.1 Suppl 1, pp. ONS-E161

Moriarity, JL.; Clatterbuck, RE. & Rigamonti, D. (1999). The natural history of cavernous malformations. *Neurosurgical Clinics of North America,* Vol.10, No.3, pp. 411-417

Nieto, J.; Hinojosa, J.; Muñoz, MJ.; Esparza, J. & Ricoy, R. (2003) Intraventricular cavernoma in pediatric age. *Childs Nervous System,* Vol.19, No.1, pp. 60-62

Nornes, H. (1973). The role of intracranial pressure in the arrest of hemorrhage in patients with ruptured intracranial aneurysm. *Journal of Neurosurgery,* Vol.39, No.2, pp. 226-234

Numaguchi, Y.; Fukui, M.; Miyake, E.; Kishikawa, T.; Ikeda, J.; Matsuura, K.; Tomonaga, M. & Kitamura, K. (1977). Angiographic manifestations of intracerebral cavernous hemangioma. *Neuroradiology* Vol.14, No.3, pp. 113-116

Oertel, JM.; Mondorf, Y. & Gaab, MR. (2009). Endoscopic third ventriculostomy in obstructive hydrocephalus due to giant basilar artery aneurysm. *Journal of Neurosurgery,* Vol.110, No.1, pp. 14-18

Ogawa, A.; Katakura, R. & Yoshimoto, T. (1990). Third ventricle cavernous angioma: report of two cases. *Surgical Neurology,* Vol.34, No.6 pp. 414-420

Ogilvy, CS.; Stieg, PE.; Awad, I.; Brown, RD.; Kondziolka, D.; Rosenwasser, R.; Young, WL. & Hademenos, G. (Stroke Council, American Stroke Association). (2001). Recommendations for the management of intracranial arteriovenous malformations: a statement for healthcare professionals from a special writing group of the Stroke Council, American Stroke Association. *Circulation,* Vol.103, No.21, pp. 2644-1657

Oka, K.; Kumate, S.; Kibe, M.; Tomonaga, M.; Maehara, F. & Higashi, Y. (1993). Aqueductal stenosis due to mesencephalic venous malformation: case report. *Surgical Neurology,* Vol.40, No.3, pp. 230-235

Ostertun, B. & Solymosi, L. (1993). Magnetic resonance angiography of cerebral developmental venous anomalies: its role in differential diagnosis. *Neuroradiology,* Vol.35, No.2, pp. 97-104

Paré, L.; Delfino, R. & Leblanc, R. (1992). The relationship of ventricular drainage to aneurysmal rebleeding. *Journal of Neurosurgery,* Vol.76, No.3, pp. 422-427

Prat, R. & Galeano, I. (2008). Endoscopic resection of cavernoma of foramen of Monro in a patient with familial multiple cavernomatosis. *Clinical Neurology Neurosurgery,* Vol.110, No.8, pp. 834-837

Ramina, R.; Ingunza, W. & Vonofakos, D. (1980). Cystic cerebral cavernous angioma with dense calcification. Case report. *Journal of Neurosurgery,* Vol.52, No.2, pp. 259-262

Raychaudhuri, R.; Batjer, HH. & Awad, IA. (2005). Intracranial cavernous angioma: a practical review of clinical and biological aspects. *Surgical Neurology,* Vol.63, No.4, pp.319-328

Reyns, N.; Assaker, R.; Louis, E. & Lejeune, JP. (1999). Intraventricular cavernomas: three cases and review of the literature. *Neurosurgery,* Vol.44, No.3, pp. 648-654

Roda, JM.; Moneo, JH.; Villarejo, FJ.; Morales, C. & Blázquez, MG. (1981). Cryptic arteriovenous malformation of the choroid plexus of the third ventricle. *Surgical Neurology,* Vol.16, No.5, pp. 353-356

Rosenørn, J.; Westergaard, L. & Hansen, PH. (1983). Mannitol-induced rebleeding from intracranial aneurysm. Case report. *Journal of Neurosurgery,* Vol.59, No.3, pp. 529-530

Saito, Y. & Kobayashi, N. Cerebral venous angiomas: clinical evaluation and possible etiology. *Radiology,* Vol.139, No.1, pp. 87-94

Sanli, M.; Ergün, R.; Gürkanlar, D. & Uluoğlu, O. (2007). Angiographically occult vascular malformation of the third ventricle. *Journal of Clinical Neuroscience,* Vol.14, No.12, pp. 1223-1225

Sanli, AM.; Cekirge, S. & Sekerci, Z. (2011). Aneurysm of the distal anterior cerebral artery radiologically mimicking a ventricular mass. *Journal of Neurosurgery,* Vol.114, No.4, pp. 1061-1064

Sato, K.; Oka, H.; Utsuki, S.; Shimizu, S.; Suzuki, S. & Fujii, K. (2006). Neuroendoscopic appearance of an intraventricular cavernous angioma blocking the foramen of monro - case report. *Neurologia Medico-Chirurgica,* Vol.46, No.11, pp. 548-551

Schubiger, O.; Valavanis, A. & Wichmann, W. (1987). Growth-mechanism of giant intracranial aneurysms; demonstration by CT and MR imaging. *Neuroradiology,* Vol.29, No.3, pp. 266-271

Sedan, R.; Peragut, JC. & Fabrizi, A. (1989). Cavernomas and stereotaxic surgery. *Neurochirurgie,* Vol.35, No.2, pp. 126-127

Shenkar, R.; Shi, C.; Check, IJ.; Lipton, HL. & Awad, IA. (2007). Concepts and hypotheses: inflammatory hypothesis in the pathogenesis of cerebral cavernous malformations. *Neurosurgery*, Vol.61, No.4, pp.693-702

Sigal, R.; Krief, O.; Houtteville, JP.; Halimi, P.; Doyon, D. & Pariente, D. (1990). Occult cerebrovascular malformations: follow-up with MR imaging. *Radiology*, Vol.176, No.3, pp. 815-819

Simard, JM.; Garcia-Bengochea, F.; Ballinger, WE.; Mickle, JP. & Quisling RG. (1986). Cavernous angioma: a review of 126 collected and 12 new clinical cases. *Neurosurgery*, Vol.18, No.2, pp. 162-172

Sinson, G.; Zager, EL.; Grossman, RI.; Gennarelli, TA. & Flamm, ES. (1995). Cavernous malformations of the third ventricle. *Neurosurgery*, Vol.37, No.1, pp. 37-42

Smith, KA.; Kraus, GE.; Johnson, BA. & Spetzler, RF. (1994). Giant posterior communicating artery aneurysm presenting as third ventricle mass with obstructive hydrocephalus. Case report. *Journal of Neurosurgery*, Vol.81, No.2, pp. 299-303

Song, WZ.; Mao, BY.; Hu, BF.; Liu, YH.; Sun, H. & Mao, Q. (2008). Intraventricular vascular malformations mimicking tumors: case reports and review of the literature. *Journal of Neurological Sciences*, Vol.266, No.1-2, pp. 63-69

Stavrinou, LC.; Stranjalis, G.; Flaskas, T. & Sakas, DE. (2009). Trigonal cavernous angioma: a short illustrated review. *Acta Neurochirurgica*, Vol.151, No.11, pp. 1517-1520

Sure, U.; Freman, S.; Bozinov, O.; Benes, L.; Siegel, AM. & Bertalanffy, H. (2005). Biological activity of adult cavernous malformations: a study of 56 patients. *Journal of Neurosurgery*, Vol.102, No.2, pp.342-347

Sze, G.; Krol, G.; Olsen, WL.; Harper, PS.; Galicich, JH.; Heier, LA.; Zimmerman, RD. & Deck, MD. (1987). Hemorrhagic neoplasms: MR mimics of occult vascular malformations. *American Journal of Roentgenology*, Vol.149, No.6, pp. 1223-1230

Tamaki, M.; Ohno, K.; Asano, T.; Niimi, Y.; Uchihara, T. & Hirakawa, K. (1994). Cryptic arteriovenous malformation of the choroid plexus of the fourth ventricle--case report. *Neurologia Medico-Chirurgica*, Vol.34, No.1, pp. 38-43

Tatagiba, M.; Schönmayr, R. & Samii, M. (1991). Intraventricular cavernous angioma. A survey. *Acta Neurochirurgica*, Vol.110, No.3-4, pp. 140-145

Tien, R.; Harsh, GR.; Dillon, WP. & Wilson, CB. (1990). Unilateral hydrocephalus caused by an intraventricular venous malformation obstructing the foramen of Monro. *Neurosurgery*, Vol.26, No.4, pp. 664-666

Tsugane, R.; Shimoda, M.; Yamaguchi, T.; Yamamoto, I. & Sato, O. (1992). Entrapment of the temporal horn: a form of focal non-communicating hydrocephalus caused by intraventricular block of cerebrospinal fluid flow--report of two cases. *Neurologia Medico-Chirurgica*, Vol.32, No.4, pp. 210-214

Voigt, K. & Yaşargil, MG. (1976). Cerebral cavernous haemangiomas or cavernomas. Incidence, pathology, localization, diagnosis, clinical features and treatment. Review of the literature and report of an unusual case. *Neurochirurgia*, Vol.19, No.2, pp. 59-68

Voldby, B. & Enevoldsen, EM. (1982). Intracranial pressure changes following aneurysm rupture. Part 3: Recurrent hemorrhage. *Journal of Neurosurgery,* Vol.56, No.6, pp. 784-789

Yagmurlu, B.; Fitoz, S.; Atasoy, C.; Erden, I.; Deda, G. & Unal, O. (2005). An unusual cause of hydrocephalus: aqueductal developmental venous anomaly. *European Radiology,* Vol.15, No.6 pp. 1159-1162

Watanabe, A.; Imamura, K. & Ishii, R. (1999). Endosaccular aneurysm occlusion withGuglielmi detachable coils for obstructive hydrocephalus caused by a large basilar tip aneurysm. Case report.*Journal of Neurosurg*ery, Vol.91, No.4, pp.675-667

Yamada, S.; Iacono, RP.; Mandybur, GT.; Anton, R.; Lonser, R.; Yamada, S. & Haugen, GE. (1999). Endoscopic procedures for resection of arteriovenous malformations. *Surgical Neurology,* Vol.51, No.6, pp. 641-649

3

Clinical Presentation of Hydrocephalus

Sadip Pant[1] and Iype Cherian[2]
[1]*University of Arkansas for Medical Sciences,*
[2]*College of Medical Sciences*
[1]*USA*
[2]*Nepal*

1. Introduction

The two key determinants of clinical presentation of hydrocephalus are the age of onset and the acuity of the rise in intracranial pressure.

In fetus, while minor degree of hydrocephalus often goes undetected, severe cases of obstructive variety present with the following features: 1 .the head is felt larger, globular and softer than the normal head 2.the head is high up and difficult to push down into pelvis 3.fetal heart sound is situated high up above the umbilicus 4.internal examination during labor may reveal widening of sutures and tense fontanelle. In breech presentation however, the diagnosis is not made until the after-coming head is arrested at the brim. In the communicating variety, often the head is of normal size at birth and its enlargement starts only at 6-12 weeks of age.

In Infancy and early childhood (prior to 2 years of age), progressive enlargement of the head is the commonest manifestation of hydrocephalus as sutures have not united firmly. Occipitofrontal circumference should be measured after 24 hours of birth when moulding and overriding of sutures have disappeared. The head continues to enlarge and appears to be disproportionately larger than the rest of the body. The head is quite heavy and the child is not able to hold it without support. The child starts becoming less playful and does not feed properly. Milestones tend to get delayed. On examination, the child's head is found to be large in proportion to the body with bossing of frontal bones giving an inverted triangular appearance to the head. Serial head circumference should be taken to identify whether it is progressive (active) or arrested hydrocephalus. The fontanelle are widely open, bulging, tense and non pulsatile and the scalp veins are engorged, strikingly so when the infant cries. Sutures are widely separated. Cracked pot sound may be heard on percussion of the head due to separation of sutures and is called "Macewen's sign".Bruits over fontanels on auscultation of skull with the bell of the stethoscope indicates vascular origin of hydrocephalus (vein of Galen aneurysm or other vascular malformation).Transillumination of skull should be done in all cases. Normally, the halo of light around the rim of the illuminator extends upto 1 cm in the occipital region and upto 2 cm in frontal region in term babies. Excessive transillumination indicates abnormal collection of fluids as in hydranencephaly where the whole skull may glow with light or Dandy Walker syndrome where posterior part of skull transilluminates owing to the fluid accumulation in the posterior fossa.

The limbs may show increased tone and brisk reflexes "spastic paraparesis". This results from stretching and distortion of paraventricular corticospinal tracts arising from leg area of motor cortex. These fibres have a longer distance to travel around the ventricles than those supplying the face and the upper limbs. However, mild spasticity and weakness of upper limbs is not uncommon particularly in advanced cases. Spine examination should be performed in all cases to look for presence of spina bifida (commonly associated with Chiari Malformation II).

Downturning of eyeballs with visibility of sclera above the iris is called 'Sunsetting Sign" and is a frequent finding. It is due to pressure on the superior quadrigeminal plate against the free edge of the tentorium causing a supranuclear paresis. It may be intermittent to begin with but later becomes continuous. Other ocular disturbances include unilateral or bilateral abducens nerve paresis, nystagmus, ptosis, strabismus and diminished papillary light responses.Optic atrophy can occur due to compression of the chiasm and optic nerves by a dilated anterior portion of the third ventricle. Papilledema is rare because rising tension is easily buffered by sutural diastasis.

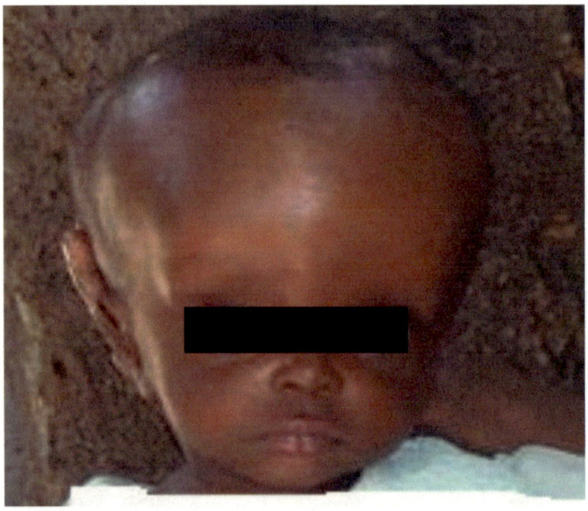

Fig. 1. Congential Hydrocephalus: Downturning of eyeballs with visibility of sclera above the iris (Sunsetting Sign).

In earlier stage, child may be quite playful, pick up the objects, put them into mouth, recognize the parents and follow light and objects. As hydrocephalus progresses , further destruction of cerebral cortex occurs, child tends to become listless , stops taking interest in the surroundings and regression of earlier achieved milestones occurs .There is unusual somnolence, persistent vomiting ,failure to thrive and visual loss. Finally a decerebrate state ensues.

In early to late childhood (2 years and above), neurological symptoms caused by increased intracranial pressure or by focal deficits referable to the primary lesion is the predominant finding and appear before any significant change in head size. The clinical picture of various space occupying lesions depend on their site of origin.A unique but rare hydrocephalic syndrome "the bobble head doll syndrome" is related to obstructive lesions in or around third ventricle and is characterized by bobbing of head forward and back involuntarily mimicking a bobble head doll. This can be inhibited voluntarily and disappears during sleep. A symptom very closely associated with head bobbing is the presence of ataxia. Several patients were reported to have difficulty in walking, running, and climbing steps because of the bobbing. One likely explanation for such symptom is interruption of the patient's ability to balance which rely on input from various sources namely, the vestibular, ocular and somatosensory due to constant bobbing. The head bobbing is a neurological phenomenon and stems from dilated third ventricle impinging on the medial aspects of the dorsomedial nucleus of the thalamus.

1.	Hydrocephalus
2.	Hydranencephaly
3.	Subdural Effusion
4.	Thickened skull bones (achondroplasia, osteopetrosis,pyknodysostosis,craniometaphyseal dysplasia, orodigitofacial dysostosis , rickets, leontiasis ossea,etc.)
5.	Cerebral Gigantism
6.	Mucopolysaccharidosis
7.	Cerebral lipidosis (gangliosidosis)
8.	Metachromatic leukodystrophy
9.	Fragile X Syndrome
10.	Porencephaly
11.	Subdural Hematoma
12.	Intracranial Tumor
13.	Glutaryl-1-Coenzyme A dehydrogenase deficiency

Table 1. D/d of Enlarged Head in Newborn, Infancy and Children

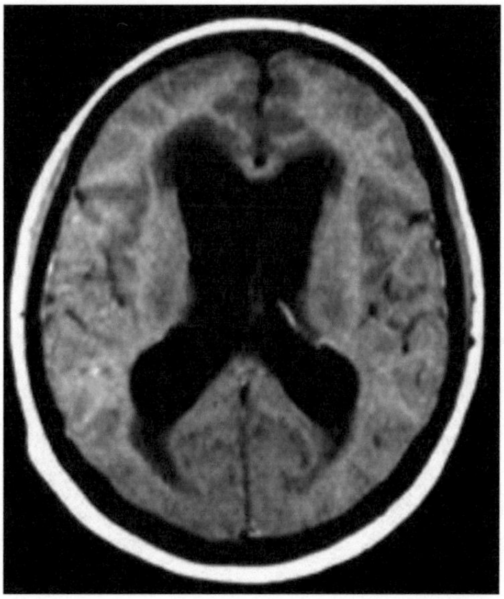

Fig. 2. CT scan of the brain at the level of basal ganglia showing enlarged lateral ventricles suggestive of hydrocephalus.

The features of raised intracranial pressure are evident in almost all instances and includes frontal headache aggravated in the morning, improving with upright posture and associated with nausea and vomiting. The cracked pot sound is prominent on skull percussion. Fundoscopy may show papilledema. Additional features seen in late group are endocrine changes including small stature, gigantism, obesity, precocious or delayed puberty, menstrual irregularities, absent secondary sexual characteristics and central diabetes insipidus. They are probably caused by compression of hypothalamic pituitary axis by an enlarged third ventricle (a particular risk in aqueductal stenosis) resulting in abnormal hypothalamic pituitary function. Spastic diplegia is common. Thought and behavior may be affected adversely. Learning disabilities are fairly common and these children are credited with better verbal IQ than performance IQ. While the severity of hydrocephalus can differ considerably between individuals, some are of average or even above-average intelligence. Patients may develop motion and visual problems, coordination problems, or may be clumsy. Perceptual motor deficits and visual spatial disorganization follow as a result of stretched corticospinal fibres of parietal and occipital cortex due to dilated posterior horns of lateral ventricles. About one in four develops epilepsy.

2. Normal Pressure Hydrocephalus

Normal Pressure Hydrocephalus (NPH) is a clinical symptom complex, characterized by the classic triad of gait abnormality, dementia and urinary incontinence (commonly referred to as "wet, wobbly and wacky").NPH occurs either as idiopathic or secondary condition, roughly in equal proportions. While NPH secondary to an identifiable cause can occur in all age groups, idiopathic NPH is most common in adults over 60 years of age without any sex predilection. These manifestations are believed to arise from dysfunction of periventricular white matter tracts, particularly those sub serving frontal lobe connections .Gait difficulty is often the first clinical manifestation. It is the effect of expansion of the ventricular system (particularly the lateral ventricles) and subsequent traction on the lumbosacral corticospinal fibers arising from the motor cortex. It is also believed to be the most responsive feature to shunting. It is classically described as “magnetic gait”; the patient's feet appear to stuck to the floor, steps are characteristically short with decreased stride length and height and a broad base. This may resemble parkinsonian gait at a glance but is distinguished by a narrow base and absence of tremor or rigidity. Postural stability is impaired, and a history of falls may be reported.

The cognitive disturbance of NPH is likely to be frontal in nature with psychomotor slowing, decreased attention and concentration, and apathy. The patient is slower in timed tasks, performs poorly on tests of divided attention and executive function, has difficulty with fluency tests, and has poor learning and better preserved recognition memory. The dementia is believed to be the consequence of stretching of frontal and limbic fibers that travel in the periventricular region. The Mini Mental State Examination may be an insensitive measure of cognitive impairment in NPH since it exhibits a frontal subcortical pattern rather than a cortical pattern and neuropsychological tests may prove to be a better tool in its characterization as well as diagnosis of coexisting dementia conditions (including Alzheimer’s dementia and vascular dementia which are also highly likely in advancing age).

The third component, urinary incontinence, often begins as urgency and frequency rather than incontinence per se. However, overtime, true urinary incontinence ensues and is accompanied by a lack of concern to urinary symptoms, reflecting its probable origin in the frontal lobe.

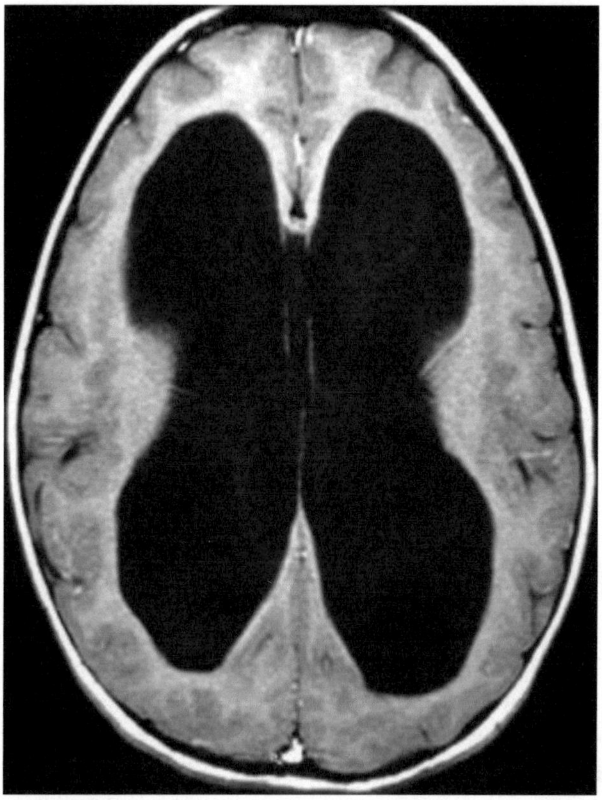

Fig. 3. Enlarged lateral ventricles with thinning out of cerebral cortex in a patient with normal pressure hydrocephalus.

Other features of NPH may include long tract signs with spasticity of lower limbs, hyperreflexia and extensor plantar responses (upper motor neuron signs). In very late stages, frontal release signs, akinetic mutism, and quadriparesis may occur.

3. References

[1] Fishman, MA. Hydrocephalus. In: Neurological Pathophysiology, Eliasson, SG, Prensky, AL, Hardin, WB (Eds), Oxford, New York 1978.

[2] Carey, CM, Tullous, MW, Walker, ML. Hydrocephalus: Etiology, Pathologic Effects, Diagnosis, and Natural History. In: Pediatric Neurosurgery, 3rd ed, Cheek, WR (Ed), WB Saunders Company, Philadelphia 1994.

[3] Chumas P, Tyagi A, Livingston J. Hydrocephalus--what's new? Arch Dis Child Fetal Neonatal Ed 2001; 85:F149.

[4] Blackburn BL, Fineman RM. Epidemiology of congenital hydrocephalus in Utah, 1940-1979: report of an iatrogenically related "epidemic". Am J Med Genet 1994; 52:123.

[5] Fernell E, Hagberg G, Hagberg B. Infantile hydrocephalus epidemiology: an indicator of enhanced survival. Arch Dis Child Fetal Neonatal Ed 1994; 70:F123.
[6] Bondurant CP, Jimenez DF. Epidemiology of cerebrospinal fluid shunting. Pediatr Neurosurg 1995; 23:254.
[7] Yasuda T, Tomita T, McLone DG, Donovan M. Measurement of cerebrospinal fluid output through external ventricular drainage in one hundred infants and children: correlation with cerebrospinal fluid production. Pediatr Neurosurg 2002; 36:22.
[8] Frawley GP, Dargaville PA, Mitchell PJ, et al. Clinical course and medical management of neonates with severe cardiac failure related to vein of Galen malformation. Arch Dis Child Fetal Neonatal Ed 2002; 87:F144.
[9] Graf WD, Born DE, Sarnat HB. The pachygyria-polymicrogyria spectrum of cortical dysplasia in X-linked hydrocephalus. Eur J Pediatr Surg 1998; 8 Suppl 1:10.
[10] Schrander-Stumpel C, Fryns JP. Congenital hydrocephalus: nosology and guidelines for clinical approach and genetic counselling. Eur J Pediatr 1998; 157:355.
[11] Fransen E, Van Camp G, Vits L, Willems PJ. L1-associated diseases: clinical geneticists divide, molecular geneticists unite. Hum Mol Genet 1997; 6:1625.
[12] Sasaki-Adams D, Elbabaa SK, Jewells V, et al. The Dandy-Walker variant: a case series of 24 pediatric patients and evaluation of associated anomalies, incidence of hydrocephalus, and developmental outcomes. J Neurosurg Pediatr 2008; 2:194.
[13] Kirkpatrick M, Engleman H, Minns RA. Symptoms and signs of progressive hydrocephalus. Arch Dis Child 1989; 64:124.
[14] Löppönen T, Saukkonen AL, Serlo W, et al. Accelerated pubertal development in patients with shunted hydrocephalus. Arch Dis Child 1996; 74:490.
[15] Rekate, HL. Treatment of Hydrocephalus. In: Pediatric Neurosurgery, 3rd ed, Cheek, WR (Ed), WB Saunders Company, Philadelphia 1994.
[16] Drake JM, Kestle JR, Milner R, et al. Randomized trial of cerebrospinal fluid shunt valve design in pediatric hydrocephalus. Neurosurgery 1998; 43:294.
[17] Langley JM, LeBlanc JC, Drake J, Milner R. Efficacy of antimicrobial prophylaxis in placement of cerebrospinal fluid shunts: meta-analysis. Clin Infect Dis 1993; 17:98.
[18] Casey AT, Kimmings EJ, Kleinlugtebeld AD, et al. The long-term outlook for hydrocephalus in childhood. A ten-year cohort study of 155 patients. Pediatr Neurosurg 1997; 27:63.
[19] Forward KR, Fewer HD, Stiver HG. Cerebrospinal fluid shunt infections. A review of 35 infections in 32 patients. J Neurosurg 1983; 59:389.
[20] Shapiro S, Boaz J, Kleiman M, et al. Origin of organisms infecting ventricular shunts. Neurosurgery 1988; 22:868.
[21] Siomin V, Cinalli G, Grotenhuis A, et al. Endoscopic third ventriculostomy in patients with cerebrospinal fluid infection and/or hemorrhage. J Neurosurg 2002; 97:519.
[22] Scarrow AM, Levy EI, Pascucci L, Albright AL. Outcome analysis of endoscopic III ventriculostomy. Childs Nerv Syst 2000; 16:442.
[23] Javadpour M, Mallucci C, Brodbelt A, et al. The impact of endoscopic third ventriculostomy on the management of newly diagnosed hydrocephalus in infants. Pediatr Neurosurg 2001; 35:131.
[24] Kulkarni AV, Drake JM, Mallucci CL, et al. Endoscopic third ventriculostomy in the treatment of childhood hydrocephalus. J Pediatr 2009; 155:254.
[25] Sacko O, Boetto S, Lauwers-Cances V, et al. Endoscopic third ventriculostomy: outcome analysis in 368 procedures. J Neurosurg Pediatr 2010; 5:68.

[26] Libenson MH, Kaye EM, Rosman NP, Gilmore HE. Acetazolamide and furosemide for posthemorrhagic hydrocephalus of the newborn. Pediatr Neurol 1999; 20:185.
[27] Whitelaw A, Kennedy CR, Brion LP. Diuretic therapy for newborn infants with posthemorrhagic ventricular dilatation. Cochrane Database Syst Rev 2001; :CD002270.
[28] International randomised controlled trial of acetazolamide and furosemide in posthaemorrhagic ventricular dilatation in infancy. International PHVD Drug Trial Group. Lancet 1998; 352:433.
[29] Haines SJ, Lapointe M. Fibrinolytic agents in the management of posthemorrhagic hydrocephalus in preterm infants: the evidence. Childs Nerv Syst 1999; 15:226.
[30] Whitelaw A. Repeated lumbar or ventricular punctures in newborns with intraventricular hemorrhage. Cochrane Database Syst Rev 2001; :CD000216.
[31] Berger A, Weninger M, Reinprecht A, et al. Long-term experience with subcutaneously tunneled external ventricular drainage in preterm infants. Childs Nerv Syst 2000; 16:103.
[32] Heep A, Engelskirchen R, Holschneider A, Groneck P. Primary intervention for posthemorrhagic hydrocephalus in very low birthweight infants by ventriculostomy. Childs Nerv Syst 2001; 17:47.
[33] Hoppe-Hirsch E, Laroussinie F, Brunet L, et al. Late outcome of the surgical treatment of hydrocephalus. Childs Nerv Syst 1998; 14:97.
[34] Klepper J, Büsse M, Strassburg HM, Sörensen N. Epilepsy in shunt-treated hydrocephalus. Dev Med Child Neurol 1998; 40:731.
[35] Bourgeois M, Sainte-Rose C, Cinalli G, et al. Epilepsy in children with shunted hydrocephalus. J Neurosurg 1999; 90:274.
[36] Caraballo RH, Bongiorni L, Cersósimo R, et al. Epileptic encephalopathy with continuous spikes and waves during sleep in children with shunted hydrocephalus: a study of nine cases. Epilepsia 2008; 49:1520.
[37] Lindquist B, Carlsson G, Persson EK, Uvebrant P. Learning disabilities in a population-based group of children with hydrocephalus. Acta Paediatr 2005; 94:878.
[38] Brookshire BL, Fletcher JM, Bohan TP, et al. Verbal and nonverbal skill discrepancies in children with hydrocephalus: a five-year longitudinal follow-up. J Pediatr Psychol 1995; 20:785.
[39] Stoll C. Problems in the diagnosis of fragile X syndrome in young children are still present. Am J Med Genet 2001; 100:110.
[40] Zvulunov A, Weitz R, Metzker A. Neurofibromatosis type 1 in childhood: evaluation of clinical and epidemiologic features as predictive factors for severity. Clin Pediatr (Phila) 1998; 37:295.
[41] Furuta T, Tabuchi A, Adachi Y, et al. Primary brain tumors in children under age 3 years. Brain Tumor Pathol 1998; 15:7.
[42] Tomita T, McLone DG. Brain tumors during the first twenty-four months of life. Neurosurgery 1985; 17:913.
[43] Nard, JA. Abnormal head size and shape. In: Gartner, JC, Zitelli, BJ. Common & Chronic Symptoms in Pediatrics, Mosby, St. Louis, 1997.
[44] Rios A. Microcephaly. Pediatr Rev 1996; 17:386.
[45] Fenichel, GM. Disorders of cranial volume and shape. In: Clinical Pediatric Neurology: A Signs and Symptoms Approach, 5th ed. Elsevier Saunders, Philadelphia 2005. p. 353.

[46] Nellhaus G. Head circumference from birth to eighteen years. Practical composite international and interracial graphs. Pediatrics 1968; 41:106.
[47] Roche AF, Mukherjee D, Guo SM, Moore WM. Head circumference reference data: birth to 18 years. Pediatrics 1987; 79:706.
[48] Rollins JD, Collins JS, Holden KR. United States head circumference growth reference charts: birth to 21 years. J Pediatr 2010; 156:907.
[49] Grummer-Strawn LM, Reinold C, Krebs NF, Centers for Disease Control and Prevention (CDC). Use of World Health Organization and CDC growth charts for children aged 0-59 months in the United States. MMWR Recomm Rep 2010; 59:1.
[50] Committee on Nutrition American Academy of Pediatrics. Failure to thrive. In: Pediatric Nutrition Handbook, 6th ed, Kleinman, RE (Ed), American Academy of Pediatrics, Elk Grove Village, IL 2009. p.601.
[51] Bushby KM, Cole T, Matthews JN, Goodship JA. Centiles for adult head circumference. Arch Dis Child 1992; 67:1286.
[52] Daymont C, Hwang WT, Feudtner C, Rubin D. Head-circumference distribution in a large primary care network differs from CDC and WHO curves. Pediatrics 2010; 126:e836.
[53] Varma, R, Williams, SD, Wessel, HB. Neurology In: Atlas of Pediatric Physical Diagnosis, 5th ed. Zitelli, BJ, Davis, HW (Eds). Mosby Elsevier, Philadelphia 2007. p. 563.
[54] Opitz JM, Holt MC. Microcephaly: general considerations and aids to nosology. J Craniofac Genet Dev Biol 1990; 10:175.
[55] Williams CA, Dagli A, Battaglia A. Genetic disorders associated with macrocephaly. Am J Med Genet A 2008; 146A:2023.
[56] Olney AH. Macrocephaly syndromes. Semin Pediatr Neurol 2007; 14:128.
[57] DeMyer W. Megalencephaly: types, clinical syndromes, and management. Pediatr Neurol 1986; 2:321.
[58] Day RE, Schutt WH. Normal children with large heads--benign familial megalencephaly. Arch Dis Child 1979; 54:512.
[59] Lorber J, Priestley BL. Children with large heads: a practical approach to diagnosis in 557 children, with special reference to 109 children with megalencephaly. Dev Med Child Neurol 1981; 23:494.
[60] Weaver DD, Christian JC. Familial variation of head size and adjustment for parental head circumference. J Pediatr 1980; 96:990.
[61] Aoki N, Oikawa A, Sakai T. Serial neuroimaging studies in Sotos syndrome (cerebral gigantism syndrome). Neurol Res 1998; 20:149.
[62] Gleeson, JG, Dobyns, WB, Plawner, L, Ashwal, S. Congenital structural defects. In: Pediatric Neurology Principles and Practice, 4th ed. Swaiman, KF, Ashwal, S, Ferriero, DM (Eds). Mosby Elsevier, Philadephia 2006. p. 399.
[63] Zahl SM, Wester K. Routine measurement of head circumference as a tool for detecting intracranial expansion in infants: what is the gain? A nationwide survey. Pediatrics 2008; 121:e416.
[64] Alvarez LA, Maytal J, Shinnar S. Idiopathic external hydrocephalus: natural history and relationship to benign familial macrocephaly. Pediatrics 1986; 77:901.
[65] Ment LR, Duncan CC, Geehr R. Benign enlargement of the subarachnoid spaces in the infant. J Neurosurg 1981; 54:504.
[66] Kumar R. External hydrocephalus in small children. Childs Nerv Syst 2006; 22:1237.

[67] Menkes, JH, Sarnat, HB, Flores-Sarnat, L. Malformations of the central nervous system. In: Child Neurology, 7th ed. Menkes, JH, Sarnat, HB, Maria, BL (Eds) Lippincott, Williams & Wilkins, Philadelphia, 2006. p.284.
[68] Hellbusch LC. Benign extracerebral fluid collections in infancy: clinical presentation and long-term follow-up. J Neurosurg 2007; 107:119.
[69] Andersson H, Elfverson J, Svendsen P. External hydrocephalus in infants. Childs Brain 1984; 11:398.
[70] Gherpelli JL, Scaramuzzi V, Manreza ML, Diament AJ. Follow-up study of macrocephalic children with enlargement of the subarachnoid space. Arq Neuropsiquiatr 1992; 50:156.
[71] Pettit RE, Kilroy AW, Allen JH. Macrocephaly with head growth parallel to normal growth pattern: neurological, developmental, and computerized tomography findings in full-term infants. Arch Neurol 1980; 37:518.
[72] Hamza M, Bodensteiner JB, Noorani PA, Barnes PD. Benign extracerebral fluid collections: a cause of macrocrania in infancy. Pediatr Neurol 1987; 3:218.
[73] Nickel RE, Gallenstein JS. Developmental prognosis for infants with benign enlargement of the subarachnoid spaces. Dev Med Child Neurol 1987; 29:181.
[74] Bosnjak V, Besenski N, Marusić-Della Marina B, Kogler A. Cranial ultrasonography in the evaluation of macrocrania in infancy. Dev Med Child Neurol 1989; 31:66.
[75] Ravid S, Maytal J. External hydrocephalus: a probable cause for subdural hematoma in infancy. Pediatr Neurol 2003; 28:139.
[76] Lago P, Rebsamen S, Clancy RR, et al. MRI, MRA, and neurodevelopmental outcome following neonatal ECMO. Pediatr Neurol 1995; 12:294.
[77] Canady AI, Fessler RD, Klein MD. Ultrasound abnormalities in term infants on ECMO. Pediatr Neurosurg 1993; 19:202.
[78] Lorch SA, D'Agostino JA, Zimmerman R, Bernbaum J. "Benign" extra-axial fluid in survivors of neonatal intensive care. Arch Pediatr Adolesc Med 2004; 158:178.
[79] The Head. In: Green, MG (Ed), Pediatric Diagnosis Interpretation of Symptoms and Signs in Children and Adolescents, 6th ed, WB Saunders, Philadelphia, 1998. p.4.
[80] Firth, HV, Hurst, JA, Hall, JG. Macrocephaly. In: Oxford Desk Reference: Clinical Genetics, 1st ed. Oxford University Press, Oxford 2005. p. 162.
[81] Smith R, Leonidas JC, Maytal J. The value of head ultrasound in infants with macrocephaly. Pediatr Radiol 1998; 28:143.
[82] Krauss JK, Halve B. Normal pressure hydrocephalus: survey on contemporary diagnostic algorithms and therapeutic decision-making in clinical practice. Acta Neurochir (Wien) 2004; 146:379.
[83] Tisell M, Höglund M, Wikkelsø C. National and regional incidence of surgery for adult hydrocephalus in Sweden. Acta Neurol Scand 2005; 112:72.
[84] Vanneste JA. Diagnosis and management of normal-pressure hydrocephalus. J Neurol 2000; 247:5.
[85] Petersen RC, Mokri B, Laws ER Jr. Surgical treatment of idiopathic hydrocephalus in elderly patients. Neurology 1985; 35:307.
[86] Black PM, Ojemann RG, Tzouras A. CSF shunts for dementia, incontinence, and gait disturbance. Clin Neurosurg 1985; 32:632.
[87] Marmarou A, Young HF, Aygok GA, et al. Diagnosis and management of idiopathic normal-pressure hydrocephalus: a prospective study in 151 patients. J Neurosurg 2005; 102:987.

[88] Hebb AO, Cusimano MD. Idiopathic normal pressure hydrocephalus: a systematic review of diagnosis and outcome. Neurosurgery 2001; 49:1166.

[89] Bech RA, Juhler M, Waldemar G, et al. Frontal brain and leptomeningeal biopsy specimens correlated with cerebrospinal fluid outflow resistance and B-wave activity in patients suspected of normal-pressure hydrocephalus. Neurosurgery 1997; 40:497.

[90] Bech RA, Waldemar G, Gjerris F, et al. Shunting effects in patients with idiopathic normal pressure hydrocephalus; correlation with cerebral and leptomeningeal biopsy findings. Acta Neurochir (Wien) 1999; 141:633.

[91] Graff-Radford NR, Godersky JC. Symptomatic congenital hydrocephalus in the elderly simulating normal pressure hydrocephalus. Neurology 1989; 39:1596.

[92] Krefft TA, Graff-Radford NR, Lucas JA, Mortimer JA. Normal pressure hydrocephalus and large head size. Alzheimer Dis Assoc Disord 2004; 18:35.

[93] McComb JG, Bradley WG Jr, Safar FG, et al. Is a large hat size hazardous to your health? AJNR Am J Neuroradiol 2004; 25:1454.

[94] Krauss JK, Regel JP, Vach W, et al. Vascular risk factors and arteriosclerotic disease in idiopathic normal-pressure hydrocephalus of the elderly. Stroke 1996; 27:24.

[95] Graff-Radford NR, Godersky JC. Idiopathic normal pressure hydrocephalus and systemic hypertension. Neurology 1987; 37:868.

[96] Ritter S, Dinh TT. Progressive postnatal dilation of brain ventricles in spontaneously hypertensive rats. Brain Res 1986; 370:327.

[97] Bradley WG Jr, Whittemore AR, Watanabe AS, et al. Association of deep white matter infarction with chronic communicating hydrocephalus: implications regarding the possible origin of normal-pressure hydrocephalus. AJNR Am J Neuroradiol 1991; 12:31.

[98] Krauss JK, Regel JP, Vach W, et al. White matter lesions in patients with idiopathic normal pressure hydrocephalus and in an age-matched control group: a comparative study. Neurosurgery 1997; 40:491.

[99] Bradley WG. Normal pressure hydrocephalus: new concepts on etiology and diagnosis. AJNR Am J Neuroradiol 2000; 21:1586.

[100] Kuriyama N, Tokuda T, Miyamoto J, et al. Retrograde jugular flow associated with idiopathic normal pressure hydrocephalus. Ann Neurol 2008; 64:217.

[101] ADAMS RD, FISHER CM, HAKIM S, et al. SYMPTOMATIC OCCULT HYDROCEPHALUS WITH "NORMAL" CEREBROSPINAL-FLUID PRESSURE.A TREATABLE SYNDROME. N Engl J Med 1965; 273:117.

[102] Lenfeldt N, Larsson A, Nyberg L, et al. Idiopathic normal pressure hydrocephalus: increased supplementary motor activity accounts for improvement after CSF drainage. Brain 2008; 131:2904.

[103] Sudarsky L, Simon S. Gait disorder in late-life hydrocephalus. Arch Neurol 1987; 44:263.

[104] Stolze H, Kuhtz-Buschbeck JP, Drücke H, et al. Comparative analysis of the gait disorder of normal pressure hydrocephalus and Parkinson's disease. J Neurol Neurosurg Psychiatry 2001; 70:289.

[105] Iddon JL, Pickard JD, Cross JJ, et al. Specific patterns of cognitive impairment in patients with idiopathic normal pressure hydrocephalus and Alzheimer's disease: a pilot study. J Neurol Neurosurg Psychiatry 1999; 67:723.

[106] Tullberg M, Hultin L, Ekholm S, et al. White matter changes in normal pressure hydrocephalus and Binswanger disease: specificity, predictive value and correlations to axonal degeneration and demyelination. Acta Neurol Scand 2002; 105:417.

[107] Sudarsky L, Ronthal M. Gait disorders among elderly patients. A survey study of 50 patients. Arch Neurol 1983; 40:740.

[108] Temml C, Haidinger G, Schmidbauer J, et al. Urinary incontinence in both sexes: prevalence rates and impact on quality of life and sexual life. Neurourol Urodyn 2000; 19:259.

[109] Savolainen S, Paljärvi L, Vapalahti M. Prevalence of Alzheimer's disease in patients investigated for presumed normal pressure hydrocephalus: a clinical and neuropathological study. Acta Neurochir (Wien) 1999; 141:849.

[110] Golomb J, Wisoff J, Miller DC, et al. Alzheimer's disease comorbidity in normal pressure hydrocephalus: prevalence and shunt response. J Neurol Neurosurg Psychiatry 2000; 68:778.

[111] Savolainen S, Hurskainen H, Paljärvi L, et al. Five-year outcome of normal pressure hydrocephalus with or without a shunt: predictive value of the clinical signs, neuropsychological evaluation and infusion test. Acta Neurochir (Wien) 2002; 144:515.

[112] Hamilton R, Patel S, Lee EB, et al. Lack of shunt response in suspected idiopathic normal pressure hydrocephalus with Alzheimer disease pathology. Ann Neurol 2010; 68:535.

[113] Malm, J, Eklund, A. Idiopathic normal pressure hydrocephalus. Practical Neurology 2006; 6:14.

[114] Barron SA, Jacobs L, Kinkel WR. Changes in size of normal lateral ventricles during aging determined by computerized tomography. Neurology 1976; 26:1011.

[115] Gyldensted C. Measurements of the normal ventricular system and hemispheric sulci of 100 adults with computed tomography. Neuroradiology 1977; 14:183.

[116] Black PM. Idiopathic normal-pressure hydrocephalus. Results of shunting in 62 patients. J Neurosurg 1980; 52:371.

[117] Thomsen AM, Børgesen SE, Bruhn P, Gjerris F. Prognosis of dementia in normal-pressure hydrocephalus after a shunt operation. Ann Neurol 1986; 20:304.

[118] Børgesen SE, Gjerris F. The predictive value of conductance to outflow of CSF in normal pressure hydrocephalus. Brain 1982; 105:65.

[119] Palm WM, Saczynski JS, van der Grond J, et al. Ventricular dilation: association with gait and cognition. Ann Neurol 2009; 66:485.

[120] Krauss JK, Droste DW, Vach W, et al. Cerebrospinal fluid shunting in idiopathic normal-pressure hydrocephalus of the elderly: effect of periventricular and deep white matter lesions. Neurosurgery 1996; 39:292.

[121] Boon AJ, Tans JT, Delwel EJ, et al. Dutch Normal-Pressure Hydrocephalus Study: the role of cerebrovascular disease. J Neurosurg 1999; 90:221.

[122] Tullberg M, Jensen C, Ekholm S, Wikkelsø C. Normal pressure hydrocephalus: vascular white matter changes on MR images must not exclude patients from shunt surgery. AJNR Am J Neuroradiol 2001; 22:1665.

[123] Tullberg M, Ziegelitz D, Ribbelin S, Ekholm S. White matter diffusion is higher in Binswanger disease than in idiopathic normal pressure hydrocephalus. Acta Neurol Scand 2009; 120:226.

[124] Bradley WG Jr, Whittemore AR, Kortman KE, et al. Marked cerebrospinal fluid void: indicator of successful shunt in patients with suspected normal-pressure hydrocephalus. Radiology 1991; 178:459.
[125] Krauss JK, Regel JP, Vach W, et al. Flow void of cerebrospinal fluid in idiopathic normal pressure hydrocephalus of the elderly: can it predict outcome after shunting? Neurosurgery 1997; 40:67.
[126] Hakim R, Black PM. Correlation between lumbo-ventricular perfusion and MRI-CSF flow studies in idiopathic normal pressure hydrocephalus. Surg Neurol 1998; 49:14.
[127] Jack CR Jr, Petersen RC, O'Brien PC, Tangalos EG. MR-based hippocampal volumetry in the diagnosis of Alzheimer's disease. Neurology 1992; 42:183.
[128] Holodny AI, Waxman R, George AE, et al. MR differential diagnosis of normal-pressure hydrocephalus and Alzheimer disease: significance of perihippocampal fissures. AJNR Am J Neuroradiol 1998; 19:813.
[129] Savolainen S, Laakso MP, Paljärvi L, et al. MR imaging of the hippocampus in normal pressure hydrocephalus: correlations with cortical Alzheimer's disease confirmed by pathologic analysis. AJNR Am J Neuroradiol 2000; 21:409.
[130] Miyoshi N, Kazui H, Ogino A, et al. Association between cognitive impairment and gait disturbance in patients with idiopathic normal pressure hydrocephalus. Dement Geriatr Cogn Disord 2005; 20:71.
[131] Graff-Radford NR, Godersky JC, Jones MP. Variables predicting surgical outcome in symptomatic hydrocephalus in the elderly. Neurology 1989; 39:1601.
[132] De Mol J. [Prognostic factors for therapeutic outcome in normal-pressure hydrocephalus. Review of the literature and personal study]. Acta Neurol Belg 1985; 85:13.
[133] Stolze H, Kuhtz-Buschbeck JP, Drücke H, et al. Gait analysis in idiopathic normal pressure hydrocephalus--which parameters respond to the CSF tap test? Clin Neurophysiol 2000; 111:1678.
[134] Wikkelsö C, Andersson H, Blomstrand C, et al. Normal pressure hydrocephalus. Predictive value of the cerebrospinal fluid tap-test. Acta Neurol Scand 1986; 73:566.
[135] Walchenbach R, Geiger E, Thomeer RT, Vanneste JA. The value of temporary external lumbar CSF drainage in predicting the outcome of shunting on normal pressure hydrocephalus. J Neurol Neurosurg Psychiatry 2002; 72:503.
[136] Kahlon B, Sundbärg G, Rehncrona S. Comparison between the lumbar infusion and CSF tap tests to predict outcome after shunt surgery in suspected normal pressure hydrocephalus. J Neurol Neurosurg Psychiatry 2002; 73:721.
[137] Malm J, Kristensen B, Karlsson T, et al. The predictive value of cerebrospinal fluid dynamic tests in patients with th idiopathic adult hydrocephalus syndrome. Arch Neurol 1995; 52:783.
[138] Chen IH, Huang CI, Liu HC, Chen KK. Effectiveness of shunting in patients with normal pressure hydrocephalus predicted by temporary, controlled-resistance, continuous lumbar drainage: a pilot study. J Neurol Neurosurg Psychiatry 1994; 57:1430.
[139] Haan J, Thomeer RT. Predictive value of temporary external lumbar drainage in normal pressure hydrocephalus. Neurosurgery 1988; 22:388.
[140] Duinkerke A, Williams MA, Rigamonti D, Hillis AE. Cognitive recovery in idiopathic normal pressure hydrocephalus after shunt. Cogn Behav Neurol 2004; 17:179.

[141] Krauss JK, Regel JP. The predictive value of ventricular CSF removal in normal pressure hydrocephalus. Neurol Res 1997; 19:357.
[142] Symon L, Dorsch NW. Use of long-term intracranial pressure measurement to assess hydrocephalic patients prior to shunt surgery. J Neurosurg 1975; 42:258.
[143] Crockard HA, Hanlon K, Duda EE, Mullan JF. Hydrocephalus as a cause of dementia: evaluation by computerised tomography and intracranial pressure monitoring. J Neurol Neurosurg Psychiatry 1977; 40:736.
[144] Stephensen H, Andersson N, Eklund A, et al. Objective B wave analysis in 55 patients with non-communicating and communicating hydrocephalus. J Neurol Neurosurg Psychiatry 2005; 76:965.
[145] Krauss JK, Droste DW, Bohus M, et al. The relation of intracranial pressure B-waves to different sleep stages in patients with suspected normal pressure hydrocephalus. Acta Neurochir (Wien) 1995; 136:195.
[146] Katzman R, Hussey F. A simple constant-infusion manometric test for measurement of CSF absorption. I. Rationale and method. Neurology 1970; 20:534.
[147] Boon AJ, Tans JT, Delwel EJ, et al. Dutch normal-pressure hydrocephalus study: prediction of outcome after shunting by resistance to outflow of cerebrospinal fluid. J Neurosurg 1997; 87:687.
[148] Meier U, Bartels P. The importance of the intrathecal infusion test in the diagnostic of normal-pressure hydrocephalus. Eur Neurol 2001; 46:178.
[149] Malm J, Lundkvist B, Eklund A, et al. CSF outflow resistance as predictor of shunt function. A long-term study. Acta Neurol Scand 2004; 110:154.
[150] Vanneste J, Augustijn P, Dirven C, et al. Shunting normal-pressure hydrocephalus: do the benefits outweigh the risks? A multicenter study and literature review. Neurology 1992; 42:54.
[151] Lins H, Wichart I, Bancher C, et al. Immunoreactivities of amyloid beta peptide((1-42)) and total tau protein in lumbar cerebrospinal fluid of patients with normal pressure hydrocephalus. J Neural Transm 2004; 111:273.
[152] Kudo T, Mima T, Hashimoto R, et al. Tau protein is a potential biological marker for normal pressure hydrocephalus. Psychiatry Clin Neurosci 2000; 54:199.
[153] Tullberg M, Rosengren L, Blomsterwall E, et al. CSF neurofilament and glial fibrillary acidic protein in normal pressure hydrocephalus. Neurology 1998; 50:1122.
[154] Tullberg M, Månsson JE, Fredman P, et al. CSF sulfatide distinguishes between normal pressure hydrocephalus and subcortical arteriosclerotic encephalopathy. J Neurol Neurosurg Psychiatry 2000; 69:74.
[155] Dixon GR, Friedman JA, Luetmer PH, et al. Use of cerebrospinal fluid flow rates measured by phase-contrast MR to predict outcome of ventriculoperitoneal shunting for idiopathic normal-pressure hydrocephalus. Mayo Clin Proc 2002; 77:509.
[156] Egeler-Peerdeman SM, Barkhof F, Walchenbach R, Valk J. Cine phase-contrast MR imaging in normal pressure hydrocephalus patients: relation to surgical outcome. Acta Neurochir Suppl 1998; 71:340.
[157] del Mar Matarín M, Pueyo R, Poca MA, et al. Post-surgical changes in brain metabolism detected by magnetic resonance spectroscopy in normal pressure hydrocephalus: results of a pilot study. J Neurol Neurosurg Psychiatry 2007; 78:760.

[158] Kristensen B, Malm J, Fagerland M, et al. Regional cerebral blood flow, white matter abnormalities, and cerebrospinal fluid hydrodynamics in patients with idiopathic adult hydrocephalus syndrome. J Neurol Neurosurg Psychiatry 1996; 60:282.
[159] Owler BK, Pickard JD. Normal pressure hydrocephalus and cerebral blood flow: a review. Acta Neurol Scand 2001; 104:325.
[160] Tedeschi E, Hasselbalch SG, Waldemar G, et al. Heterogeneous cerebral glucose metabolism in normal pressure hydrocephalus. J Neurol Neurosurg Psychiatry 1995; 59:608.
[161] Pujari S, Kharkar S, Metellus P, et al. Normal pressure hydrocephalus: long-term outcome after shunt surgery. J Neurol Neurosurg Psychiatry 2008; 79:1282.
[162] Sand T, Bovim G, Grimse R, et al. Idiopathic normal pressure hydrocephalus: the CSF tap-test may predict the clinical response to shunting. Acta Neurol Scand 1994; 89:311.
[163] Gustafson L, Hagberg B. Recovery in hydrocephalic dementia after shunt operation. J Neurol Neurosurg Psychiatry 1978; 41:940.
[164] Raftopoulos C, Deleval J, Chaskis C, et al. Cognitive recovery in idiopathic normal pressure hydrocephalus: a prospective study. Neurosurgery 1994; 35:397.
[165] Fisher CM. The clinical picture in occult hydrocephalus. Clin Neurosurg 1977; 24:270.
[166] Hughes CP, Siegel BA, Coxe WS, et al. Adult idiopathic communicating hydrocephalus with and without shunting. J Neurol Neurosurg Psychiatry 1978; 41:961.
[167] Czosnyka Z, Czosnyka M, Richards HK, Pickard JD. Laboratory testing of hydrocephalus shunts -- conclusion of the U.K. Shunt evaluation programme. Acta Neurochir (Wien) 2002; 144:525.
[168] Ringel F, Schramm J, Meyer B. Comparison of programmable shunt valves vs standard valves for communicating hydrocephalus of adults: a retrospective analysis of 407 patients. Surg Neurol 2005; 63:36.
[169] Boon AJ, Tans JT, Delwel EJ, et al. Dutch Normal-Pressure Hydrocephalus Study: randomized comparison of low- and medium-pressure shunts. J Neurosurg 1998; 88:490.
[170] Weiner HL, Constantini S, Cohen H, Wisoff JH. Current treatment of normal-pressure hydrocephalus: comparison of flow-regulated and differential-pressure shunt valves. Neurosurgery 1995; 37:877.
[171] Raftopoulos C, Massager N, Balériaux D, et al. Prospective analysis by computed tomography and long-term outcome of 23 adult patients with chronic idiopathic hydrocephalus. Neurosurgery 1996; 38:51.
[172] Malm J, Kristensen B, Stegmayr B, et al. Three-year survival and functional outcome of patients with idiopathic adult hydrocephalus syndrome. Neurology 2000; 55:576.
[173] Lundkvist B, Eklund A, Kristensen B, et al. Cerebrospinal fluid hydrodynamics after placement of a shunt with an antisiphon device: a long-term study. J Neurosurg 2001; 94:750.

4

Interpretation of Cerebrospinal Fluid Parameters in Children with Hydrocephalus

Daniel Fulkerson
Indiana University School of Medicine/Riley Hospital for Children
Goodman Campbell Brain and Spine, Indianapolis, Indiana
USA

1. Introduction

Cerebrospinal fluid (CSF) is an ultrafiltrate of plasma formed by active, ATP-dependent pumps located predominantly in the choroidal epithelium. CSF is continuously produced and absorbed, turning over approximately 3-4 times per day. CSF normally is colorless, odorless, and contains very few cells. Compared to serum, CSF is low in protein, glucose, potassium and calcium, but high in sodium, magnesium, and chloride.(Burt 1993) Reference values for "normal" CSF levels are shown in Table 1.

CSF may be collected through a spinal puncture, ventricular access device or drain, or from a shunt "tap" in evaluating a child for shunt failure or infection. This chapter addresses some basic scenarios where interpretation of the CSF sample may guide clinical decision-making

Cerebrospinal Fluid Parameter:	Value:
Leukocytes	< 4/mL
Lymphocytes	60-70%
Monocytes	30-50%
Polymorphonuclear leukocytes	0%
Eosinophils	0%
Red Blood Cells	0
Protein	20-50 mg/dL
Glucose	40-70 mg/dL

Table 1. Normal Cerebrospinal Fluid values in adults

2. CSF cell counts in children with shunts

Children may have different CSF counts compared to adults. For example, healthy neonates may have leukocytes in the CSF in the absence of infection or neuropathology.(Smith, Garges et al. 2008) Portnoy and Olson evaluated the CSF from 371 children who were proven to *not* have CNS infection or pathology (seizures). They found 1-3 WBC in 25% of all children and 1-10 WBC in 5% of normal neonates.(Portnoy and Olson 1985) Ahmed et al. found a mean of 7.3 WBC/mm^3 in non-infected neonates, with a range of 0 –

130/mm^3.(Ahmed, Hickey et al. 1996) (Shah, Shofer et al. 2005) Other authors have noted a wide variability of CSF cell counts in children with or without infection.(Garges, Moody et al. 2006)

The presence of a shunt may alter the chemistry and cell levels. Lenfestey et al. examined the CSF cell levels for 181 neonates with either a VP shunt or CSF reservoir and compared them to a group of neonates without ventricular catheters.(Lenfestey, Smith et al. 2007) There was no significant difference in baseline WBC between the groups. Neonates with a ventricular catheter and infection had a mean WBC count of 150 cells/mm^3.

3. Intraventricular hemorrhage of prematurity

Premature, low-birth weight neonates have a risk of intraventricular hemorrhage. Approximately 57-85% of patients with hemorrhage will develop post-hemorrhagic hydrocephalus (PHH). The complication rate for shunts in these children is high due to an immature immune system, medical co-morbidites, and often thin, tenuous skin.

Many premature children will undergo temporizing procedures prior to placement of a definitive shunt. Temporizing procedures include serial lumbar or ventricular punctures, placement of a ventricular-subgaleal shunt, or placement of a ventricular access device (VAD). These measures allow removal of CSF while the child grows.

The clinician is often faced with a decision of how to interpret data from sample of CSF prior to placing the shunt. Given the prior intraventricular hemorrhage, the CSF may contain elevated levels of red blood cells (RBC), white blood cells (WBC), and protein levels. There is a persistent concern that elevation of cell or protein levels may affect the survivability of a shunt.

There are few laboratory studies evaluating the physical properties of CSF in relation to its cell and protein content. CSF normally has a similar viscosity to water, however its physical properties may be altered by high levels of cells or protein.(Brydon, Hayward et al. 1995) Brydon et al. studied the properties of 126 CSF samples from patients with hydrocephalus of various etiologies. They found that the viscosity of CSF differed from water by 1.4%. At supraphysiologic protein contents, the difference in viscosity was only approximately 6%.(Brydon, Hayward et al. 1995; Brydon, Hayward et al. 1995) In a separate publication, they also demonstrated that CSF protein levels did not impair shunt function, although an elevated RBC count did. An acceptable level of RBCs for safe shunt function was not defined.(Brydon, Bayston et al. 1996) Bloomfield et al. examined the physical properties of CSF by sampling 23 patients undergoing cranial surgery.(Bloomfield, Johnston et al. 1998) In their model, CSF viscosity also did not differ significantly from water over a range of protein contents. Baird et al. studied the effects of fluid with varying concentrations of protein or RBC in the function of a PS Medical (Medtronic, Inc.) valve. They found that protein did not affect valve function but that large numbers of RBCs led to valve failure.(Baird, Farner et al. 2002) Sainte-Rose et al. found no effect on Orbis Sigma valves with solutions containing up to 25 g of protein/liter.(Sainte-Rose, Hooven et al. 1987)

Brydon et al. performed clinical studies after the aforementioned laboratory work. They concluded that an elevated CSF protein count did not statistically increase the risk of shunt complications.(Brydon, Hayward et al. 1996) There are studies evaluating shunting after aneurysmal subarachnoid hemorrhage in adults. Both Rammos et al. and Kang et al. found that shunt malfunction was not statistically related to CSF protein or RBC counts.(Kang, Park et al. ; Rammos, Klopfenstein et al. 2008)

It is important to note that results found in adults do not necessarily translate to the preterm child. The brain of a preterm infant significantly differs from that of an adult in the degree of myelination and thus brain compliance. The overall risk of shunt failure in an adult is generally low, however the risk in a preterm infant is high.

We studied 58 low birth-weight, premature infants who developed PHH.(Fulkerson, Vachhrajani et al.) The CSF samples taken within 2 weeks prior to shunt insertion are shown in Table 2. Note that all these children had high numbers of RBCs and WBCs.

Of these 58 patients, ten (17.2%) had shunt failure within 3 months of insertion and nine (15.5%) suffered shunt infection. Both the failure and infection rate were higher for children with PHH compared to our overall rates for all children over the study period. A statistical analysis was performed to see if the shunt failure or infection rate was related to cell count or protein level prior to shunt insertion. Previous case reports have attributed shunt failure to high cell or protein levels.(Foltz and Shurtleff 1963; Lorber and Bhat 1974; Wise and Ballard 1976; Taylor and Peter 2001) Some authors recommend delaying shunt insertion until arbitrary CSF levels are reached. However, we found no statistical relationship of shunt infection or shunt failure with levels of CSF RBCs, WBCs, or protein levels at the time of shunt insertion.(Fulkerson, Vachhrajani et al.) Therefore, the timing of shunt placement should be based on the child's gestational age, weight, and overall clinical condition.

CSF Parameter:	Value:
RBC/mm3	3103.5 ± 9102.4
WBC/mm3	168.8 ± 1163.6
Protein (MG/DL)	211.1 ± 158.7
Glucose (MG/DL)	26.3 ± 12.7

Table 2. Cerebrospinal fluid values (mean ± standard deviation) of 58 low birth weight-premature infants prior to shunt insertion

4. CSF eosinophilia

As stated earlier, small numbers of leukocytes may be found in the CSF in children. The majority of these are lymphocytes or monocytes; eosinophils are normally absent. Eosinophils are granulocytes produced in the bone marrow and normally found in mucosa. They have a myriad of functions associated with hypersensitivity and inflammatory reactions. Bosch and Oehmichen examined 10,000 qualitative CSF cytological preparations and found eosinophilia in less than 1%. Given the overall rarity of eosinophils, the authors concluded that their presence was pathologic.(Bosch and Oehmichen 1978)

The finding of CSF eosinophils has been associated with allergy, intrathecal antibiotic administration, parasitic infestation, neurosyphilis, and fungal or tuberculosis infection.(Kessler and Cheek 1959; Bosch and Oehmichen 1978; Traynelis, Powell et al. 1988; Snow and Kossovsky 1989; Vinchon, Vallee et al. 1992; Niggemann, Bauer et al. 1997; Lo Re and Gluckman 2003) It has also been found in patients with hypersensitivity reactions to a shunt, predominately in older tubing materials.(Traynelis, Powell et al. 1988; Jimenez, Keating et al. 1994)

While eosinophils are normally absent in patients without shunts, their presence is relatively common after shunt placement. We followed CSF samples after initial shunt placement in 300 children.(Fulkerson and Boaz 2008) We identified eosinophilia in 93 of the 300 (31%) patients who underwent placement of their initial shunt. Statistical analysis identified that the risk factors for eosinophilia included a history of intraventricular hemorrhage of prematurity, younger age at shunt insertion, CSF leakage, infection, use of intrathecal antibiotics, and blood in the cerebrospinal fluid.

Shunted patients may have eosinophils in the absence of infection. Eosinophilia occurred within one month of shunt insertion in 69.2% (average 14.6 ± 8.7 days) and was transient in 95% of cases. We found two strong correlations with non-infectious eosinophilia: CSF leakage and intraventricular blood.

There was a statistical relationship of eosinophilia with CSF leakage or fluid accumulation under the skin. This was especially true in patients with the largest numbers of eosinophils

Figure 1 illustrates the clinical course of a 3-month-old male with a shunt infection. The shunt was removed (Day 0) and an external ventricular drain (EVD) was placed. He has a small eosinophilic reaction to the initial infection. He had a leakage of CSF around the drain site (Day 9 - first vertical line). The eosinophil counts rose dramatically after the leak. He suffered a second leak (Day 15 - second vertical line) and again, the eosinophils rise. This suggests that the eosinophilia is more a reaction rather than a cause of malfunction.

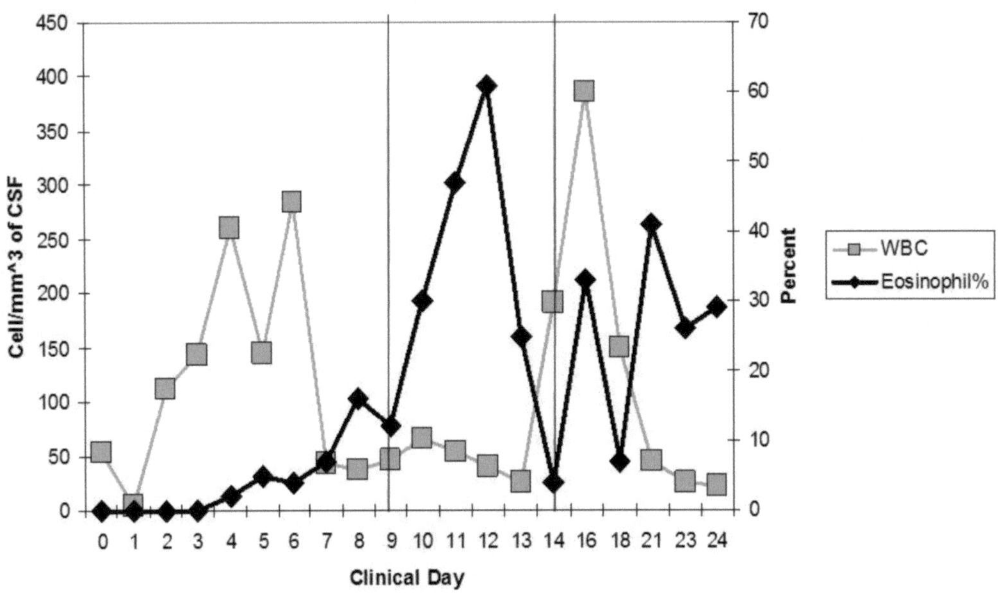

Fig. 1. **Clinical course of 3-month old with shunt infection.** The patient had leakage of CSF on Day 9 and 15. The number and percentage of eosinophils rose after these two events.(Reprinted with permission from *Journal of Neurosurgery:Pediatrics* 1: 288-295, 2008)

The second correlation of CSF eosinophilia is with the presence of intraventricular blood. We found a statistically significant relationship between eosinophilia and a CSF sample with greater than 100 RBC/mm^3.

The intraventricular space is relatively protected. Inflammatory cells are normally not present. CSF leakage exposes this immunologically privileged area to a space with inflammatory cells. Hemorrhage may bring these immunogens into the ventricular space. Eosinophils are known to migrate to areas rich in fibroblasts and enhance tissue remodeling through release of numerous cytokines.(Munitz and Levi-Schaffer 2004) Eosinophils interact with endothelial cells and enhance angiogenesis through growth factors. (Rothenberg 1998; Munitz and Levi-Schaffer 2004)

In our series, patients with CSF eosinophilia had a higher incidence of shunt malfunction compared to the general shunted population. This has also been reported by other authors. (Tung, Raffel et al. 1991) In these patients, the valve or catheter may be blocked with inflammatory debris. Eosinophils are known to propagate many inflammatory responses through secretion of chemicals involved in up-regulating adhesion systems and cellular trafficking.(Rothenberg 1998) This likely promotes the attraction and adhesion of cells, contributing to shunt blockage. The need for shunt revision after initial placement was statistically correlated with the total number and percentage of eosinophils in this series.

5. Shunt infection

Approximately 5-8% of newly placed shunts will become infected.(Drake, Kestle et al. 1998) Clinical signs of infection include shunt failure, fever, abdominal pain, and wound dehiscence. Diagnosis of a shunt infection comes from the appropriate clinical scenario with a positive CSF bacterial culture. The treatment of shunt infection generally includes surgical removal of all existing shunt hardware, temporary CSF diversion, and antibiotics. However, the culture results may not be known for a number of days to weeks. The treating physician may need to make clinical decisions based on interpretation of the CSF sample.

The most common bacterial organisms causing shunt infection are coagulase-negative *Staphylococci* and *Staphylococcus aureus*. Other potential pathogens include *Propionibacterium acnes*, Streptococcal species, and gram-negative organism (*E. coli, P. aeruginosa, Klebsiella* species, and *Enterobacter* species). CSF samples will often show a rise in the WBC count with a predominance of polymorphonuclear leukocytes (PMNs) in patients with infection from these pathogens.

The WBC count that is diagnostic of infection is unknown.(Kestenbaum, Ebberson et al. ; Garges, Moody et al. 2006; Lenfestey, Smith et al. 2007) Previous authors have used a level of 100 WBC/mm3 as a level indicative of infection.(Lan, Wong et al. 2003; Lenfestey, Smith et al. 2007) However, the WBC count in shunt infections is variable. Conen et al. examined 78 shunt infections in patients over 12 years old. While 80% of patient had a CSF leukocyte count greater than 5 x 10^6 cells/mm^3, a "normal" cell count occurred in approximately 20% of infections.(Conen, Walti et al. 2008) Other markers for infection have been studied, including tumor necrosis factor-α, various interleukin concentrations, (Asi-Bautista, Heidemann et al. 1997) and polymerase chain reaction for amplification of bacterial DNA.

(Banks, Bharara et al. 2005) While these show promise, there is not yet widespread acceptance.

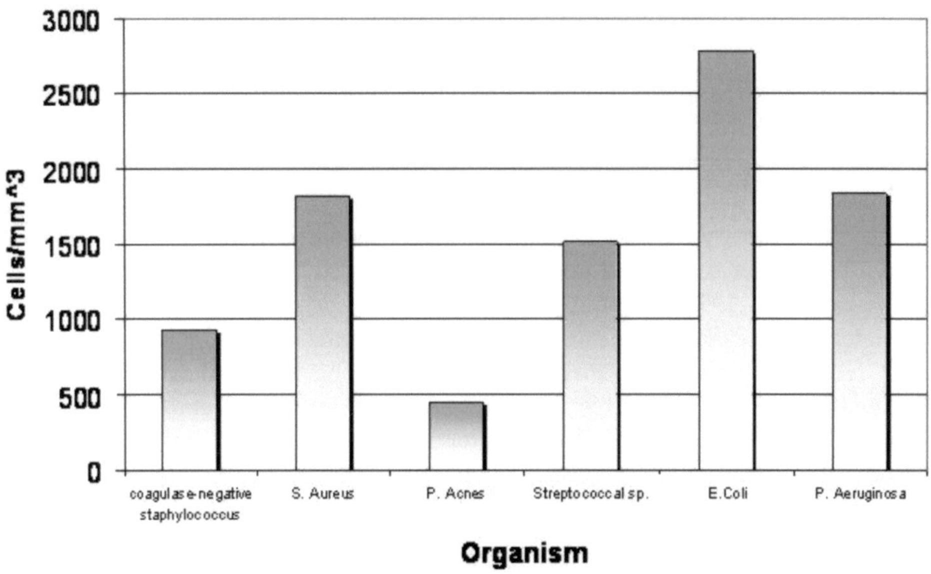

Fig. 2. **Average White Blood Cells (WBC) on diagnosis of shunt infection.** The number of leukocytes varies with infecting organism, with higher numbers for gram-negative pathogens, and low levels for *P. acnes*. (Reprinted with permission from *Journal of Neurosurgery: Pediatrics* 1:288-295, 2008)

The levels of CSF WBC and the differential percentage of PMNs, lymphocytes, monocytes and eosinophils vary depending on the infecting organism (Figure 2). A case example is shown in Figure 3. This figure shows the cell count in a child who presented with a shunt infection with *P. acnes*. Note the high eosinophil count shown in Figure 3A. The child became secondarily infected with *N. flavum*, a gram-negative organism. He spiked a very high WBC count which was predominantely PMNs (Figure 3B). His infection cleared and a new shunt was placed. Unfortunately, the new shunt also became infected with coagulase-negative staphylococcus. He had a moderate WBC reaction with a higher percentage of PMNs and lymphocytes.

We evaluated 105 patients with shunt infection. The WBC count and differential of these 105 patients is shown in Table 3. Gram-negative organisms cause an extremely high WBC count with a predominance of PMNs. In our analysis, a diffential percentage of greater than 62% PMNs was most suggestive of a gram-negative infection. Therefore, the treating physician may consider choosing an antibiotic regimen that covers gram-negative organisms in a patient with clinical signs of shunt infection and a CSF sample with a high WBC count with > 62% PMNs.

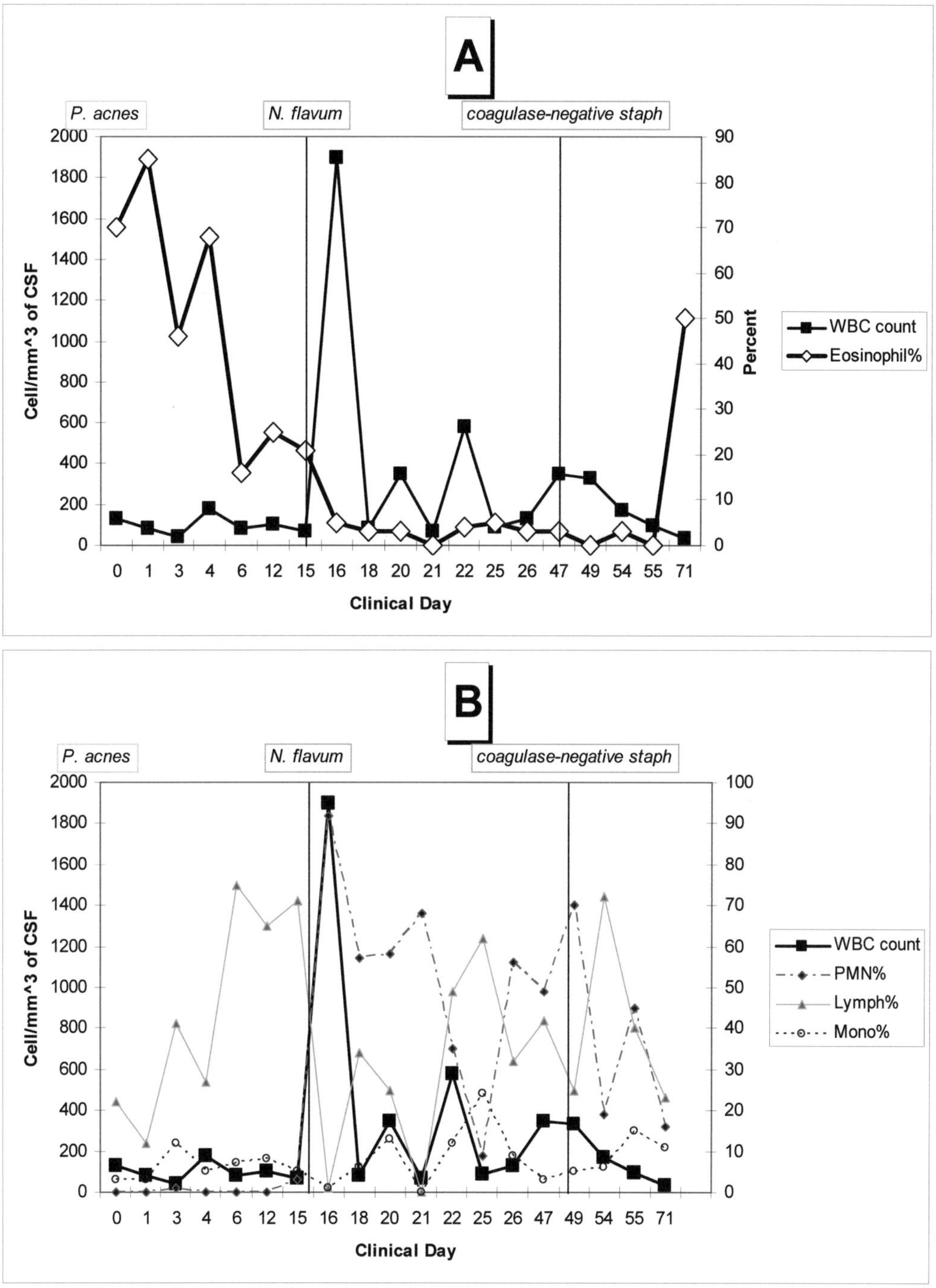

Fig. 3. CSF reaction in patient with three shunt infections with *P. acnes, N. flavum*, and coagulase-negative staphylococcus. (Reprinted with permission from *Journal of Neurosurgery: Pediatrics* 1: 288-295, 2008)

Organism:	Initial WBC count (cells/mm^3):	PMN (%)	Lymphocyte (%)	Monocyte (%)	Eosinophil (%)
Coagulase-negative *Staphylococci*	387.9 ± 652.8	48.3 ± 31.6	28.7 ± 24.9	19.4 ± 16.1	3.3 ± 4.0
S. aureus	574.6 ± 1539.0	56.1 ± 26.3	16.6 ± 15.8	22.9 ± 17.3	5.1 ± 6.8
P. acnes	110.8 ± 163.9	18.0 ± 38.0	37.2 ± 29.0	33.0 ± 32.7	14.4 ± 24.8
Streptococcal sp.	913.9 ± 1190.9	66.7 ± 41.9	16.7 ± 20.1	16.6 ± 19.6	3.5 ± 4.0
Gram-negative sp.	1618.0 ± 3165.9	69.3 ± 31.6	11.9 ± 12.0	15.6 ± 23.1	6.9 ± 13.2

Table 3. Average white blood cell count and differential based on infecting organism

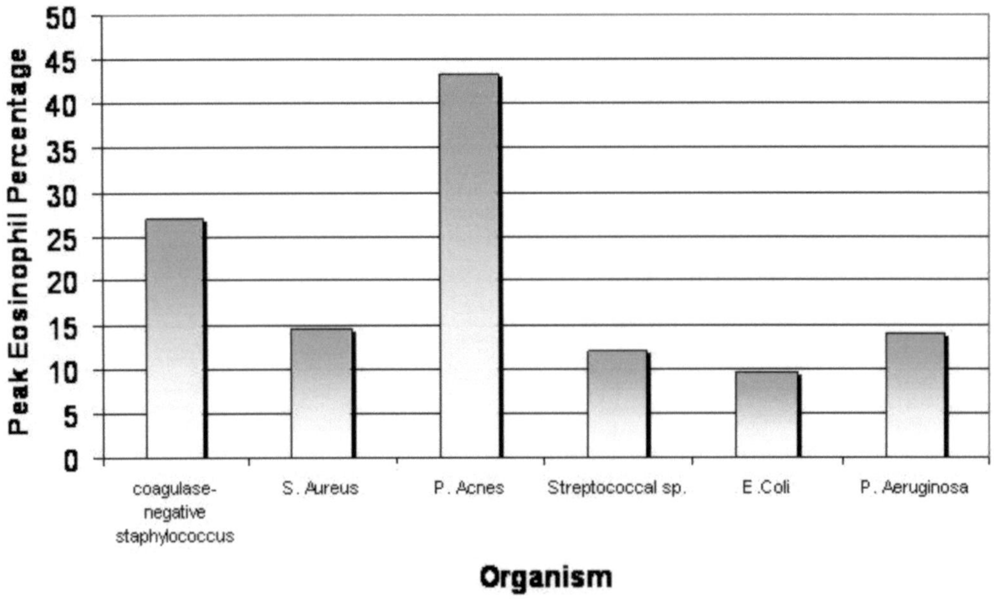

Fig. 4. Peak eosinophil differential percentage of the CSF leukocyte count related to the infecting organism in shunt infections. *P. acnes* infections have a significantly higher eosinophil percentage compared to other pathogens. (Reprinted with permission from *Journal of Neurosurgery: Pediatrics* 1: 288-295, 2008)

More indolent organisms cause less of a CSF reaction. *P. acnes* is a gram-positive, anaerobic diphtheroid that is part of the normal skin flora. This organism may cause shunt infection, however the CSF has a significantly lower WBC compared to other organisms. The diagnosis of *P. acnes* infection may be challenging, as culture growth generally requires anaerobic preparation and extended incubation times (up to 2 weeks).(Rekate, Ruch et al. 1980) *P. acnes* infections have a characteristically high percentage of eosinophils (Figure 4).

The clinician should suspect *P. acnes* in the patient with clinical signs of shunt infection, but with a CSF WBC count < 16 with the presence of eosinophils.

The CSF reaction to infection is similar among all organisms. There is an initial predominance of PMNs, although this is lower in *P. acnes*. This is followed by a rise in monocytes and lymphocytes, with possible influx of eosinophils. The total WBC trends towards zero by two weeks with successful treatment of the shunt infection.

6. Conclusions

Interpretation of CSF samples in children with shunts may help guide clinical decision-making.

Children with hydrocephalus resulting from intraventricular hemorrhage of prematurity are at a higher risk of shunt malfunction and infection compared to other shunted patients. They often have elevated levels of protein in their CSF, however, this is not statistically correlated with subsequent shunt malfunction.

CSF eosinophils may be rarely associated with allergic reactions. Eosinophils are found in up to 31% of patients with a newly placed shunt. Children with eosinophils in the CSF have a higher risk of shunt malfunction. Eosinophilia may be caused by exposure of the immunologically privileged intraventricular space with the skin or blood.

Eosinophils are also seen commonly in children with shunt infections. In addition to the presence of eosinophils, examination of the distribution of CSF leukocytes may provide information in evaluating children with shunt infection. Some pathogens, such as gram-negative organims cause a very high WBC count with a predominance of PMNs. Others, such as *P. acnes*, have a low WBC count but a high percentage of eosinophils. This is clinically relevant because *P. acnes* may require a longer incubation time with anaerobic culture preparation for diagnosis.

7. References

Ahmed, A., S. M. Hickey, et al. (1996). "Cerebrospinal fluid values in the term neonate." *Pediatr Infect Dis J* 15(4): 298-303.

Asi-Bautista, M. C., S. M. Heidemann, et al. (1997). "Tumor necrosis factor-alpha, interleukin-1 beta, and interleukin-6 concentrations in cerebrospinal fluid predict ventriculoperitoneal shunt infection." *Crit Care Med* 25(10): 1713-6.

Baird, C., S. Farner, et al. (2002). "The effects of protein, red blood cells and whole blood on PS valve function." *Pediatr Neurosurg* 37(4): 186-93.

Banks, J. T., S. Bharara, et al. (2005). "Polymerase chain reaction for the rapid detection of cerebrospinal fluid shunt or ventriculostomy infections." *Neurosurgery* 57(6): 1237-43; discussion 1237-43.

Bloomfield, I. G., I. H. Johnston, et al. (1998). "Effects of proteins, blood cells and glucose on the viscosity of cerebrospinal fluid." *Pediatr Neurosurg* 28(5): 246-51.

Bosch, I. and M. Oehmichen (1978). "Eosinophilic granulocytes in cerebrospinal fluid: analysis of 94 cerebrospinal fluid specimens and review of the literature." *J Neurol* 219(2): 93-105.

Brydon, H. L., R. Bayston, et al. (1996). "The effect of protein and blood cells on the flow-pressure characteristics of shunts." *Neurosurgery* 38(3): 498-504; discussion 505.

Brydon, H. L., R. Hayward, et al. (1995). "Physical properties of cerebrospinal fluid of relevance to shunt function. 1: The effect of protein upon CSF viscosity." *Br J Neurosurg* 9(5): 639-44.

Brydon, H. L., R. Hayward, et al. (1995). "Physical properties of cerebrospinal fluid of relevance to shunt function. 2: The effect of protein upon CSF surface tension and contact angle." *Br J Neurosurg* 9(5): 645-51.

Brydon, H. L., R. Hayward, et al. (1996). "Does the cerebrospinal fluid protein concentration increase the risk of shunt complications?" *Br J Neurosurg* 10(3): 267-73.

Burt, A. M. (1993). *Textbook of Neuroanatomy*. Philadelphia, Pennsylvania, W.B. Saunders Company.

Conen, A., L. N. Walti, et al. (2008). "Characteristics and treatment outcome of cerebrospinal fluid shunt-associated infections in adults: a retrospective analysis over an 11-year period." *Clin Infect Dis* 47(1): 73-82.

Drake, J. M., J. R. Kestle, et al. (1998). "Randomized trial of cerebrospinal fluid shunt valve design in pediatric hydrocephalus." *Neurosurgery* 43(2): 294-303; discussion 303-5.

Foltz, E. L. and D. B. Shurtleff (1963). "Five-Year Comparative Study of Hydrocephalus in Children with and without Operation (113 Cases)." *J Neurosurg* 20: 1064-79.

Fulkerson, D. H. and J. C. Boaz (2008). "Cerebrospinal fluid eosinophilia in children with ventricular shunts." *J Neurosurg Pediatr* 1(4): 288-95.

Fulkerson, D. H., S. Vachhrajani, et al. "Analysis of the risk of shunt failure or infection related to cerebrospinal fluid cell count, protein level, and glucose levels in low-birth-weight premature infants with posthemorrhagic hydrocephalus." *J Neurosurg Pediatr* 7(2): 147-51.

Garges, H. P., M. A. Moody, et al. (2006). "Neonatal meningitis: what is the correlation among cerebrospinal fluid cultures, blood cultures, and cerebrospinal fluid parameters?" *Pediatrics* 117(4): 1094-100.

Jimenez, D. F., R. Keating, et al. (1994). "Silicone allergy in ventriculoperitoneal shunts." *Childs Nerv Syst* 10(1): 59-63.

Kang, D. H., J. Park, et al. "Early ventriculoperitoneal shunt placement after severe aneurysmal subarachnoid hemorrhage: role of intraventricular hemorrhage and shunt function." *Neurosurgery* 66(5): 904-8; discussion 908-9.

Kessler, L. A. and W. R. Cheek (1959). "Eosinophilia of the cerebrospinal fluid of noninfectious origin: report of 2 cases." *Neurology* 9(5): 371-4.

Kestenbaum, L. A., J. Ebberson, et al. "Defining cerebrospinal fluid white blood cell count reference values in neonates and young infants." *Pediatrics* 125(2): 257-64.

Lan, C. C., T. T. Wong, et al. (2003). "Early diagnosis of ventriculoperitoneal shunt infections and malfunctions in children with hydrocephalus." *J Microbiol Immunol Infect* 36(1): 47-50.

Lenfestey, R. W., P. B. Smith, et al. (2007). "Predictive value of cerebrospinal fluid parameters in neonates with intraventricular drainage devices." *J Neurosurg* 107(3 Suppl): 209-12.

Lo Re, V., 3rd and S. J. Gluckman (2003). "Eosinophilic meningitis." *Am J Med* 114(3): 217-23.

Lorber, J. and U. S. Bhat (1974). "Posthaemorrhagic hydrocephalus. Diagnosis, differential diagnosis, treatment, and long-term results." *Arch Dis Child* 49(10): 751-62.

Munitz, A. and F. Levi-Schaffer (2004). "Eosinophils: 'new' roles for 'old' cells." *Allergy* 59(3): 268-75.

Niggemann, B., A. Bauer, et al. (1997). "Latex allergy as a cause of eosinophilia in cerebrospinal fluid in a child with a ventricular shunt." *J Allergy Clin Immunol* 100(6 Pt 1): 849-50.

Portnoy, J. M. and L. C. Olson (1985). "Normal cerebrospinal fluid values in children: another look." *Pediatrics* 75(3): 484-7.

Rammos, S., J. Klopfenstein, et al. (2008). "Conversion of external ventricular drains to ventriculoperitoneal shunts after aneurysmal subarachnoid hemorrhage: effects of site and protein/red blood cell counts on shunt infection and malfunction." *J Neurosurg* 109(6): 1001-4.

Rekate, H. L., T. Ruch, et al. (1980). "Diphtheroid infections of cerebrospinal fluid shunts. The changing pattern of shunt infection in Cleveland." *J Neurosurg* 52(4): 553-6.

Rothenberg, M. E. (1998). "Eosinophilia." *N Engl J Med* 338(22): 1592-600.

Sainte-Rose, C., M. D. Hooven, et al. (1987). "A new approach in the treatment of hydrocephalus." *J Neurosurg* 66(2): 213-26.

Shah, S. S., F. S. Shofer, et al. (2005). "Significance of extreme leukocytosis in the evaluation of febrile children." *Pediatr Infect Dis J* 24(7): 627-30.

Smith, P. B., H. P. Garges, et al. (2008). "Meningitis in preterm neonates: importance of cerebrospinal fluid parameters." *Am J Perinatol* 25(7): 421-6.

Snow, R. B. and N. Kossovsky (1989). "Hypersensitivity reaction associated with sterile ventriculoperitoneal shunt malfunction." *Surg Neurol* 31(3): 209-14.

Taylor, A. G. and J. C. Peter (2001). "Advantages of delayed VP shunting in post-haemorrhagic hydrocephalus seen in low-birth-weight infants." *Childs Nerv Syst* 17(6): 328-33.

Traynelis, V. C., R. G. Powell, et al. (1988). "Cerebrospinal fluid eosinophilia and sterile shunt malfunction." *Neurosurgery* 23(5): 645-9.

Tung, H., C. Raffel, et al. (1991). "Ventricular cerebrospinal fluid eosinophilia in children with ventriculoperitoneal shunts." *J Neurosurg* 75(4): 541-4.

Vinchon, M., L. Vallee, et al. (1992). "Cerebro-spinal fluid eosinophilia in shunt infections." *Neuropediatrics* 23(5): 235-40.

Wise, B. L. and R. Ballard (1976). "Hydrocephalus secondary to intracranial hemorrhage in premature infants." *Childs Brain* 2(4): 234-41.

5

Management of Hydrocephalus

Parvaneh Karimzadeh
*Pediatric Neurology Department,
Shahid Beheshti University of Medical Sciences,
Pediatric Neurology Research Center,
Tehran
Iran*

1. Introduction

Hydrocephalus is a problem in which there is an excessive contains of cerebrospinal fluid (CSF) and dilates cerebral ventricles.

Regardless of etiology, early detection and early intervention of this condition is very important to prevent brain insult and normal development of children.

Decrease of this volume accumulation and pressure maintain normal chemical balance and normal function of blood-brain barrier.

In progressive symptomatic hydrocephalus patients have the symptom of intra cranial hypertension.

2. Surgical management

If there is obstructive or non-communicating hydrocephalus removal the obstruction is preferred.

In progressive symptomatic hydrocephalus surgical intervention such as shunting of cerebrospinal fluid to facilitate absorption of CSF is required.

Most patients need mechanical extra cranial shunt system for redirect cerebrospinal fluid circulation into peritoneal cavity, right atrium and pleural cavity.

3. Ventriculoperitoneal shunting

A ventriculoperitoneal shunt (VP) is used most commonly for cerebrospinal fluid diversion.

The abdomen should have the ability for absorption of the fluid. Shunts cause cerebrospinal fluid to flow unidirectional under a valve system. Pressures required enough energy to overcome valve resistance and can be used in patients with different pressure requirements.

The ventricular catheter can be placed from the coronal approach. In this approach most neurosurgeons prefer parieto-occipital catheters. The proximal catheter tip should lie anterior to choroid plexus and in the frontal horn of the lateral ventricles.

4. Complications

Common causes for failure are: infection, obstruction, over drainage, disconnection and loculated cerebrospinal fluid collection (1).

For evaluation of shunt malformation continuous intra cranial monitoring is useful. Main complication of this type of treatment is infection and the most important causative agents of infection are staphylococcus epidermitis (58% to 88.9%) , Staphylococcus aureus (12-40%), gram negative bacilli (9-22%), entrobacteria, klebsiella pneumonia and pseudomonas aeroginosa. These can cause severe complications such as cognitive and neurological deficits (1-4).

If infection causes impairment of the shunting mechanism, removal and new shunting system are necessary.

Prophylactic antibiotics during shunting decrease the incidence of infection.

As there is a great preponderance of the skin agents in these infections considering of Vancomycin plus third or fourth generation Cephalosporin like cefteriaxon as empiric treatment until cultures are obtained is an appropriate treatment.

Dysfunction of the hydrocephalus valve is also another serious cause of complication and it's a result of the obstruction of proximal catheter.

Over drainage of CSF is another long term complication of cerebrospinal fluid shunting. This complication and obstruction need more surgery.

5. Ventriculoatrial shunting

This procedure usually is the first choice for patients who are unable to have abdominal distal catheters. It is a high risk procedure with possibility of serious long term complications such as renal failure or thrombosis of great vein.

An incision is made across the anterior border of the sternocloidomastoid muscle to expose the jugular vein. Alternately, the shunt can be placed in the common facial vein just as it enters the jugular vein. Once the jugular vein is isolated with ligatures, the vein is tied off distally.

A small opening is then made into the jugular vein to pass the shunt into the right atrium of the heart. Ventriculo-atrial shunts may occlude due to thrombus formation, if the distal end moves out of the atrium (4-5).

6. Endoscopic Third Ventriculostomy (ETV)

ETV is an alternative therapy to cerebrospinal fluid shunting in selected patients.

This method is a selective surgical management in patients with congenital aqueduct stenosis.

Also ventriculostomy is useful for patients with intracranial cysts and local cerebrospinal fluid collection.

Overall the failure rate of different shunt is approximately 40% in the first year after surgery (6).

It is a minimally invasive procedure which is used in children with obstructive hydrocephalus (such as aqueduct stenosis or tumor) that have normal or near normal spinal fluid as an alternative to shunt revision (7-8).

The goal of ventriculostomy is to create an opening in the floor of the third ventricle to subarachnoid space, usually the trapped fluid begin to absorb right after the opening, in that case there is no need for further interventions.

This surgery takes only one hour and the neurosurgeon uses a tiny camera and a minute surgical instrument and will follow the child regularly after undergoing ETV to make sure of normal intracranial pressure and no complications occur. Third ventriculostomy is divided into several stages. After general anesthesia is induced, the patient is placed supine with the head in the neutral position on a doughnut pillow. The head is then elevated approximately 30° to minimize excessive CSF loss and entry of air. A coronal burr hole is placed 3 cm lateral to the midline and just anterior to the coronal suture.

The stages of this operation are:

- finding and entering the foramen of Munro
- Inspecting the floor of the third ventricle
- Perforating the floor of the third ventricle
- Enlarging this perforation
- Inspecting the prepontine cistern (9)
- **Advantages**
- No foreign objects (shunt tubing and valve) implanted in the body, minimizing the risk of infection.
- Fewer incisions cause less discomfort.
- A lower long term complication rate compared to a shunt.
- **Disadvantages**
- The chances of improving may be lower in comparison with shunting
- Although very unlikely, there is a risk of serious complications with ETV compared to a shunt operation.

7. Complications

Neurosurgeons have accepted Endoscopic third ventriculostomy as a choice procedure for the treatment of obstructive hydrocephalus especially in children.

The success of the procedure depends on the cause of hydrocephalus and past complications.

The most common complications of endoscopic third ventriculostomy are fever and bleeding. The use of a cold light source and a monopolar coagulation in the confined volume of the third ventricle can increase CSF temperatures to high levels, sometimes causing fever. Attempts to perforate the ventricular floor can lead to bleeding, as can damage to ventricular walls or perforation of the basilar artery.

Fever up to 40`C within 3 days after ventriculostomy within clinical or laboratory tests of meningitis , meningitis with fever and clinical & positive findings of CSF, occurrence of very mild hemorrhage from free edge of stoma, mild hemorrhage from ependymal veins , moderate to severe intraventricular hemorrhage were considered as the most common complications.

Short-term memory loss is another potential complication of endoscopic third ventriculostomy, since the procedure may affect the hypothalamus, which is responsible for memory. However, given time, an individual usually recovers from any short-term memory loss following endoscopic third ventriculostomy.

Other Complications of ETV could leakage of CSF, bradycardia, loss of thirst, increased appetite, subdural hematoma, injury to periventricular structures such as hypothalamus which can result diabetes inspidus.(7)

According to Canadian Pediatric Neurosurgery Study Group about the Canadian experience in Endoscopic third ventriculostomy (in children) age has a significant effect on outcome in pediatric patients.

Canadian pediatric neurosurgery study group evaluated age, sex, etiology of hydrocephalus and history of previous surgery and finally found failure rates are particularly high in young infants, therefore, this procedure in neonates and early infants should be carefully considered (8).

8. Factors associated with outcomes in ETV

The outcome of this procedure remains controversial regards to etiology, age and long term complications.

The most controversial issue is the lower age limit for affectivity of this procedure.

The best results were reported in patients with posterior fossa tumor or pineal glioma . The next priority is the cases with Aqueductal stenosis.

Fewer good outcomes were seen in post hemorrhagic hydrocephalus and in chronic cases with hydrocephalus.

Also patients with myelomeningocele and post meningitis hydrocephalus had poor outcomes (9).

9. Non surgical management

Non surgical management is treatment of symptomatic hydrocephalus and includes the temporary use of medications to decrease CSF production such as Acetazolamide or Isossorbide which produce hyper osmotic diuresis and increases CSF absorption (10).

In premature infants hydrocephalus may develop as a result of intraventricular hemorrhage. This intraventricular hemorrhage causes obstruction of arachnoid granulations by production of materials reminder from break down of hemorrhage. Shunting has high morbidity in premature infants.

Multiple other interventions have been considered. One of these interventions is lumbar punctures.

Repeated lumbar punctures CSF are a common non surgical management in premature infants to periventricular dilation after periventricular hemorrhage. They believe removal of CSF with blood and protein (approximately 10 to 15 ml/kg) causes normal resorption of CSF to prevent the development of hydrocephalus after periventricular hemorrhage. Despite few studies support this method, other studies revealed the repeated lumbar puncture did not reduce the need for shunting of cerebrospinal fluid and also this method did not decrease the likelihood of dead or disability in these patients.

Some studies showed a higher incidence of cerebrospinal fluid infections in those premature infants who received repeated lumbar punctures for intraventricular hemorrhage (11).

In this procedure the child is getting immobile and a minute needle is placed in Childs lower back and the CSF is removed.

Some studies recommend cerebrospinal fluid tapping in specific situations and by some expert physicians; they consider a sufficient quantity of CSF for these premature infants (about 10-15 ml/kg).

Other studies have examined direct ventricular drainage in patients with rapidly progressive ventriculomegaly who their brain ventricles are too small to shunt the ventriculoperitoneal shunt placement (12-13).

It has the relative risks for shunt placement, death disability and multiple disabilities were similar for repeated lumbar punctures.

In progressive hydrocephalus serial lumbar punctures may be needed until the infant is large enough for permanent placement.

10. Rehabilitation

Regardless of different surgical management patients with hydrocephalus have some disabilities such as: learning disorder, behavioral problems, and speech delay.

Early intervention with different methods of rehabilitation is necessary for non surgical management of patients with hydrocephalus.

Successful shunting is usually related to more obvious and rapid improvements in rehabilitation efforts and rapid improvements in rehabilitation efforts (14).

11. Physical therapy interventions

Physical therapy goals for child with hydrocephalus appropriates functional skills and reducing secondary impairment such as contractures, fractures and obesity which could interfere with developmental skills .the physiotherapist can work with child in home hospital or clinic depending on the age and medical conditions.

12. Fetal ventriculomegaly and hydrocephalus

Fetal ventriculomegaly is a relatively common finding on second trimester obstetrical ultrasound examination (15). Most experts define fetal ventriculomegaly as a lateral ventricular atrial measurement of greater than 15mm.Ventriculomegaly is "isolated" when the fetus has no other anomalies (15-16). The prevalence of ventriculomegaly is less than 2 percent, but reports vary widely within that range (17).

The preferred diagnostic technique for assessing ventriculomegaly is ultrasound measurement of the diameter of the lateral ventricles at the level of the atria. The ventricle should be measured in the axial plane, at the level of the frontal horns and cavum septi pellucidi.

The outcome of ventriculomegaly depends on several factors including the actual size of the ventricles, whether or not there are any other findings on the ultrasound, such as agenesis of the corpus callosum, and the results of the amniocentesis. In general, the outcome is worse when the ventricles are larger, the amniocentesis is abnormal, or there are other problems seen on the ultrasound.

The best outcome is typically observed when the fetus' ventricles are only mildly enlarged (measure between 10-15 millimeters in size), and when there are no other problems seen on the ultrasound, and when genetic testing results are normal—this is called "Isolated Mild Ventriculomegaly". The most common effect in the child is developmental delay. This seems to be related to the size of the ventricles.

13. References

[1] Lima MM, Pereira CU, Silva AM. Infecçóes em dispositivos neurológicos implant veis em crianças e adolescentes.Arq Neuropsiquiatr 2007; 65(1):118-123.
[2] Paiva WS, et al. Management of the ventriculoperitoneal shunt infections Rev Panam Infectol 2010;12(3):43-47.
[3] Lima MM, Pereira CU, Silva AM. Infecçóes em dispositivosneurológicos implant veis em crianças e adolescentes. Arq Neuropsiquiatr 2007; 65(1):118-123.
[4] Raza Rizvi, Qudsia Anjum. Hydrocephalus in Children .J Pak Med Assoc Vol. 55, No. 11, November 2005.
[5] Hydrocephalus surgery. copied 2010 available at URL:http://hydrocephalus.allanch.dk.
[6] Drake JM, Kestle JR, Milner R,et al.Randomized trial of cerebrospinal fluid shunt valve design in pediatric hydrocephalus,Neurosurgery 1998;43:294.
[7] Marvin A fishman, MD.Hydrocephalus.2011 available at URL: http://uptodate.com.
[8] George I. Jallo, M.D., Karl F. Kothbauer, M.D., and I. Rick Abbott, M.D. Endoscopic Third Ventriculostomy: Technique Neurosurg Focus. 2005; 19(6)
[9] Drake, James M.F. Endoscopic Third Ventriculostomy in padiatric patients, The 25 Canadian Experience, Neurosurgery , May 2007, 60(5) 881-886
[10] Alberto J Espay, MD; available at URL: http://emedicine.medscape.com/article/1135286-treatment Updated: Apr 27, 2010.
[11] Whitelaw A. Repeated lumbar or ventricular punctures in newborns with intraventricular hemorrhage. Cochrane Database Syst Rev 2001;CD000216.
[12] Berger A, Weninger M, Reinprecht A, et al. Long-term experience with subcutaneously tunneled external ventricular drainage in preterm infants. Childs Nerv Syst 2000; 16:103.
[13] Heep A, Engelskirchen R, Holschneider A, Groneck P. Primary intervention for posthemorrhagic hydrocephalus in very low birthweight infants by ventriculostomy. Childs Nerv Syst 2001; 17:47.
[14] Bontke CF, Zasler ND, Boake C. Rehabilitation of the head-injured patient. In: Narayan RK, Wilberger JE, Povlishock JT, eds. *Neurotrauma*. New York, NY: McGraw-Hill; 1996:841-58.
[15] Griffiths PD, Reeves MJ, Morris JE, et al. A prospective study of fetuses with isolated ventriculomegaly investigated by antenatal sonography and in utero MR imaging. AJNR Am J Neuroradiol 2010; 31:106.
[16] Davis GH. Fetal hydrocephalus. Clin Perinatol 2003; 30:531.
[17] Partington MD. Congenital hydrocephalus. Neurosurg Clin N Am 2001; 12:737.

6

Complications Associated with Surgical Treatment of Hydrocephalus

Takeshi Satow, Masaaki Saiki and Takayuki Kikuchi
Department of Neurosurgery, Shiga Medical Center for Adults
Japan

1. Introduction

Excessive accumulation of cerebrospinal fluid (CSF) in the brain is a condition known as hydrocephalus. It may cause a life-threatening increase in intracranial pressure (ICP). Nonsurgical treatment of hydrocephalus includes continuous CSF drainage, repetitive lumbar punctures (Lim et al., 2009), or osmotic diuretics such as mannitol or glycerol, but their effects are transient and limited. Surgical treatment is needed to resolve the critical condition caused by increased ICP.

Hydrocephalus can be classified as communicating or obstructive (non-communicating). In selecting surgical treatment, it is important to judge which is involved. Communicating hydrocephalus occurs when CSF flow is not blocked at any part of the passages connecting the ventricles. In obstructive hydrocephalus, CSF flow is blocked along one or more narrow passages between the ventricles. Hydrocephalus is treated by surgical insertion of a shunt system, such as a ventriculoperitoneal shunt (VP shunt), lumboperitoneal shunt (LP shunt) or ventriculoatrial shunt (VA shunt). The LP shunt should not be used in patients with obstructive hydrocephalus, because it can induce tentorial herniation leading to death. A limited number of patients with obstructive hydrocephalus are candidates for third ventriculostomy by neuroendoscope. Below, we review articles focusing on complications associated with various types of CSF diversion procedure.

2. Complications associated with any shunts

Surgical techniques for treatment of hydrocephalus are well established, but are associated with a relatively high incidence of complications (Blount et al., 1993, Kang & Lee, 1999). Complications associated with shunt procedures include infection, malfunction (obstruction or disconnection) and silicone allergy, and overdrainage.

Infection of the shunt system is a troublesome and common complication. It is a major cause of morbidity and mortality in the treatment of hydrocephalus. The incidence of CSF shunt infection is approximately 2 – 22% in most neurosurgical units throughout the world (Schoenbaum et al., 1975, Mayhall et al., 1984, Spanu et al., 1986, Patir et al., 1992). The use of an antibiotic-impregnated shunt (AIS, impregnated with rifampicin and clindamycin) has been reported recently to reduce the incidence of shunt infection (Govender et al., 2003, Sciubba et al., 2005, Pattavilakom et al., 2007). AIS use is not common, however, so that it is difficult to determine the efficacy of AIS in preventing shunt infection (Steinbok et al., 2010).

Moreover, a systematic review by Ratilal et al. (2008) found that systemic prophylactic antibiotics prevented shunt infection better than AIS. There have been investigations of the effect of more simple techniques, focusing on intraoperative sterile conditions such as intraoperative irrigation (Hayashi et al., 2008, 2010), changing gloves before handling the shunt catheter (Sørensen et al., 2008, Rehman et al., 2010) or a double-gloving strategy (Tulipan & Cleves, 2006), and antimicrobial suture wound closure (Rozzelle et al., 2008). Where AIS is unavailable, we recommend the systemic administration of antibiotics, generous intraoperative irrigation and double-gloving.

Shunt malfunction is another common problem following CSF shunting. It leads to various symptoms including headache, nausea and vomiting, visual disturbance, seizures, changes in intellect or personality, disturbance of consciousness and sudden death. The ventricular side is reportedly obstructed more often (Cozzens & Chandler, 1997). Disconnection at any point of the shunt system is first investigated by plain radiograph and/or CT (Fig.1).

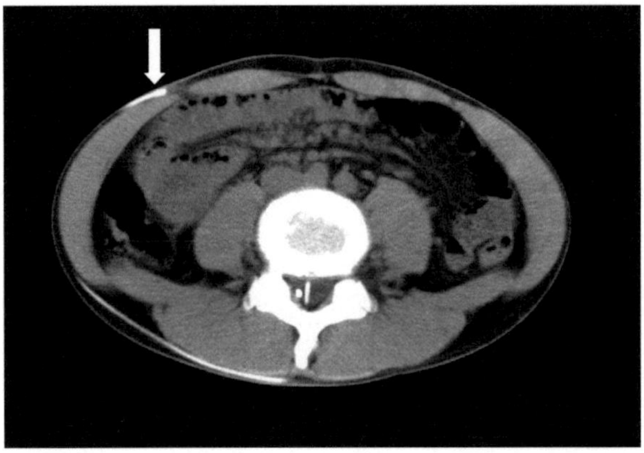

Fig. 1. CT scan of the abdomen

A patient with a previous LP shunt placement presented with it malfunctioning. CT showed it had disconnected where the catheter entered the peritoneal cavity (arrow).

Recently a programmable shunt valve has been used to control the CSF flow. Breakage of the programmable pressure valve is difficult to diagnose by plain radiograph or CT, however. Since the tract of shunt tube becomes calcified in patients harboring a shunt system for a long period, making diagnosis of its disconnection difficult, it might be advisable to carry out shuntgraphy to locate the occlusion of the shunt system. CSF infection must then be investigated. Fibrous tissue generated by long-lasting contact of the ventricular catheter with the choroid plexus can lead to its occlusion. High CSF cell count and protein levels are believed to be a cause of shunt malfunction, although not in all cases (Fulkerson et al., 2011). Even without infection, an allergic reaction to the shunt catheter occasionally leads to shunt malfunction (Jimenez et al., 1994, Hussain et al., 2005, Bezerra et al., 2011). In such cases, prolonged use of corticosteroid or replacement of the shunt system with a polyurethane-based system (Hussain et al., 2005) is appropriate.

In shunt malfunction, there have been numerous reports of malfunctions of the distal catheter (peritoneal tube). When malfunction at the distal catheter is suspected, plain radiograph and CT scan are performed. Bowel perforation (Fig.2) (Abu-Dalu et al., 1983, Sathyanarayana et al., 2000, Vinchon et al., 2006) and intra-abdominal pseudocyst formation

(Rainov et al., 1994; Anderson et al., 2003) are known to be a cause of distal catheter malfunction.

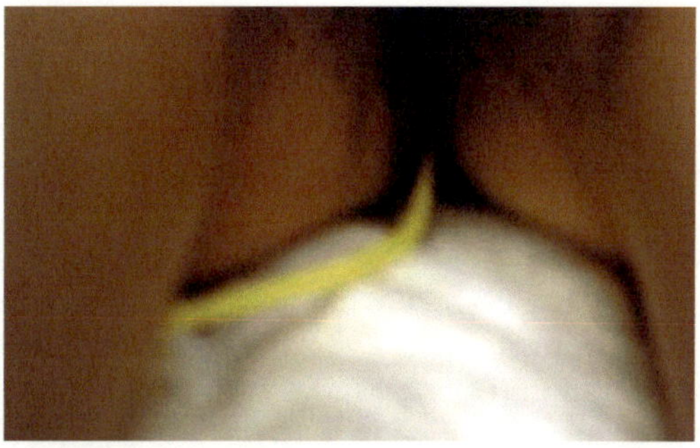

Fig. 2. Photograph of a patient with bowel perforation of a VP shunt.
The peritoneal side of the catheter extruded from the anus. The shunt system was removed surgically. The peritoneal catheter was cut at the point where it perforated into the rectum, and the extruded distal catheter was pulled out from the side of the anus.

Latent infection could give rise to complications of this sort. In such cases, we carry out tentative externalization of the ventricular catheter after removing the peritoneal catheter and repairing the fistula point if necessary. Even without evidence of infection, we have occasionally experienced patients in whom a shunt of this sort has not been functional from the start (unnecessary shunt). Clearly it is important to consider the indication for CSF shunt before any implantation. Protrusion or migration of a peritoneal catheter has also been reported from other sites, including the heart (Fewel & Garton, 2004), pleural cavity (Doh et al., 1995), stomach (Alonso-Vanegas et al., 1994), a gastrostomy wound (Chan et al., 2003), mouth (Berhouma et al., 2008), scrotum (Oktem et al., 1998), umbilicus (Wani et al., 2002, Kanojia et al., 2008) and lumbar region (Kanojia et al., 2008). Also, very rare cases of knot formation of a peritoneal catheter, leading to obstruction of the shunt as well as small-bowel, have been reported (Starreveld et al., 1998, Woerdeman & Hanlo, 2006, Eftekhar & Hunn, 2008).
Constipation is often observed in bed-ridden patients. Infrequently it is a cause of shunt malfunction, due to increased intra-abdominal pressure (Powers et al., 2006, Martínez-Lage et al., 2008). Treatment of constipation could improve the neurological condition of such patients. Constipation should not be forgotten as a cause of shunt malfunction prior to revision surgery.
The sections below review complications associated with particular treatment methods.

3. Complication associated with particular shunts

3.1 Ventriculoperitoneal shunt (VP shunt)

VP shunt is the most common procedure for treating hydrocephalus. Various reported complications derive from the VP shunt. As the VP shunt system is longer than the LP shunt or VA shunt, we speculate that migration is unlikely to occur in association with a VP shunt. Many reports (Ammar & Nasser, 1995, Acharya et al., 2002, Nadkarni et al., 2007, Chen et al., 2011) have found an upward migration of a VP shunt, however. Even in VP shunt implantation, firm fixation is recommended, particularly at the rectus abdominis fascia.

Pneumocephalus (Kawajiri et al., 1994, Villarejo et al., 1998, Barada et al., 2009) and pneumoventricle (Perrin & Bernstein, 2005) have been reported as a complication of VP shunt. This overdrainage complication seems to occur in association with VP shunt and also in other shunt operations. It is believed that this complication arises when a shunt is implanted in patients whose paranasal sinus is left open. Consequently, it is important to investigate the possibility of open paranasal sinuses, particularly when patients undergo shunt placement after a head injury or previous cranial surgeries involving the paranasal sinuses.

In patients with a brain tumor who underwent VP shunt, peritoneal dissemination of the tumor can take place (Berger et al., 1991, Newton et al., 1992, Rickert et al., 1998).

As in other cranial surgeries, patients with a ventricular catheter have a 5.5% risk of seizure in the first year after the operation (Dan & Wade, 1986). The efficacy of prophylactic use of anticonvulsants has never been established in patients undergoing shunt surgery, however. In addition, epileptic seizure could be a manifestation of shunt malfunction (Johnson et al., 1996).

Very rarely, superficial siderosis of the central nervous system (Fig.3) has been reported after VP shunt (Satow et al., 2010). This might be caused by repeated long-lasting contact of the ventricular catheter with the choroid plexus. Transient improvement of neurological symptoms such as ataxia was observed following prescription of corticosteroid. In such cases, replacement of the VP shunt by a lumboperitoneal shunt might be necessary.

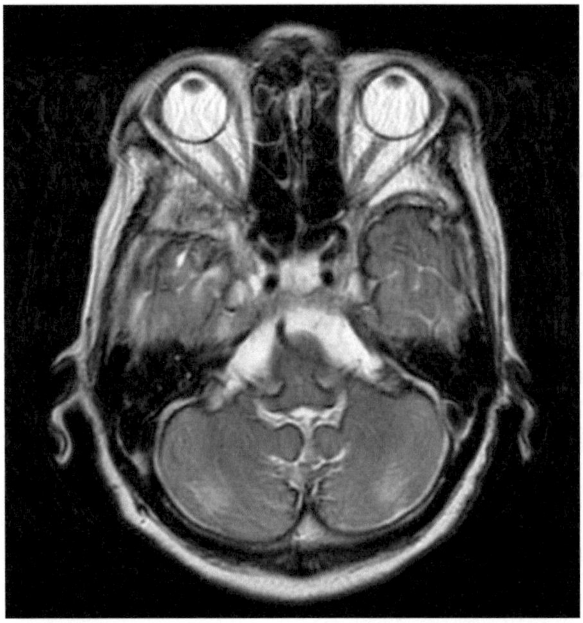

Fig. 3. MRI of the brain showing superficial siderosis after VP shunt (T2-weighted sequence)

A patient with normal pressure hydrocephalus underwent VP shunt placement. About 2 years after the operation, new symptoms developed including ataxia and hearing disturbance. MRI showed a rim of low-intensity enveloping the surface of the brain stem and cerebellum, which is the characteristic appearance of superficial siderosis of the central nervous system.

3.2 Lumboperitoneal shunt (LP shunt)

Lumboperitoneal shunt (LP shunt) is performed in patients with communicating hydrocephalus. It is also performed for the treatment of CSF fistula, idiopathic intracranial hypertension (Burgett et al., 1997) and slit-ventricle syndrome (Le et al., 2002). Complications such as infection and malfunction were reportedly lower in LP shunt than VP shunt (Aoki, 1990).

Acute subdural hematoma after minor head trauma is reported in about 2% of patients with LP shunt (Kamiryo et al., 2003). LP shunt is cautiously indicated for patients who do not live independently on a daily basis and who are prone to fall. Acquired Chiari malformation is a well-known complication after LP shunt (Payner et al., 1994, Wang et al., 2007). These complications are a manifestation of overdrainage. Complications due to overdrainage could be prevented by introducing a pressure control valve for the LP shunt (Wang et al., 2007).

Proximal migration of LP shunts have been reported (Yoshida et al., 2000, Satow et al., 2001, Rodrigues et al., 2005). Defects in the fixation device or increased intraabdominal pressure are believed to be a cause of proximal migration of the LP shunt. Recently, programmable shunt systems have become available for LP shunt (Toma et al., 2010), and these might act as an anchor to prevent migration of the LP shunt.

LP shunt surgery does not include cranial procedures, which causes surgeons to believe it is a safer treatment. However, it should be kept in mind that various serious complications can occur after LP shunt.

3.3 Ventriculoatrial shunt (VA shunt)

VA shunt has recently been performed on rare occasions. A distal shunt catheter is inserted into the right atrium via the facial vein or internal jugular vein. Consequently, once infection of the shunt system occurs, septicemia develops. Chronic infection of a VA shunt results in an immune-complex-mediated glomerulonephritis, called "shunt nephritis" (Sticker et al., 1968). This serious complication is caused by a skin commensal organism such as *Staphylococcus epidermidis* or other bacteria, and it requires revision of the shunt system. Very rarely, pulmonary hypertension caused by venous thrombus formation has been reported as a complication of VA shunt (Piatt & Hoffman, 1989, Tonn et al., 2005, Kluge et al., 2010); this could be lethal. As there are fatal cardiopulmonary complications associated with VA shunt, it should be used only in patients whose peritoneal cavity is not suitable for the placement of a distal shunt catheter.

3.4 Endoscopic third ventriculostomy

Endoscopic third ventriculostomy (ETV) is indicated and effective for obstructive hydrocephalus (Hellwig et al., 2005, Schroeder et al., 2007). Some authors have reported the use of ETV for communicating hydrocephalus (Gangemi et al., 2004, 2008, Hailong et al., 2008). The procedure did not need foreign materials such as a shunt catheter, so the incidence of infection is considered to be low. Moreover, in patients with shunt malfunction caused by infection of the shunt, ETV and removal of the shunt system are recommended.

Fatal complications have been also reported, including high-frequency tachypnea (Bernard et al., 2010), late failure (Drake et al., 2006, Lipina et al., 2007), and subarachnoid hemorrhage due to injury to the basilar artery (Schroeder et al., 1999, 2002). Although rare, overdrainage complication involving chronic subdural hematoma or fluid collection has also been reported (Kim et al., 2004, Sqaramella et al., 2004). An overdrainage complication manifesting acute subdural hematoma can occur, leading to death (Fig. 4).

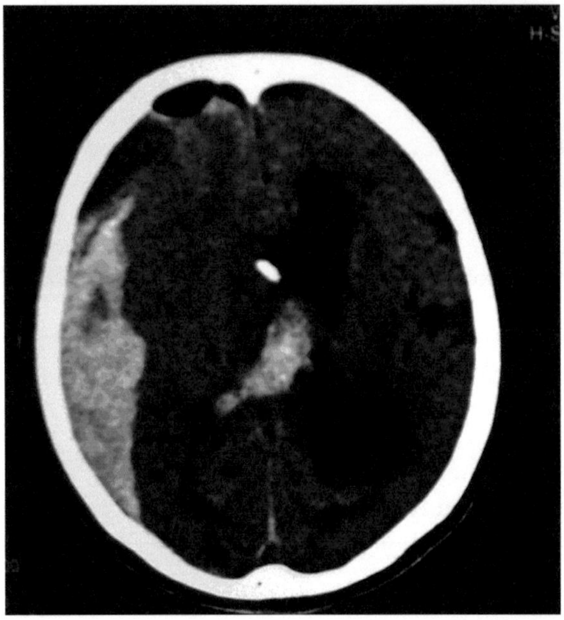

Fig. 4. Acute subdural hematoma (ASDH) after ETV for obstructive hydrocephalus due to brain stem hemorrhage.
One day after ETV, the patient developed dilation of pupils more on the right side. CT disclosed ASDH on the right side. When ETV was performed, external ventricular drainage was placed because of the likelihood of early failure of the ventriculostomy. Although ventricular drainage remained nonfunctioning, ASDH developed as an overdrainage complication of ETV. At surgical evacuation of the hematoma, the bleeding point was confirmed as a cortical artery around the sylvian fissure, far from the puncture point of the ETV.

4. Conclusion

In this article we have reviewed various complications associated with CSF diversion procedures, which are performed routinely in neurosurgical practice for the treatment of hydrocephalus. There appear to be numerous ways of preventing those complications, developed by various physicians, as described in this article. In the literature of general surgery, complications associated with operation have usually been considered underreported (Wanzel et al., 2000). It is important to report these ways so as to reduce the rate of complication in this common neurosurgical operation.

5. References

Abu-Dalu, K., Pade, D., Hadani, M., & Sahar, A. (1983). Colonic complications of ventriculoperitoneal shunts. *Neurosurgery,* Vol.13, pp. 167-169.

Acharya, R., Bhutani, A., Saxena, H., & Madan, VS. (2002). Complete migration of ventriculoperitoneal shunt into the ventricle. Neurol Sci, Vol.23, pp. 75-77.

Alonso-Vanegas, M., Alvarez, JL., Delgado, L., Mendizabal, R., Jiménez, JL., & Sanchez-Cabrera, JM. (1994). Gastric perforation due to ventriculo-peritoneal shunt. *Pediatr Neurosurg,* Vol.21, pp. 192-194.

Ammar, A., & Nasser, M. (1995). Intraventricular migration of VP shunt. *Neurosurg Rev,* Vol.18, pp. 293-295.

Anderson, CM., Sorrells, DL., & Kerby, JD. (2003). Intra-abdominal pseudocysts as a complication of ventriculoperitoneal shunts: a case report and review of the literature. *Curr Surg,* Vol.60, pp. 338-340.

Aoki N. (1990). Lumboperitoneal shunt: clinical applications, complications, and comparison with ventriculoperitoneal shunt. *Neurosurgery,* Vol.26, pp. 998-1003.

Barada, W., Najjar, M., & Beydoun, A. (2009). Early onset tension pneumocephalus following ventriculoperitoneal shunt insertion for normal pressure hydrocephalus: a case report. *Clin Neurol Neurosurg,* Vol.111, pp. 300-302.

Berger, MS., Baumeister, B., Geyer, JR., Milstein, J., Kabev, PM., & LeRoux, PD. (1991). The risks of metastases from shunting in children with primary central nervous system tumors. *J Neurosurg,* Vol.74, pp. 872-877.

Berhouma, M., Messerer, M., Houissa, S., & Khaldi, M. (2008). Transoral protrusion of a peritoneal catheter: a rare complication of ventriculoperitoneal shunt. *Pediatr Neurosurg,* Vol.44, pp. 169-171.

Bernard, R., Vallee, F., Mateo, J., Marsella, M., George, B., Payen, D., & Chibbaro, S. (2010). Uncntrollable high-frequency tachypnea: a rare and nearly fatal complication of endoscopic third ventriculostomy: case report and literature review. *Minim Invasive Neurosurg,* Vol.53, pp. 270-272.

Bezerra, S., Frigeri, TM., Severo, CM., Santana, JC., & Graeff-Teixeira, C. (2011). Cerebrospinal fluid eosinophilia associated with intraventricular shunts. *Clin Neurol Neurosurg,* Vol.113, pp. 345-349.

Blount, JP., Campbell, JA., & Haines, SJ. (1993). Complications in ventricular cerebrospinal shunting. *Neurosurg Clin N Am,* Vol.4, pp. 633-656.

Burgett, RA., Purvin, VA., & Kawasaki, A. (1997). Lumboperitoneal shunting for pseudotumor cerebri. *Neurology,* Vol.49, pp. 734-739.

Chan, Y., Datta, NN., Chan, KY., Rehman, SU., Poon, CY., & Kwok, JC. (2003). Extrusion of the peritoneal catheter of a VP shunt system through a gastrostomy wound. *Surg Neurol,* Vol.60, pp. 68-69.

Chen, HH., Riva-Cambrin, J., Brockmeyer, DL., Walker, ML., & Kestle, JR. (2011). Shunt failure due to intracranial migration of BioGlide ventricular catheter. *J Neurosurg Pediatr,* Vol.7, pp. 408-412.

Cozzens, JW., & Chandler, JP. (1997). Increased risk of distal ventriculoperitoneal shunt obstruction associated with slit valves or distal slits in the peritoneal catheter. *J Neurosurg,* Vol.87, pp. 682-686.

Dan, NG., & Wade, MJ. (1986). The incidence of epilepsy after ventricular shunting procedures. *J Neurosurg,* Vol.65, pp. 19-21.

Doh, JW., Bae, HG., Lee, KS., Yun, IG., & Byun, BJ. (1995). Hydrothorax from intrathoracic migration of a ventriculoperitoneal shunt catheter. *Surg Neurol,* Vol.43, pp.340-343.

Drake, J., Chumas, P., Kestle, J., Pierre-Kahn, A., Vinchon, M., Brown, J., Pollack, IF., & Arai, H. (2006). Late rapid deterioration after endoscopic third ventriculostomy: additional cases and review of the literature. *J Neurosurg,* Vol.105 (2 Suppl), pp. 118-126.

Eftekhar, B., & Hunn, A. (2008). Ventriculoperitoneal shunt blockage due to spontaneous knot formation in the peritoneal catheter. Case report. *J Neurosurg Pediatr,* Vol.1, pp. 142-143.

Fewel, ME., & Garton, HJ. (2004). Migration of distal ventriculoperitoneal shunt catheter into the heart. Case report and review of the literature. *J Neurosurg,* Vol.100 (2 Suppl Pediatrics), pp. 206-211.

Fulkerson, DH., Vachhrajani, S., Bohnstedt, BN., Patel, NB., Patel, AJ., Fox, BD., Jea, A., & Boaz, JC. (2011). Analysis of the risk of shunt failure or infection related to cerebrospinal fluid cell count, protein level, and glucose levels in low-birth-weight premature infants with posthemorrhagic hydrocephalus. *J Neurosurg Pediatr,* Vol.7, pp. 147-151.

Gangemi, M., Maiuri, F., Buonamassa, S., Colella, G., & de Divitiis, E. (2004). Endoscopic third ventriculostomy in idiopathic normal pressure hydrocephalus. *Neurosurgery,* Vol.55, pp. 129-134.

Gangemi, M., Maiuri, F., Naddeo, M., Godano, U., Mascari, C., Broggi, G., & Ferroli, P. (2008). Endoscopic third ventriculostomy in idiopathic normal pressure hydrocephalus: an Italian multicenter study. *Neurosurgery,* Vol.63, pp. 62-67.

Govender, ST., Nathoo, N., & van Dellen, Jr. (2003). Evaluation of an antibiotic-impregnated shunt system for the treatment of hydrocephalus. *J Neurosurg,* Vol.99, pp. 831-839.

Hailong, F., Guangfu, H., Haibin, T., Hong, P., Yong, C., Weidong, L., & Dongdong, Z. (2008). Endoscopic third ventriculostomy in the management of communicating hydrocephalus: a preliminary study. *J Neurosurg,* Vol.109, pp. 923-930.

Hayashi, T., Shirane, T., Kato, T., & Tominaga, T. (2008) Efficacy of intraoperative wound irrigation for preventing shunt infection. *J Neurosurg Pediatr,* Vol.2, pp. 25-28.

Hayashi, T., Shirane, R., Yokosawa, M., Kimiwada, T., & Tominaga, T. (2010). Efficacy of intraoperative irrigation with saline for preventing shunt infection. *J Neurosurg Pediatr,* Vol.6, pp. 273-276.

Hellwig, D., Grotenhuis, JA., Tirakotai, W., Riegel, T., Schulte, DM., Bauer, BL., & Bertalanffy, H. (2005). Endoscopic third ventriculostomy for obstructive hydrocephalus. *Neurosurg Rev,* Vol.28, pp. 1-34

Hussain, NS., Wang, PP., James, C., Carson, BS., & Avellino, AM. (2005). Distal ventriculoperitoneal shunt failure caused by silicone allergy. Case report. *J Neurosurg,* Vol.102, pp. 536-539.

Javadpour, M., May, P., & Mallucci, C. (2003). Sudden death secondary to delayed closure of endoscopic third ventriculostomy. *Br J Neurosurg,* Vol.17, pp. 266-269.

Jimenez, DF., Keating, R., & Goodrich, JT. (1994). Silicone allergy in ventriculoperitoneal shunts. *Childs Nerv Syst,* Vol.10, pp. 59-63.

Johnson, DL., Conry, J., & O'Donnell, R. (1996). Epileptic seizure as a sign of cerebrospinal fluid shunt malfunction. *Pediatr Neurosurg,* Vol.24, pp. 223-227.

Kamiryo, T., Hamada, J., Fuwa, I., & Ushio, Y. (2003). Acute subdural hematoma after lumboperitoneal shunt placement in patients with normal pressure hydrocephalus. *Neurol Med Chir (Tokyo)*, Vol.43, pp. 197-200.

Kang, JK., & Lee, IW. (1999). Long-term follow-up of shunting therapy. *Childs Nerv Syst*, Vol.15, pp. 711-717.

Kanojia, R., Sinha, SK., Rawat, J., Wakhlu, A., Kureel, S., & Tandon, R. (2008). Unusual ventriculuperitoneal shunt extrusion: experience with 5 cases and review of the literature. *Pediatr Neurosurg*, Vol.44, pp. 49-51.

Kawajiri, K., Matsuoka, Y., & Hayazaki, K. (1994). Brain tumor complicated by pneumocephalus following cerebrospinal fluid shunting-two case reports. *Neurol Med Chir (Tokyo)*, Vol.34, pp. 10-14.

Kim, BS., Jallo, GI., Kothbauer, K., & Abbott, IR. (2004). Chronic subdural hematoma as a complication of endoscopic third ventriculostomy. *Surg Neurol*, Vol.62, pp. 64-68.

Kluge, S., Baumann, HJ., Regelsberger, J., Kehler, U., Gliemroth, J., Koziej, B., Klose, H., & Meyer, A. (2010). Pulmonary hypertension after ventriculoatrial shunt implantation. *J Neurosurg*, Vol.113, pp. 1279-1283.

Le, H., Yamini, B., & Frim, DM. (2002). Lumboperitoneal shunting as a treatment for slit ventricle syndrome. *Pediatr Neurosurg*, Vol.36, pp. 178-182.

Lim, TS., Yong, SW., & Moon, SY. (2009). Repetitive lumbar punctures as treatment for normal pressure hydrocephalus. *Eur Neurol*, Vol.62, pp. 293-297.

Lipina, R., Palecek, T., Requli, S., & Kovarova, M. (2007). Death in consequence of late failure of endoscopic third ventriculostomy. *Childs Nerv Syst*, Vol.23, pp. 815-819.

Martínez-Lage, JF., Martos-Tello, JM., Ros-de-San Pedro, J., & Almagro, MJ. (2008). Severe constipation: an under-appreciated cause of VP shunt malfunction: a case-based update. *Childs Nerv Syst*, Vol.24, pp. 431-435.

Mayhall, CG., Archer, NH., Lamb, VA., Spadora, AC., Baggett, JW., Ward, JD., & Narayan, RK. (1984). Ventriculostomy-related infections. A prospective epidemiologic study. *N Engl J Med*, Vol.310, pp. 553-559.

Nadkarni, TD., Menon, RK., Dange, NN., Desai, KI., & Goel, A. (2007). Cranial migration of complete ventriculoperitoneal shunt assembly. *J Clin Neurosci*, Vol.14, pp. 92-94.

Newton, HB., Rosenblum, MK., & Walker, RW. (1992). Extraneural metastases of infratentorial glioblastoma multiforme to the peritoneal cavity. *Cancer*, Vol.69, pp. 2149-2153.

Oktem, IS., Akdemir, H., Koç, K., Menkü, A., Tucer, B., Selçuklu, A., & Turan, C. (1998). Migration of abdominal catheter of ventriculoperitoneal shunt into the scrotum. *Acta Neurochir (Wien)*, Vol.140, pp.167-170.

Patir, R., Mahapatra, AK., & Banerju, AK. (1992). Risk factors in postoperative neurosurgical infection. A prospective study. *Acta Neurochir (Wien)*, Vol.119, pp. 80-84.

Pattavilakom, A., Xenos, C., Bradfield, O., & Danks, RA. (2007). Reduction in shunt infection using antibiotic impregnated CSF shunt catheters: an Australian prospective study. *J Clin Neurosci*, Vol.14, pp. 526-531.

Payner, TD., Prenger, E., Berger, TS., & Crone, KR. (1994). Acquired Chiari malformations: incidence, diagnosis, and management. *Neurosurgery*, Vol.34, pp. 429-434.

Perrin, RG., & Bernstein, M. (2005). Tension pneumoventricle after placement of a ventriculoperitoneal shunt: a novel treatment strategy. Case report. *J Neurosurg,* Vol.102, pp. 386-388.

Piatt, JH. Jr, & Hoffman, HJ. (1989). Cor pulmonale: a lethal complication of ventriculoatrial CSF diversion. *Childs Nerv Syst,* Vol.5, pp. 29-31.

Powers, CJ., George, T., & Fuchs, HE. (2006). Constipation as a reversible cause of ventriculoperitoneal shunt failure. Report of two cases. *J Neurosurg,* Vol.105 (3 Suppl), pp. 227-230.

Rainov, N., Schobess, A., Heidecke, V., & Burkert, W. (1994). Abdominal CSF pseudocysts in patients with ventriculo-peritoneal shunts. Report of fourteen cases and review of the literature. *Acta Neurochir (Wien),* Vol.127, pp. 73-78.

Ratilal, B., Costa, J., & Sampaio, C. (2008). Antibiotic prophylaxis for surgical introduction of intracranial venricular shunts: systematic review. *J Neurosurg Pediatr,* Vol.1, pp. 48-56.

Rehman, AU., Rehman, TU., Bashir, HH., & Gupta, V. (2010). A simple method to reduce infection of ventriculoperitoneal shunts. *J Neurosurg Pediatr,* Vol.5, pp. 569-572.

Rickert, CH., Reznik, M., Lenelle, J., & Rinaldi, P. (1998) Shunt-related abdominal metastasis of cerebral teratocarcinoma: report of an unusual case and review of the literature. *Neurosurgery,* Vol.42, pp. 1378-1382.

Rodrigues, D., Nannapaneni, R., Behari, S., Prasad, M., Herwadkar, A., Gerber, CJ., & Mitchell, P. (2005). Proximal migration of a lumboperitoneal unishunt system. *J Clin Neurosci,* Vol.12, pp. 838-841.

Rozzelle, CJ., Leonardo, J., & Li, V. (2008). Antimicrobial suture wound closure for cerebrospinal fluid shunt surgery: a prospective, double-blinded, randomized controlled trial. *J Neurosurg Pediatr,* Vol.2, pp. 111-117.

Sathyanarayana, S., Wylen, EL., Baskaya, MK., & Nanda, A. (2000). Spontaneous bowel perforation after ventriculoperitoneal shunt surgery: case report and a review of 45 cases. *Surg Neurol,* Vol.54, pp. 388-396.

Satow, T., Motoyama, Y., Yamazoe, N., Isaka, F., Higuchi, K., & Nabeshima, S. (2001). Migration of a lumboperitoneal shunt catheter into the spinal canal-case report. *Neurol Med Chir (Tokyo),* Vol.41, pp. 97-99.

Satow, T., Yamada, S., Yagi, M., & Saiki, M. (2010). Superficial siderosis of the central nervous system after ventriculoperitoneal shunt. *J Neurosurg,* Vol. 113, pp. 93-96.

Schoenbaum, SC., Gardner, P., & Shillito, J. (1975). Infections of cerebrospinal fluid shunts: epidemiology, clinical manifestations, and therapy. *J Infect Dis,* Vol.131, pp. 443-452.

Schroeder, HW., Warzok, RW., Assaf, JA., & Gaaf, MR. (1999). Fatal subarachnoid hemorrhage after endoscopic third ventriculostomy. Case report. *J Neurosurg,* Vol.90, pp. 153-155.

Schroeder, HW., Niendorf, WR., & Gaaf, MR. (2002). Complications of endoscopic third ventriculostomy. *J Neurosurg,* Vol.96, pp. 1032-1040.

Schroeder, HW., Oertel, J., & Gaab, MR. (2007). Endoscopic treatment of cerebrospinal fluid pathway obstructions. *Neurosurgery,* Vol.60(2 Suppl 1), pp. ONS44-51.

Sciubba, DM., Stuart, RM., McGirt, MJ., Woodworth, GF., Samdani, A., Carson, B., & Jallo, GI. (2005). Effect of antibiotic-impregnated shunt in decreasing the incidence of shunt infection in the treatment of hydrocephalus. *J Neurosurg,* Vol.103 (2 Suppl), pp. 131-136.

Spanu, G., Karussos, G., Adinolfi, D., & Bonfanti, N. (1986). An analysis of cerebrospinal fluid shunt infections in adults. A clinical experience of twelve years. *Acta Neurochir (Wien),* Vol.80, pp. 79-82.

Sqaramella, E., Castelli, G., & Sotgiu, S. (2004). Chronic subdural collection after endoscopic third ventriculostomy. *Acta Neurochir (Wien),* Vol.146, pp. 529-530.

Starreveld, Y., Poenaru, D., & Ellis, P. (1998). Ventriculoperitoneal shunt knot: a rare cause of bowel obstruction and ischemia. *Can J Surg,* Vol.41, pp. 239-240.

Steinbok, P., Milner, R., Agrawal, D., Farace, E., Leung, GK., Ng, I., Tomita, T., Wang, E., Wang, N., Wong, GK., & Zhou, LF. (2010). A multicenter multinational registry for assessing ventriculoperitoneal shunt infections for hydrocephalus. *Neurosurgery,* Vol.67, pp.1303-1310.

Sticker, GB., Shin, MH., Burke, EC., Holley, KE., Miller, RH., & Segar, WE. (1968). Diffuse glomerulonephritis associated with infected ventriculoatrial shunt. *N Engl J Med,* Vol.279, pp. 1077-1082.

Sørensen, P., Ejlertsen, T., Aaen, D., & Poulsen, K. (2008). Bacterial contamination of surgeons gloves during shunt insertion: a pilot study. *Br J Neurosurg,* Vol.22, pp.675-677.

Toma, AK., Dherijha, M., Kitchen, ND., & Watkins, LD. (2010). Use of lumboperitoneal shunts with the Strata NSC valve: a single-center experience. *J Neurosurg,* Vol.113, pp. 1304-1308.

Tonn, P., Gilsbach, JM., Kreitschmann-Andermahr, I., Franke, A., & Blindt, R. (2005). A rare but life-threatening complication of ventriculo-atrial shunt. *Acta Neurochir (Wien),* Vol.147, pp. 1303-1304.

Tulipan, N., & Cleves, MA. (2006). Effect of an intraoperative double-gloving strategy on the incidence of cerebrospinal fluid shunt infection. *J Neurosurg,* Vol.104 (1 Suppl), pp. 5-8.

Villarejo, F., Carceller, F., Alvarez, C., Bencosme, J., Pérez Díaz, C., Goldman, L., & Pascual, A. (1998). Pneumocephalus after shunting for hydrocephalus. *Childs Nerv Syst,* Vol.14, pp. 333-337.

Vinchon, M., Baroncini, M., Laurent, T., & Patrick, D. (2006). Bowel perforation caused by peritoneal shunt catheters: diagnosis and treatment. *Neurosurgery,* Vol.58 (1 Suppl), pp. ONS 76-82.

Wang, VY., Barbaro, NM., Lawton, MT., Pitts, L., Kunwar, S., Parsa, AT., Gupta, N., & McDermott, MW. (2007). Complications of lumboperitoneal shunts. *Neurosurgery,* Vol.60, pp. 1045-1048.

Wani, AA., Ramzan, A., & Wani, MA.. (2002). Protrusion of a peritoneal catheter through the umblicus: an unusual complication of a ventriculoperitoneal shunt. *Pediatr Surg Int,* Vol.18, pp. 171-172.

Wanzel, KR., Jamieson, CG., & Bohnen, JM.. (2000). Complications on a general surgery service: incidence and reporting. *Can J Surg,* Vol.43, pp. 113-117.

Woerdeman, PA., & Hanlo, PW. (2006). Ventriculoperitoneal shunt occlusion due to spontaneous intraabdominal knot formation in the catheter. Case report. *J Neurosurg,* Vol.105 (3 Suppl), pp. 231-232.

Yoshida, S., Masunaga, S., Hayase, M., & Oda, Y. (2000). Migration of the shunt tube after lumboperitoneal shunt-two case reports. *Neurol Med Chir (Tokyo),* Vol.40, pp. 594-596.

7

External Ventricular Drain Infections

Anderson C.O. Tsang and Gilberto K.K. Leung
The University of Hong Kong
Hong Kong

1. Introduction

The insertion of ventricular catheter is one of the most commonly performed procedures in neurosurgery. External ventricular drainage (EVD) is a reliable, accurate and cost-effective means of monitoring intracranial pressure (ICP) in acute traumatic brain injuries, subarachnoid hemorrhages, hemorrhagic and ischemic strokes. Another indication for EVD is the need for temporary cerebrospinal fluid (CSF) diversion for the treatment of acute hydrocephalus caused by intraventricular hemorrhages (IVH), infective meningitis, and space occupying lesions that obstruct CSF flow such as intracerebral hematomas and tumors. Under these circumstances, EVD serves to monitor disease progression and response to treatment until the offending pathology resolves or is dealt with definitively. As a means of CSF diversion, EVD has the advantage over permanent shunting in that CSF drainage is controlled and monitored. It can also be used as an access to the ventricles for intraventricular fibrinolysis treatment in IVH, antibiotics instillation in ventriculitis, and the performance of ventriculography (Gaberel, et al., 2011). However, EVD is only a temporizing measure for the treatment of hydrocephalus. If permanent CSF diversion is required, conversion into an internalized system using, for example, ventriculo-peritoneal shunting is necessary.

2. Surgical procedure

Depending on the available expertise and facilities, EVD may be performed by neurosurgeons, general surgeons, emergency physicians or intensivists in the operating theatre or in the ward (Ehtisham, et al., 2009). Under aseptic conditions, a scalp incision is made over the insertion site. Commonly, the Kocher's point is used which is located 2.5 cm lateral to the midline (or at the mid-pupillary line), 11 cm posterior to the nasion. To avoid the motor cortex, it should be at least one cm anterior to the coronal suture. A burr hole is then performed. After opening the dura, a ventricular catheter is passed into the ipsilateral lateral ventricle transcerebrally. This may be done free-handedly or under the guidance of ultrasound or stereotaxy. After confirming CSF drainage, the distal end of the catheter is tunneled subcutaneously and allowed to exit the skin approximately 5-cm away from the burr hole site. The catheter is connected to a closed external drainage system with an attached ICP monitoring transducer. Other authorities may elect to close the ventricular catheter with a subcutaneous reservoir without skin tunneling or externalization of the catheter. CSF drainage is achieved post-operatively by percutaneous needle puncture of the reservoir. In general, prophylactic antibiotics would be given perioperatively. Post-operative antibiotics may be given depending on individual surgeons' preferences or protocols. The implications of these variations in practices will be discussed later.

3. External ventricular drain infection

Complications arising from EVD include hemorrhage, misplacement, dislodgement, disconnection, blockage, and, most significantly, infection. EVD-related infections may lead to further serious complications such as ventriculitis, meningitis, cerebritis, brain abscess and subdural empyema. These complications can cause profound neurological damages, significant morbidities and mortalities. Even when successfully treated, EVD-related infections may impair rehabilitation progress and negatively affect the overall prognosis of the initial conditions. An infected EVD contraindicates immediate permanent shunting and may therefore delay definitive CSF diversion. It significantly prolongs hospital stay and increases cost. Lyke et al calculated the cost of treatment and hospital stay days of a patient with ventriculitis to be as high as US$85,674.27 and 30.8 days (95% CI, 23.9–37.7, *P*=.009), respectively, compared with $55,339.21 and 22.6 days (95% CI, 19.1–26.0, *P*=.03) in those without ventriculitis. Patients in the infected group also suffered from more severe neurological damages (RR 5.33, 95% CI, 1.18–32.5) (Lyke, et al., 2001). EVD-related infections require immediate and prolonged treatment once detected. Empirical antibiotics with good CSF penetration should be given to cover the common offending organisms. The commonly used agents are cephalosporins and rifampicin. Intraventricular vancomycin may be used for resistant organisms. Revision of the EVD at a different site should be considered if CSF diversion or ICP monitoring is still required (Beer, et al., 2009).

3.1 Mechanisms of infection

The presence of an EVD essentially externalizes the intra-cranial cavity and ventricular system, and is a potential route for retrograde infection. The ventricular catheter as an indwelling foreign body is prone to bacterial colonization that may result from other unrelated sources such as systemic bacteremia. The current opinion is that EVD-related infections may arise from either (i) inoculation of skin flora during insertion, and/or (ii) contamination and colonization of the drainage system during the post-operative period, with subsequent retrograde infections (Lo, et al., 2007). The risk of inoculation is related to the sterility of the insertion procedure. It may increase with repeated revisions due to elective replacement or other clinical indications. The risk of colonization and contamination is affected by the manipulation of the drainage system, EVD maintenance protocol, and the technique of insertion (Hetem, et al., 2010). The mechanism is likely to be multifactorial and varies between individual patients.

3.2 Definition of infection

There is to date no universally accepted definition for EVD-related infection. Most authorities defined EVD-related meningitis or ventriculitis as the presence of a positive CSF microbiological culture (Lo, et al., 2007; Mayhall, et al., 1984; Schade, et al., 2005). CSF culture growing commensal organisms without other signs of infection such as altered

CSF chemistry, meningism, systemic sepsis, or the perceived need for antibiotic therapy, are considered by many to represent colonization of the EVD only rather than a genuine infection (Lozier, et al., 2008). This definition has been modified from the respective criteria set by the Centers for Disease Control and Prevention (Horan, 2004). Meanwhile some authorities adopt a more stringent definition of infection that requires the presence CSF pleiocytosis and biochemical changes (elevated CSF protein and/or decreased glucose), together with the presence of a positive CSF culture (Pfisterer, et al., 2003). Because of the varied definitions, the reported incidences of EVD-related infections ranged widely from 0 to 27% with a mean of 8.8% (Lozier, et al., 2008). This makes risk factors analysis, and the comparisons between different preventive and management protocols difficult.

3.3 Bacteriology

Coagulase-negative *Staphylococcus* is consistently reported to be the most common bacteria isolated in patients with EVD-related infections, accounting for up to 47% of infected cases (Zabramski, et al., 2003). Other common organisms include *Enterococcus, Enterobacter* and *Staphylococcus aureus*. This pattern coincides with that of the usual skin flora and hospital environment although the bacteriology may also be influenced by the presence of different nosocomial microorganisms in different institutions. Gram-positive organisms are classically associated with ventriculitis, and some centers, including the author's institution, noted that ventriculitis associated with EVD were not uncommonly caused by gram-negative bacteria such as *Klebsiella*. This is postulated to be a nosocomial colonization caused by prolonged hospital stay and the selection pressure from prophylactic antibiotics targeting gram-positive organisms (Lyke, et al., 2001).

3.4 Risk factors

Many studies have been conducted to indentify risk factors for EVD-related infections. Critical reviews of these published series have identified several important factors which will be discussed in the following sections (Dasic, et al., 2006; Hoefnagel, et al., 2008; Lozier, et al., 2008).

3.4.1 Subarachnoid hemorrhage (SAH) and Intraventricular hemorrhage (IVH)

The majority of published series reported statistically significant higher incidence of EVD-related infections in patients with SAH or IVH when compared with patients with non-hemorrhagic pathologies (Hoefnagel, et al., 2008; Stenager, et al., 1986). This has been postulated to be the result of frequent manipulations of the drainage system for flushing blocked EVD, the infusion of fibrinolytic agents, and the higher chance of EVD revision in these subgroups of patient with hemorrhages (Hoefnagel, et al., 2008). In a review by Lozier et al, the risk of infection was found to be 6 to 10% higher in patients with hemorrhages (Lozier, et al., 2008).

3.4.2 Craniotomy and other neurosurgical procedures

The conduction of craniotomies or other neurosurgical procedures were found to be a risk factor for EVD-related infections when compared with patients who had received EVD alone. Holloway et al studied 584 patients of whom 211 had undergone neurosurgical procedures other than the insertion of EVD. The infection rate in this group of patients was 15.2%, compared with 7.8% in the EVD-only group (Holloway, et al., 1996). Mayhall et al also reported that 68% of patients with EVD-related infections had other neurosurgical procedures performed, while only 40% non-infected patients did (P =0.02) (Mayhall, et al., 1984).

3.4.3 Venue of insertion and skill level of surgeon

Many authorities advocated the operating theatre as a preferred venue for EVD insertion (Bader, et al., 1995). However, Roitberg et al, and Lo et al, demonstrated separately that inserting EVDs in the intensive care units, emergency rooms or neurosurgical wards was not inferior in terms of infection risks or other complications (Lo, et al., 2007; Roitberg, et al., 2001). The location of insertion did not appear to affect the risk of infection provided that strict aseptic technique was used. There was also no significant difference amongst EVDs that were performed by neurosurgical trainees, consultants or neurointensivists (Ehtisham, et al., 2009; Lo, et al., 2007).

3.4.4 Duration of drainage

The literature was very much divided on the issue of whether and how the duration of external CSF drainage may affect the risk of infection. A recent multivariate analysis of seven series with a total of 2199 EVDs in 2113 patients demonstrated no association between the risk of infection and the duration of drainage (Lozier, et al., 2002). The timing of EVD-related infections appeared to follow a normal distribution during the first five post-operative days, and the majority of infections occurred between day two and day 11. Lo et al postulated that these early infections may arise from initial inoculations, which developed into detectable infections after variable incubation periods of around five days (Hetem, et al., 2010). A delayed peak of infection has also been observed after day 20, but the small number of reported cases rendered confirmation difficult (Winfield, et al., 1993).

Based on the belief that the risk of infection would increase with prolonged EVD, some authorities have advocated elective revisions of EVD after a fixed interval of, say, five days. However, the review by Park et al on 595 patients with EVD insertions found that the daily infection rates would plateau after day 4 post-insertion, and remain steady beyond day 10 (Park, et al., 2004). In reported series that adopted the practice of regular elective EVD revisions, revisions were not found to decrease infection rate significantly, and may actually increase it (Lo, et al., 2007; Wong, et al., 2002). Current evidence indicates that although the duration of drainage is an independent risk factor for EVD-related infections, routine revision of EVD in the absence of other clinical indications is not recommended. It is, however, prudent and logical to minimize the duration of drainage and to remove the catheter as soon as it is safe and feasible to do so.

3.4.5 Manipulation of the EVD system

Manipulations and opening of the otherwise closed EVD system for CSF sampling or flushing may introduce microorganisms and potentially cause infection. Aucoin et al reported a 6% increase in relative risk of infection for patients whose EVD was flushed with bacitracin solution (Aucoin, et al., 1986). A previously published report by the present authors also demonstrated intraventricular urokinase infusion as one of the risk factors for infection (Leung, et al., 2007). Historically, CSF was sampled routinely and indeed daily in some centers in an attempt to pick up early infections. This practice has been shown to increase the risk of infection; decreasing the frequency of CSF sampling to once every 3 days was associated with a lower incidence of ventriculitis (OR 0.44, 95% CI 0.22-0.88, p = 0.02) (Williams, et al., 2011). CSF sampling should be performed when there is clinical suspicion of infection but routine sampling is no longer encouraged (Korinek, et al., 2005).

In our center, we adopt a minimal-touch technique in handling EVD systems. If CSF sampling or infusion of intraventricular medication is required, we employ strict hand hygiene protocol, sterile gloving, and disinfection of the 3-way connector site with povidone-iodine before breaching the drainage system. Although it is difficult to demonstrate conclusively the benefit of these practices, many authorities in the literature support this logical awareness of strict hygiene in their EVD maintenance protocol (Korinek, et al., 2005; Leverstein-van Hall, et al., 2010). CSF leakage around the site of EVD has been identified as another major risk factor (Korinek, et al., 2005; Leverstein-van Hall, et al., 2010; Lyke, et al., 2001). Lyke et al reported that CSF leakage conferred a significant risk for ventriculitis (OR, 7.33; 95% CI, 1.05–37.47; P=.003) (Lyke, et al., 2001). Meticulous suturing of skin after EVD removal and better coupling of catheter size and dural puncture hole may effectively reduce the risk of infection (Korinek, et al., 2005). Interestingly, accidental disconnection, dislodgement or changes in the components of the system were not found to increase infection risks.

3.4.6 Prophylactic antibiotics

Antibiotic prophylaxis is a widely used strategy to prevent EVD-related infections. There is, however, no consensus as to what and for how long it should be given. As demonstrated by a recent survey by McCarthy et al, responders in Europe favored a single dose of antibiotics given immediately before the operation, while those from Asia and North America tend to cover also the whole period of post-operative drainage (McCarthy, et al., 2010). In a meta-analysis by Sonabend et al, the use of prophylactic antibiotics was found to significantly reduce the risk of EVD- related infections, but the authors also noted that the available data were of suboptimal quality, and that there were wide variations in the types of antibiotics used and the definitions of infection (Sonabend, et al., 2011).

Several randomized controlled trials (RCT) have been conducted to investigate the prolonged use of prophylactic antibiotics. In one study, co-trimoxazole given for the whole lifespan of an EVD did not result in a lower infection rate (Blomstedt, 1985). Another study found that the prolonged use of ampicillin/sulbactam and aztreonam resulted in a lower infection rate compared with a single dose of perioperative ampicillin/sulbactam. However the former was associated with infections caused by resistant organisms such as methicillin-resistant *Staphylococcus aureus,* and gram-negative organisms such as *Pseudomonas* or *Klebsiella* (Poon, et al., 1998). The role of prolonged systemic antibiotics and the best regimens are yet to be defined.

Apart from systemic antibiotics, some investigators have described the possible beneficial effect of prophylactic intraventricular antibiotics. Ragel et al demonstrated that using prophylactic intraventricular vancomycin and gentamicin together with systemic antibiotics significantly decreased the risk of infection in shunted patients (Ragel, et al., 2006). Whether this beneficial effect can be translated to EVD remains to be confirmed.

3.4.7 Coated ventricular catheter

The potential roles of coated EVD catheter have received a lot of attention and research effort in recent years. The underlying rationale is that coating the surface of the catheter with special materials or antibiotics may decrease bacterial colonization and thus prevent infection. The findings were controversial depending on the coating material used. One RCT did not show any benefit with the use of hydrogel-coated catheters presoaked in bacitracin solution (Kaufmann, et al., 2004). Silver-coated catheters were first used in central venous line with equivocal results (Bach, et al., 1999; Kalfon, et al., 2007). Thereafter, two retrospective analyses have been conducted using silver nanoparticle-impregnated catheters for EVD. Both studies showed significant reduction in infection rates and a trend of reduced bacterial colonization despite the studies' small sample sizes (Fichtner, et al., 2010; Lackner, et al., 2008).

Antibiotics-impregnated catheter is an important development. To date, two RCTs and 3 observational studies have been conducted to investigate the efficacy of antibiotics-impregnated catheters. Zabramski et al studied minocycline/rifampicin-coated catheters (M/R catheters) in a RCT involving 149 cases of M/R catheters and 139 controls with standard silastic catheters. Both groups received systemic antibiotics throughout the lifespan of the EVD. The infection rate in the M/R catheter group was 1.3% compared with 9.6% in the standard EVD group ($P<0.0012$) (Zabramski, et al., 2003). Sonabend et al pooled the data of the above RCT with other studies for a meta-analysis, and demonstrated a risk ratio of 0.19 (95%CI 0.07-0.52) for EVD-related infections in patients with antibiotics-impregnated catheters (Sonabend, et al., 2011). A more recent RCT by Abla et al compared the efficacy of M/R catheters and clindamycin/rifampicin-impregnated catheters (C/R catheters). A total of 129 patients were randomized into receiving either M/R or C/R catheters in a 3-monthly rotation. The mean duration of EVD was 12.7 and 11.8 days in the M/R and C/R groups, respectively. A single dose of perioperative cefuroxime was given to 45% of M/R group and 55% of C/R group patients. The study demonstrated a remarkable 0% infection rate in both groups of patients (Abla, et al., 2011). Only one patient showed a minimal growth of *Staphylococcus epidermidis* in one culture broth, with the culture in another broth, blood agar, gram stain being negative for the same CSF specimen. The potential side-effects of these catheters include allergy to the impregnated antibiotics and the selection of resistant organisms. To date, there have been no reports of antibiotics-impregnated catheters increasing the risk of selection of resistant organisms. A drawback of these catheters is the relaively high cost which may prevent its adoption world-wide.

3.4.8 Subcutaneous catheter tunnel

Historically, one major development was the tunneling technique which created a subcutaneous tract between the burr hole and catheter exit site. Freidman et al first proposed subcutaneous tunneling of the EVD catheter, and reported an infection rate of 0% in a series of 100 patients (Friedman & Vries, 1980). Similar principle of preventing ascending infection has been applied to the design of indwelling intravenous catheters and, indeed, intravenous Broviac catheter has been described for cerebrospinal fluid (CSF) drainage. Although infection continued to be reported with the tunneling technique, the latter has become standard neurosurgical practice. Since then this practice has been widely adopted in the majority of neurosurgical centers. The idea was further elaborated by Khanna et al who advocated the construction of a long subcutaneous tunnel which exits over the anterior chest or abdominal wall. His group demonstrated an inverse relationship between tunnel length and infection rate (Khanna, et al., 1995). The rationale of this extended-tunnel technique was that bacterial contamination of the ventricular catheter at the site of skin penetration would act an important source of ascending infection, and that removing this site from the central nervous system would reduce the risk of infection. The disadvantages of this long-tunnel EVD include the presence of a large dead space that is theoretically prone to blockage, and the requirement of general anesthesia for the removal of the system. In our center we have previously used long-tunnel EVD which will be disucssed in the next section.

4. Extended-tunnel EVD

The procedure is performed with prophylactic antibiotics cover using intravenous cefazoline (2 grams) or co-trimoxazole (960 mg). A standard burr hole is made at the Kocher's point or posterior parietal region. An extended subcutaneous tunnel measuring 40 to 50 cm was developed from the burr hole site down to the anterior chest wall using a metallic trocar. Ventricular puncture is performed and the ventricular catheter is connected to a distal silastic catheter through an interposing Rickham CSF reservoir (Codman, Medos, Switzerland). The distal catheter is then passed down the subcutaneous tunnel and exits through the chest wall. The distal catheter is then connected to a closed external drainage system. No antibiotic is given post-operatively unless indicated for CSF or systemic infections. When CSF drainage is no longer required, removal of the catheter system is performed at the cranial end under general anesthesia. Alternatively, the distal catheter can be divided and plugged off over the chest wall under local anesthesia.

4.1 Patient outcome

We have reviewed 114 patients who have previously received the extended-tunnel EVD at our institution. There were 61 men and 53 women, ranging in age from 4 months to 90 years old (mean age = 52.6 years). The mean duration of CSF drainage was 20 days (median = 13 days). Fourteen patients received more than one EVD which yielded a total of 133 procedures. Thirty (22.6%) cases started with prior infections and 103 (77.4%) were infection-free at the time of insertion. Within the latter group, new infections developed in seven cases, yielding an overall infection rate of 6.8%. The mean time to infection was 9.7 days (median = 5.0 days). A trend of increasing daily infection risk could be observed during the first five days. It remained relatively low and constant in the second week and then increased again after the 14th day. Only intraventricular injection of urokinase was identified as a weakly significant risk factor (relative risk = 4.78, 95% confidence interval = 0.96 - 23.89, p = 0.039). Gender, age, primary neurosurgical diagnosis, immunodeficiency, diabetes mellitus, use of steroids, recent craniotomy, systemic sepsis at the time of and after 'long EVD' insertion were not found to be statistically significant risk factors of infection.

Prior to the above study period, both conventional and the extended-tunnel EVDs may be used according to individual surgeons' preferences. During this early phase, there was a total of 158 EVDs performed, including 33 (20.9%) long-EVDs. There were a total of 9 infections, yielding an overall infection rate of 5.8%. The infection rates for long- and conventional EVDs were similar at 6.25% and 5.65%, respectively (p=0.896). Operation time, emergency versus elective operations, operating surgeons, age of patient, nature of disease, and duration of drainage were not found to be significant risk factors for infections. Diabetes mellitus and immunosuppression were found to be significantly associated with infections, with odd ratios of 5.39 (95% C.I.=1.33-21.86) and 6.71 (95% C.I.=1.14-39.46), respectively. Overall, our findings indicated that the extended-tunnel techqniue was associated with a similar risk of infection as the conventional EVD. Although some authorities may continue to advocate the extended-tunnel technique, there is no evidence to show that it adds any distinct advantage, and we have since stopped using the technique.

5. Protocol-driven practice

Some authorities have demonstrated that adhering to a predefined protocol of EVD insertion and maintenance that incorporates evidence-based measures as discussed above would significantly reduce the risk of EVD-related infections. Infection rates have been halved by strictly following a protocol involving aseptic insertion, use of prophylactic antibiotics, subcutaneous tunneling, no routine EVD revision, and minimal manipulation such as CSF sampling; violation of the protocol was associated with increased infection rate (Dasic, et al., 2006; Korinek, et al., 2005; Leverstein-van Hall, et al., 2010). Current evidence indicates that a strict EVD protocol should be adopted in neurosurgical centers. A protocol should cover the following aspects:

Insertion of EVD

- performed in the operating theatre whenever possible, with a minimal number of attending staff
- performed in a dedicated clean treatment room if the procedure has to be done outside the operating theatre, with the surgeon and the assisting nurse dressed in sterile gown and gloves after proper hand hygiene measures
- prophylactic antibiotics to cover skin flora before incision
- shampoo the entire scalp with betadine, and disinfect with iodine alcohol
- tunneling the catheter subcutaneously for at least five cm
- covering the wound with sterile dressing

Maintenance of EVD

- respecting the close system as far as possible
- avoid CSF sampling unless infection is clinically suspected
- disinfect the connector and adopt strict aseptic technique if any breach of the system is needed
- no routine EVD revision

Removal of EVD

- aseptic condition and disinfect site with povidone-iodine/alcohol
- suture wound carefully to minimize CSF leakage

6. Conclusion

EVD is a commonly performed neurosurgical procedure for the treatment of a variety of neurosurgical conditions including hydrocephalus. It is a useful and reliable temporizing method for ICP monitoring and the controlled release of CSF. Infection is a major and serious complication of EVD that may cause significant morbidities and even mortalities. Several risk factors of EVD-related infections have been identified and preventive measures aimed at reducing these factors have been developed. These include the use of prophylactic systemic antibiotics, antibiotics-coated catheters and subcutaneous catheter tunnelling. EVD that incorporate extended subcutaneous of over 30 cm have been used without the anticipated advantage of being able to reduce infection rates. The causation of EVD-related infections is likely to be multifactorial. Adopting a clearly defined protocol which addresses various aspects of insertion and maintenance is likely to be the effective approach to minimize the occurrence of EVD-related infections.

7. References

Abla, A. A., Zabramski, J. M., Jahnke, H. K., Fusco, D., & Nakaji, P. (2011). Comparison of two antibiotic-impregnated ventricular catheters: a prospective sequential series trial. *Neurosurgery, 68*(2), 437-442; discussion 442.

Aucoin, P. J., Kotilainen, H. R., Gantz, N. M., Davidson, R., Kellogg, P., & Stone, B. (1986). Intracranial pressure monitors. Epidemiologic study of risk factors and infections. *Am J Med, 80*(3), 369-376.

Bach, A., Eberhardt, H., Frick, A., Schmidt, H., Bottiger, B. W., & Martin, E. (1999). Efficacy of silver-coating central venous catheters in reducing bacterial colonization. *Crit Care Med, 27*(3), 515-521.

Bader, M. K., Littlejohns, L., & Palmer, S. (1995). Ventriculostomy and intracranial pressure monitoring: in search of a 0% infection rate. *Heart Lung, 24*(2), 166-172.

Beer, R., Pfausler, B., & Schmutzhard, E. (2009). Management of nosocomial external ventricular drain-related ventriculomeningitis. *Neurocritical care, 10*(3), 363-367.

Blomstedt, G. C. (1985). Results of trimethoprim-sulfamethoxazole prophylaxis in ventriculostomy and shunting procedures. A double-blind randomized trial. *J Neurosurg, 62*(5), 694-697.

Dasic, D., Hanna, S. J., Bojanic, S., & Kerr, R. S. (2006). External ventricular drain infection: the effect of a strict protocol on infection rates and a review of the literature. *British journal of neurosurgery, 20*(5), 296-300.

Ehtisham, A., Taylor, S., Bayless, L., Klein, M. W., & Janzen, J. M. (2009). Placement of external ventricular drains and intracranial pressure monitors by neurointensivists. *Neurocritical care, 10*(2), 241-247.

Fichtner, J., Guresir, E., Seifert, V., & Raabe, A. (2010). Efficacy of silver-bearing external ventricular drainage catheters: a retrospective analysis. *Journal of neurosurgery, 112*(4), 840-846.

Friedman, W. A., & Vries, J. K. (1980). Percutaneous tunnel ventriculostomy. Summary of 100 procedures. *J Neurosurg, 53*(5), 662-665.

Gaberel, T., Magheru, C., Parienti, J. J., Huttner, H. B., Vivien, D., & Emery, E. (2011). Intraventricular Fibrinolysis Versus External Ventricular Drainage Alone in Intraventricular Hemorrhage: A Meta-Analysis. *Stroke.*

Hetem, D. J., Woerdeman, P. A., Bonten, M. J., & Ekkelenkamp, M. B. (2010). Relationship between bacterial colonization of external cerebrospinal fluid drains and secondary meningitis: a retrospective analysis of an 8-year period. *Journal of neurosurgery, 113*(6), 1309-1313.

Hoefnagel, D., Dammers, R., Ter Laak-Poort, M. P., & Avezaat, C. J. (2008). Risk factors for infections related to external ventricular drainage. *Acta neurochirurgica, 150*(3), 209-214; discussion 214.

Holloway, K. L., Barnes, T., Choi, S., Bullock, R., Marshall, L. F., Eisenberg, H. M., et al. (1996). Ventriculostomy infections: the effect of monitoring duration and catheter exchange in 584 patients. *J Neurosurg, 85*(3), 419-424.

Horan TC, G. R. (2004). *Surveillance of nosocomial infections.* Philadelphia.

Kalfon, P., de Vaumas, C., Samba, D., Boulet, E., Lefrant, J. Y., Eyraud, D., et al. (2007). Comparison of silver-impregnated with standard multi-lumen central venous catheters in critically ill patients. *Crit Care Med, 35*(4), 1032-1039.

Kaufmann, A. M., Lye, T., Redekop, G., Brevner, A., Hamilton, M., Kozey, M., et al. (2004). Infection rates in standard vs. hydrogel coated ventricular catheters. *Can J Neurol Sci, 31*(4), 506-510.

Khanna, R. K., Rosenblum, M. L., Rock, J. P., & Malik, G. M. (1995). Prolonged external ventricular drainage with percutaneous long-tunnel ventriculostomies. *J Neurosurg, 83*(5), 791-794.

Korinek, A. M., Reina, M., Boch, A. L., Rivera, A. O., De Bels, D., & Puybasset, L. (2005). Prevention of external ventricular drain--related ventriculitis. *Acta neurochirurgica, 147*(1), 39-45; discussion 45-36.

Lackner, P., Beer, R., Broessner, G., Helbok, R., Galiano, K., Pleifer, C., et al. (2008). Efficacy of silver nanoparticles-impregnated external ventricular drain catheters in patients with acute occlusive hydrocephalus. *Neurocritical care, 8*(3), 360-365.

Leung, G. K., Ng, K. B., Taw, B. B., & Fan, Y. W. (2007). Extended subcutaneous tunnelling technique for external ventricular drainage. *British journal of neurosurgery, 21*(4), 359-364.

Leverstein-van Hall, M. A., Hopmans, T. E., van der Sprenkel, J. W., Blok, H. E., van der Mark, W. A., Hanlo, P. W., et al. (2010). A bundle approach to reduce the incidence of external ventricular and lumbar drain-related infections. *J Neurosurg, 112*(2), 345-353.

Lo, C. H., Spelman, D., Bailey, M., Cooper, D. J., Rosenfeld, J. V., & Brecknell, J. E. (2007). External ventricular drain infections are independent of drain duration: an argument against elective revision. *J Neurosurg, 106*(3), 378-383.

Lozier, A. P., Sciacca, R. R., Romagnoli, M. F., & Connolly, E. S., Jr. (2002). Ventriculostomy-related infections: a critical review of the literature. *Neurosurgery, 51*(1), 170-181; discussion 181-172.

Lozier, A. P., Sciacca, R. R., Romagnoli, M. F., & Connolly, E. S., Jr. (2008). Ventriculostomy-related infections: a critical review of the literature. *Neurosurgery, 62 Suppl 2*, 688-700.

Lyke, K. E., Obasanjo, O. O., Williams, M. A., O'Brien, M., Chotani, R., & Perl, T. M. (2001). Ventriculitis complicating use of intraventricular catheters in adult neurosurgical patients. *Clin Infect Dis, 33*(12), 2028-2033.

Mayhall, C. G., Archer, N. H., Lamb, V. A., Spadora, A. C., Baggett, J. W., Ward, J. D., et al. (1984). Ventriculostomy-related infections. A prospective epidemiologic study. *N Engl J Med, 310*(9), 553-559.

McCarthy, P. J., Patil, S., Conrad, S. A., & Scott, L. K. (2010). International and specialty trends in the use of prophylactic antibiotics to prevent infectious complications after insertion of external ventricular drainage devices. *Neurocritical care, 12*(2), 220-224.

Park, P., Garton, H. J., Kocan, M. J., & Thompson, B. G. (2004). Risk of infection with prolonged ventricular catheterization. *Neurosurgery, 55*(3), 594-599; discussion 599-601.

Pfisterer, W., Muhlbauer, M., Czech, T., & Reinprecht, A. (2003). Early diagnosis of external ventricular drainage infection: results of a prospective study. *J Neurol Neurosurg Psychiatry, 74*(7), 929-932.

Poon, W. S., Ng, S., & Wai, S. (1998). CSF antibiotic prophylaxis for neurosurgical patients with ventriculostomy: a randomised study. *Acta Neurochir Suppl, 71*, 146-148.

Ragel, B. T., Browd, S. R., & Schmidt, R. H. (2006). Surgical shunt infection: significant reduction when using intraventricular and systemic antibiotic agents. *J Neurosurg, 105*(2), 242-247.

Roitberg, B. Z., Khan, N., Alp, M. S., Hersonskey, T., Charbel, F. T., & Ausman, J. I. (2001). Bedside external ventricular drain placement for the treatment of acute hydrocephalus. *British journal of neurosurgery, 15*(4), 324-327.

Schade, R. P., Schinkel, J., Visser, L. G., Van Dijk, J. M., Voormolen, J. H., & Kuijper, E. J. (2005). Bacterial meningitis caused by the use of ventricular or lumbar cerebrospinal fluid catheters. *J Neurosurg, 102*(2), 229-234.

Sonabend, A. M., Korenfeld, Y., Crisman, C., Badjatia, N., Mayer, S. A., & Connolly, E. S., Jr. (2011). Prevention of ventriculostomy-related infections with prophylactic antibiotics and antibiotic-coated external ventricular drains: a systematic review. *Neurosurgery, 68*(4), 996-1005.

Stenager, E., Gerner-Smidt, P., & Kock-Jensen, C. (1986). Ventriculostomy-related infections--an epidemiological study. *Acta neurochirurgica, 83*(1-2), 20-23.

Williams, T. A., Leslie, G. D., Dobb, G. J., Roberts, B., & van Heerden, P. V. (2011). Decrease in proven ventriculitis by reducing the frequency of cerebrospinal fluid sampling from extraventricular drains. *J Neurosurg*.

Winfield, J. A., Rosenthal, P., Kanter, R. K., & Casella, G. (1993). Duration of intracranial pressure monitoring does not predict daily risk of infectious complications. *Neurosurgery, 33*(3), 424-430; discussion 430-421.

Wong, G. K., Poon, W. S., Wai, S., Yu, L. M., Lyon, D., & Lam, J. M. (2002). Failure of regular external ventricular drain exchange to reduce cerebrospinal fluid infection: result of a randomised controlled trial. *J Neurol Neurosurg Psychiatry, 73*(6), 759-761.

Zabramski, J. M., Whiting, D., Darouiche, R. O., Horner, T. G., Olson, J., Robertson, C., et al. (2003). Efficacy of antimicrobial-impregnated external ventricular drain catheters: a prospective, randomized, controlled trial. *J Neurosurg, 98*(4), 725-730.

8

Role of Endoscopy in Management of Hydrocephalus

Nasser M. F. El-Ghandour
Department of Neurosurgery, Faculty of Medicine, Cairo University
Egypt

1. Introduction

Management of hydrocephalus is the most beneficial indication for endoscopy. To cure hydrocephalus and thereby render an individual shunt independent is a great achievement. The standard and the most commonly performed endoscopic procedure is endoscopic third ventriculostomy. However, the field of neuroendoscopy is prepared to extend itself beyond just the ventriculostomy procedure. The neuroendoscope plays other important roles in the management of hydrocephalus.

Although the literature is focusing mainly on the role of endoscopic third ventriculostomy in the treatment of aqueduct stenosis, the indications for endocopy continues to increase rapidly. With increasing experience, and improved endoscopic instruments, another important role of endoscopy has been emerged in approaching intraventricular tumors which may be completely removed without microsurgical brain dissection (Gaab & Schroeder, 1998). In addition to tumor removal it is usually possible to restore obstructed cerebrospinal fluid pathways using the same approach by performing ventriculostomies, septostomies or stent implantation (Oka et al., 1994).

The goal of this chapter is to present the role of endoscopy in the management of hydrocephalus. The following chapter gives a comprehensive review about the indications, outcome, complications, and advantages of endoscopy. Various procedures which can be performed endoscopically for the management of hydrocephalus will be discussed.

2. Historical perspectives

Endoscopy was introduced in the neurosurgical speciality at the beginning of this century. In 1910, L'Espinasse used the cystoscope to perform the first registered endoscopic procedure. He explored the lateral ventricle and coagulated the choroid plexus in 2 infants with hydrocephalus (Walker, 2001). In 1918, Walter Dandy started his work on endoscopy using a nasal speculum to inspect the ventricles. He performed choroid plexectomy under direct visualization for the treatment of hydrocephalus. The light source was a head mirror and transillumination was used through the thin cortical mantle of hydrocephalic patient. Four of his five patients did not survive this operation probably due to massive intraventricular bleeding (Dandy 1918).

In 1923, Jason Mixter reported the first endoscopic third ventriculostomy procedure (Mixter 1923). Although it appeared to be a successful procedure and communication was documented by dye studies, there was no available long-term follow-up. The procedure of endoscopic third ventriculostomy did not become widely popular, as surgeons chose instead to perform open procedures via subfrontal or subtemporal craniotomies. In 1935, Scarff described his initial results after using a novel endoscope equipped with a mobile cauterizing electrode, an irrigation system that prevented collapse of the ventricle, and a movable operating tip which was used to perforate the floor of the third ventricle (Scarff 1935). In 1947, McNickle described a percutaneous method of performing third ventriculostomy in patients of both obstructive and communicating hydrocephalus, he reported a success rate that was superior to Dandy's open approach (McNickle 1947).

In 1952, Nulsen and Spitz reported the first treatment of hydrocephalus by using ventricular shunt placement, beginning the era of ventricular cerebrospinal fluid shunting and the end of initial era of neuroendoscopy (Nulsen & Spitz 1952). The birth of ventricular shunting in 1952 pushed endoscopy further into the backward. Despite the numerous reports that demonstrated the potential utility of neuroendoscopy, the field never gained popularity in general neurosurgical practice. This was attributed to the poor magnification and illumination at that time which made neuroendoscopy difficult and unreliable. Although the development of ventricular shunting was considered to be a landmark in the treatment of hydrocephalus, it brought with it a high incidence of complications such as shunt malfunction, infection, migration, and overdrainage. Recognition of the complications associated with ventriculoperitoneal and ventriculoatrial shunting stimulated neurosurgeons to investigate new treatment options and to reuse old ones that existed before ventricular shunts began to be used.

Technical advances in the development of endoscopic lenses and instruments such as bipolar diathermy, irrigation and laser, have led neurosurgeons to begin again to consider the field of neuroendoscopy. With the improved imaging capability of the endoscope, the interest of endoscopic third ventriculostomy for treatment of obstructive hydrocephalus was renewed. Currently endoscopic third ventriculostomy is the primary procedure used to treat obstructive hydrocephalus caused by benign aqueductal stenosis or compressive periaqueductal mass lesions. The endoscopic third ventriculostomy procedure has recently been reported to be superior to ventricular shunt placement for hydrocephalus caused by pineal region tumors (Yamini et al., 2004), tectal gliomas (Li et al., 2005), and posterior fossa tumors (El-Ghandour, 2011). This procedure was subsequently proposed as the primary surgical approach for the treatment of hydrocephalus in these cases.

3. Indications of endoscopy

3.1 Aqueductal stenosis

In noncommunicating hydrocephalus, there is an obstruction to the passage of cerebrospinal fluid from the ventricular system into the subarachnoid space. The classic example is aqueductal stenosis, in which there is enlargement of the lateral and third ventricles without enlargement of the fourth ventricle. If an opening is created in the third ventricle proximal to the site of obstruction (endoscopic third ventriculostomy), then the cerebrospinal fluid can escape into the subarachnoid space and bypass the obstruction. If there is no co-existing blockage in the subarachnoid space, cerebrospinal fluid can be absorbed into the venous system and the hydrocephalus can be treated without using a ventriculoperitoneal shunt.

The ideal candidates for endoscopic third ventriculostomy are those patients who have developed aqueductal stenosis or occlusion and became symptomatic later on in life. These patients are more likely to have a functional communication between the subarachnoid space and venous system, as they were presumably able to absorb their cerebrospinal fluid before the aqueduct became obstructed. There is no simple noninvasive study to predict which patients can benefit from endoscopic third ventriculostomy. We need a study which can demonstrate both the stenosis or obstruction of aqueduct as well as efficient passage of cerebrospinal fluid from the subarachnoid space into the venous system.

Currently, the best available imaging modality is the MR imaging, which delineates the anatomy of the aqueduct of Sylvius, the size of the third ventricle, and location of the basilar artery. Moreover, MR imaging can be used to obtain a noninvasive cerebrospinal fluid flow study, using a two-dimensional phase contrast technique which is gated to the cardiac cycle. Such a study (flow gated MR imaging) can be used preoperatively to confirm the diagnosis of aqueductal stenosis, and postoperatively to confirm patency of the third ventriculostomy without the need for intraventricular injection of a contrast agent.

3.2 Fourth ventricular outlet obstruction

Hydrocephalus resulting from fourth ventricular outlet obstruction is commonly observed in infants and young children, due to either infection or intraventricular hemorrhage. Both conditions cause an inflammatory response with arachoniditis and scar tissue formation, leading to secondary obstruction of the foramina of Magendie and Luschka. Because the associated hydrocephalus is obstructive in nature due to obstruction occuring at the level of the foramen magnum, it is amenable to cerebrospinal fluid diversion by endoscopic third ventriculostomy. However, the underlying pathological process that results in scarring of the subarachnoid space plays a considerable role in determining the overall outcome of the procedure. The extent of adhesions in the basal cisterns is directly correlated with failure of endoscopic third ventriculostomy.

For this reason, some authors advocate endoscopic transaqueductal exploration of the fourth ventricular outlet foramina (Longatti et al., 2006; Mohanty et al., 2008). A thin transparent membrane is sometimes found stretched across the foramen of Magendie and obstructing the flow of cerebrospinal fluid, and membrane fenestration is performed. Nevertheless, diagnostic accuracy is of paramount importance, particularly in differentiating this condition from the noninflammatory obstruction of the outlet of the fourth ventricle which is often seen with other neurological conditions, such as Chiari malformation, basilar invagination, and other craniocervical junction anomalies. In these cases, the obstruction of fourth ventricular outlet is due to crowding in the region of the foramen magnum, and no membranous obstruction has been encountered in direct exploration.

3.3 Complex hydrocephalus

3.3.1 Uniloculated hydrocephalus

Hydrocephalus may occur in association with loculated collection of cerebrospinal fluid. The lateral ventricle may become trapped by obstruction at the foramina of Monro which results in an isolated lateral ventricle. Arachnoid and ependymal cysts as well as congenital malformations may contribute to ventricular isolation. When the lateral ventricle is trapped by scar at the foramen of Monro, the endoscope can be used to unblock the ventricle by fenestrating the septum pellucidum (septum pellucidotomy). The septum contains relatively avascular tissue, and a generous septostomy can be performed using a fiberoptic laser, taking care to avoid injury of the fornices or the corpous callosum (Cohen, 1996).

Isolated fourth ventricle is a rare complication observed in patients with ventricular shunts placed to treat hydrocephalus that developed after inflammatory disease such as infection or hemorrhage. This unusual condition arises when two events occur at the same time: collapse of the aqueduct following reduction of transtentorial pressure gradient, and blockage of cerebrospinal fluid at the outlet of the fourth ventricle or at the basal cisterns (Oi & Matsumoto, 1986). In such cases, shunt placement in the lateral ventricle decreases supratentorial pressure and also reduces the pressure keeping the aqueduct open, which occasionally leads to collapse of the aqueduct of Sylvius. Meanwhile, cerebrospinal fluid continues to be produced in the fourth ventricle and make its marked enlargement. Surgical management of isolated fourth ventricle is problematic, and sometimes results in patients undergoing multiple surgeries until the situation is well controlled (Shin et al., 2000).

3.3.2 Multiloculated hydrocephalus

The ventricular system may become trabeculated and encysted following germinal matrix hemorrhage or infection. The ventricular system is converted into multiple cavities or loculations which are isolated from each other by multiple membranes. When a loculated collection of cerebrospinal fluid occurs in association with hydrocephalus, conventional treatment often entails inserting shunt catheters into more than one compartment. Endoscopic fenestration techniques can be used to simplify the treatment of loculated hydrocephalus, permitting the use of a single shunt to drain multiple compartments and sometimes avoiding or eliminating the need for shunt (El-Ghandour, 2006, 2008). Contrast CT ventriculography is useful to confirm noncommunication of the compartments preoperatively, and the study can be repeated postoperatively to confirm patency of the fenestrations.

3.4 Normal pressure hydrocephalus

The use of endoscopic third ventriculostomy for treating normal pressure hydrocephalus was first suggested in 1999 by Mitchel and Mathew in a series of four patients (Mitchel & Mathew, 1999). One year later, Meier et al reported a series of 48 patients with idiopathic normal pressure hydrocephalus (Meire et al., 2000) treated by insertion of a ventriculoperitoneal shunt (37 cases) or endoscopic third ventriculostomy (11 cases). It has been reported, that patients with a pathologically increased resistance to cerebrospinal fluid outflow in the lumbar infusion test should be treated by endoscopic third ventriculostomy. Nevertheless, Fiorindi et al 2004, reported a low success rate (21%) of endoscopic third ventriculostomy in a series of 14 patients (Fiorindi et al., 2004).

In 2008, Gangemi et al reported the largest group of patients with idiopathic normal pressure hydrocephalus (110 patients), treated in four italian neurosurgical centers which routinely use endoscopic third ventriculostomy for treating this form of hydrocephalus.

Postoperative clinical improvement was encountered in 76 patients (69.1%) among the median follow-up duration of 6.5 years (Gangemi et al., 2008). It is not exactly well known why endoscopic third ventriculostomy results in clinical improvement in patients with idiopathic normal pressure hydrocephalus who do not have obstruction of the cerebrospinal fluid pathways and show normal or slightly increased cerebrospinal fluid pressure.

It was always believed that chronic hydrocephalus results from cerebrospinal fluid malabsorption owing to hindrance of cerebrospinal fluid circulation. Nevertheless, the modern theory considers hydrocephalus as ventricular enlargement caused by increased regional force directed from the ventricle toward the subarachnoid space, defined as transmantle pulsatile stress, which results in decreased compliance of the brain tissue and ventricular enlargement. Weakening and enlargement of the ventricles may also result from loss of elasticity of the ventricular walls owing to periventricular ischemic lesions (Bradley et al., 1991). According to this theory, chronic hydrocephalus is not caused by decreased cerebrospinal fluid absorption, but rather by decreased intracranial compliance.

Endoscopic third ventriculostomy increases the systolic outflow from the ventricles and decreases the intraventricular pulse pressure, thus decreasing the width of the ventricles. This would dilate the compressed vessels and increase intracranial compliance. The dilated capillaries will facilitate increased blood flow and cerebrospinal fluid absorption (Greitz, 2004). An irreversible loss of brain compliance may explain the failure of endoscopic third ventriculostomy in patients where clinical history is too long and who experienced clinical onset of dementia. In these cases, the preoperative brain involvement is likely more important (Gangemi et al., 2008).

3.5 Intraventricular tumors

3.5.1 Lateral ventricular tumors

The majority of lateral ventricular tumors are benign or low grade lesions (e.g. gliomas). Tumors of the frontal horn may cause blockage of the foramen of Monro, which results in unilateral hydrocephalus. The endoscope can be used to take biopsy or remove the lesion and restore obstructed cerebrospinal fluid pathways. If restoration of the foramen of Monro is not achieved after tumor removal, the ventricle can be unblocked by fenestration of the septum pellucidum (septum pellucidotomy). In case of very small ventricle, the endoscopic method might not be possible, since there is inadequately working space for manipulation of the instruments. The tumor must be removed microsurgically via transcortical or transcallosal approach.

3.5.2 Third ventricular tumors

Many tumors may occur within the third ventricle such as colloid cysts, astrocytomas, and ependymomas, and in the pineal region, such as germinomas, pineocytomas, pineoblastomas. Tumors located in the third ventricle are the most difficult to expose and remove. Such tumors usually obstruct one or both foramina of Monro and result in obstructive hydrocephalus. Accordingly, the aim of endoscopic surgery is reconstitution of cerebrospinal fluid pathways with prevention of recurrent obstruction, and establishment of a histological diagnosis. Neuronavigation is especially helpful for patients without ventriculomegaly and for tumors located in the posterior part of the third ventricle.

The most common third ventricular tumor operated by endoscopy is colloid cyst. Approaching a third ventricular colloid cyst is an excellent application of endoscopic technology to surgery within the ventricular system. The endoscope is an ideal instrument for exploration of fluid-filled cavities, and the intraventricular location of colloid cysts make them accessible for the endoscopic approach. The surgical removal of colloid cysts has traditionally been difficult, with a high percentage of postoperative complications.

Ventriculoperitoneal shunting should not be considered a treatment option because it does not provide a cure, frequently requires bilateral ventricular catheters, and is susceptible to malfunction and infection (Lewis & Crone, 1998). Microsurgery permits radical removal of the cyst wall and minimizes the likelihood of recurrence. However, even in very experienced hands, microsurgery implies up to 27% postoperative morbidity. The microsurgical transcortical approach is associated with a higher rate of postoperative seizures than transcortical introduction of the endoscope into the lateral ventricle. Among 190 patients operated by the endoscopic procedure through a transcortical burr hole, no postoperative seizures have occurred. The transcortical burr hole approach is fast, easy, and safe due to well-known landmarks (Gaab & Schroeder, 1998).

The more direct microsurgical transcalloal approach to the third ventricle, avoids cortical disruption. However, it carries many risks such as sagittal sinus thrombosis, venous infarction from dissection of bridging veins, damage to the pericallosal arteries, and injury to the fornix with permanent memory loss (Jeeves et al., 1979). Many reports stress the operative simplicity and low complication rate of the stereotactic approach to colloid cysts. However the initial enthusiasm for stereotactic aspiration has been tempered by its lack of success in treating some patients, lack of intraoperative visual control (i.e. blind procedure) and the high recurrence rate (up to 80%) because the cyst wall could not be resected or even widely fenestrated (Mathiesen et al., 1993). Endoscpopic surgery provides a balanced middle ground between microsurgery and stereotactic aspiration. It permits wide fenestration of the capsule and aspiration of the cyst contents under direct vision, with minimal disruption of the cortex and other normal brain structures. Resection of the cyst wall can also be performed using the endoscopic procedure (Abdou & Cohen, 1998).

Colloid cysts located in the anterior third ventricle with a large lateral ventricle are the easiest to remove endoscopically. A large ventricular system allows for more maneuverability, facilitates the endoscopic procedure markedly, and obviates the need for any guidance procedures such as stereotaxy or neuronavigation which makes the procedure more lengthy and sophisticated (El-Ghandour, 2009).

If the ventricles are small, then intraoperative ultrasound or stereotactic guidance may be required to cannulate the lateral ventricle. If there is asymmetry in the lateral ventricular system, then the approach is done through the largest frontal horn. If the patient has undergone previous shunting and has small ventricular system, the patient is admitted to the hospital, the shunt is externalized, and the drain is clamped inorder to dilate the ventricular system (Lewis & Crone, 1998).

3.5.3 Fourth ventricular tumors

The posterior fossa is a common site for various tumors to occur during childhood. It was estimated that they comprise 54-60% of childhood brain tumors. Medulloblastoma represents approximately 20% of all childhood central nervous system tumors (Polednak & Flannery, 1995). Ependymoma represents approximately 10% of all reported primary intracranial tumors in children (Farwell et al., 1977). Medulloblastomas and ependymomas are often complicated by the development of hydrocephalus due to obstruction of the fourth ventricle. Children are very sensitive to intracranial pressure elevation and thus management of hydrocephalus has the highest priority and should be performed prior to any surgical treatment of the posterior fossa tumor itself. It is claimed that precraniotomy shunt provides improvement in the patient's physiological condition, a "slack posterior fossa" and a smooth postoperative course (Albright & Reigel, 1977; Raimondi & Tomita, 1981). The development of hydrocephalus in children with posterior fossa tumors is one of the main factors influencing the outcome. In one series, the operative mortality was decreased with preoperative shunting (Albright & Reigel, 1977).

Placement of permanent shunt was the "golden" standard treatment over years. However, the technological advances and changes in the availability of neuroimaging systems have resulted in establishing an earlier diagnosis. This, coupled with the extensive list of potential complications associated with ventricular shunting in this patient population, resulted in another strategy of treatment recommending the use of corticosteroid therapy, early surgery and external ventricular drainage (Papo et al., 1982). Nevertheless, external ventricular drainage is associated with a significant risk of infection and hemorrhage. Moreover, such treatment might not be appropriate for young children with advanced hydrocephalus because these patients usually need a permanent diversion procedure.

It was estimated that children who have advanced hydrocephalus and children who are younger than 3 years of age had persistant hydrocephalus which required a postoperative shunt in about 80% of cases (Epstein, 1993). Approximately, one third of patients overall, will eventually require placement of a shunt (Lee et al., 1994). Many factors have been reported to be associated with required shunt placement including a young age (< 10 years), midline tumors, more severe ventricular enlargement at diagnosis, incomplete tumor resection, cerebrospinal fluid-related infection, prolonged use of external ventricular drainage, cadaveric dural grafts, and persistent pseudomeningocele (Culley et al., 1994).

As long-term survival becomes more frequent in children with posterior fossa tumors, issues pertaining to the quality of life, such as postoperative shunt dependency becomes increasingly important and must be taken into consideration. It has been mentioned that following tumor excision, the obstructive component of the hydrocephalus is relieved in most of the patients, and the flow of cerebrospinal fluid will be restored, thus the shunt will be no more necessary, but the patient now becomes shunt dependent (El-Ghandour, 2011).

Taking all these factors into consideration, a search for a better treatment option should be expected. The obstructive nature of the hydrocephalus associated with posterior location of the tumor, makes internal cerebrospinal fluid diversion to be a promising alternative. The rational basis of endoscopic third ventriculostomy is provided by the obstructive nature of hydrocephalus due to presence of blockage of cerebrospinal fluid pathways at the level of fourth ventricle outlets or at the aqueduct of Sylvius. It has been mentioned that obstructive hydrocephalus secondary to posterior fossa tumors in children with good absorption of cerebrospinal fluid from the subarachnoid space is a good selection for endoscopic third ventriculostomy (El-Ghandour, 2011).

Endoscopic third ventriculostomy creates a communication between the ventricular system and the subarachnoid space at the level of the third ventricle. There is only one comparative study in the literature which compares both procedures; endoscopic third ventriculostomy and ventriculoperitoneal shunt in the treatment of obstructive hydrocephalus due to midline posterior fossa tumors in children. The author reported superiority of the endoscopic third ventriculostomy over shunting because of the shorter duration of surgery, the lower incidence of morbidity, the absence of mortality, the lower incidence of procedure failure, and the significant adventage of not becoming shunt dependant (El-Ghandour, 2011).

It is worthy to mention, that in selected cases of fourth ventricular tumors, biopsy can be also taken endoscopically through the enlarged aqueduct of Sylvius. However, these tumors are rarely amenable to endoscopic resection because of the limited space within the ventricle (Gaab & Schroeder, 1998).

4. Endoscopic procedures

4.1 Endoscopic third ventriculostomy

Endoscopic third ventriculostomy is the standard and the most commonly performed endoscopic procedure. As with any other surgical procedure, appropriate patient selection is essential for successful outcome. Patients who present with classical signs of noncommunicating hydrocephalus are ideal candidates. Unquestionably, patients with aqueduct stenosis (congenital or acquired) are the best candidates. Although initially the role of endoscopy has been limited to performing endoscopic third ventriculostomy in patients with congenital aqueductal stenosis, the indications for this procedure are increasing rapidly. Any patient presenting with a lesion causing obstruction of cerebrospinal fluid outflow at the aqueduct of Sylvius is a candidate for this procedure (Jimenez 1998). Such lesions include primary or secondary (metastatic) neoplasms of the midbrain, pons, medulla, posterior fossa tumors or cysts, pineal region tumors, posterior third ventricular lesions, or ventricular exophytic thalamic gliomas (Ray et al., 2005; El-Ghandour, 2011).

Another group of patients who can benefit from this procedure are those who present with obstructive hydrocephalus secondary to arachnoid cysts of the deep cisternal system (quadrigeminal plate or ambient system). Many published studies have included patients with variety of symptoms, including those with communicating hydrocephalus (Jones et al.,1990), and idiopathic normal pressure hydrocephalus (Gangemi et al., 2008). There is much argument about spina bifida patients, whether considered to be candidates for such procedure or not. These patients have significantly abnormal ventricular anatomy and commonly present with a thick third ventricular floor, a small narrow foramen of Monro, and a large massa intermedia (Jimenez, 1998).

Selection criteria remain the most controversial aspect of this procedure. The reason for this is that there is no single or combined examination which can relatively predict who will benefit from this operation. Cerebrospinal fluid infusion studies may help to select more suitable patients, but false negative results can occur because the absorptive mechanisms may take several hours or even days to accommodate for increased load of cerebrospinal fluid, whereas the study itself extends over a significantly shorter time (Pudenz 1981).

Similarly, cerebrospinal fluid isotope clearance studies should theoretically accurately predict the ability of the arachnoid villi to absorb cerebrospinal fluid. However, it also suffers from high false negative results, thereby denying some potentially suitable candidates the opportunity to remain shunt independent. To support this contention, clinically, some patients require several weeks before their symptoms resolve and their imaging improves. This implication is that the subarachnoid space needs time to accommodate for the increased cerebrospinal fluid load (Teo, 1998).

Surgical Technique

Following induction of general anesthesia, the patient is placed supine with the head slightly flexed. A standard midpupillary coronal burr hole is used, but optimum localization can be achieved by projecting the best angle to the floor of the third ventricle using preoperative coronal and sagittal T1-weighted MR imaging. The frontal horn is cannulated with a # 14-french peel-away sheath and stylet. After withdrawal of the stylet, a 2 mm-diameter rigid lens (wide-angle, straight-forward, 0 degree) with angled eye piece and working channel diameter of 3 mm, is inserted. The choroid plexus is identified and followed anteriorly to the foramen of Monro. The endoscope is advanced into the third ventricle through the foramen of Monro. Once the third ventricle is entered, the mammillary bodies are usually visualized as well as the tuber cinereum and the infundibular recess. Sometimes, the tuber cinereum has become thin and semitransparent, allowing identification of the basilar artery.

Several methods are used to create the fenestration on the floor of the third ventricle such as using the tip of rigid endoscope, small blunt probes, tip of a transluminal angioplasty balloon catheter, tip of a contact laser fiber or bipolar electrode. An avascular area in the floor of the third ventricle anterior to the mammillary bodies is chosen for fenestration, with care taken to avoid injury of the basilar artery or any of its branches. The opening is then enlarged gently by inflating the balloon of a # 3 french angioplasty balloon catheter in a relatively atraumatic fashion. It is generally agreed that the opening should be 5-6 mm in diameter inorder to prevent its reclosure. However, it is also well known that it is the constant flow of cerebrospinal fluid through the fenestration that keeps it open and working. In other words, it is the pressure gradient between the third ventricle and the interpeduncular cistern, which exists in case of noncommunicating hydrocephalus, that prevents the ventriculostomy from reclosure.

If extensive trabeculations are encountered, the fenestration has to be extended to include all these trabeculae. Not uncommonly, a small amount of venous bleeding may be observed from the edges of the ventriculostomy. This type of bleeding usually stops with gentle irrigation or with reinflation of the balloon for 1-2 minutes. Navigation inside the interpeduncular cistern is done to confirm successful creation of the ventriculostomy. The endoscope and peel-away sheath are then removed. Unless there has been significant bleeding, an external ventricular drain is not necessary, although some surgeons leave it in place for 24-48 hours. This is done to monitor the intracranial pressure; the drain is removed once the intracranial pressure has normalized. The wound is closed in a standard fashion. If there are no complications, the patient can be discharged within 24-48 hours.

4.2 Choroid plexectomy

This treatment option is controversial and is not used nowadays by most neurosurgeons. Those patients who have a choroid plexus papilloma or who produce an abnormally high amount of cerebrospinal fluid, may benefit from this procedure. Choroid plexectomy appears to be indicated in a small group of patients who have normal communications and intact absorptive mechanisms, but do not have the capacity to cope with an overwhelming load of cerebrospinal fluid (Teo,1998).

Surgical Technique

The patient is placed in the prone position and bilateral occipital burr holes are placed 3 cm from the midline at the level of the lambdoid sutures. The rigid endoscope is introduced into the lateral ventricle and the choroid plexus is coagulated using monopolar, bipolar, or Nd:YAG (neodymium-yttrium-aluminum-garnet) laser coagulation. Access to all three horns of the lateral ventricle is possible through this approach. Care should be taken not to coagulate the choroidal arteries, as this may result in retrograde occlusion of the proximal perforating vessels.

4.3 Endoscopic opening of foramen of Magendie

This procedure is used in the treatment of patients with obstructive hydrocephalus due to fourth ventricular outlet obstruction caused by idiopathic stenosis or membranous occlusion of the foramina of Magendie and Luschka (Longatti et al., 2006; Mohanty et al., 2008).

Surgical Technique

The patient is placed supine and general anesthesia is induced. The frontal horn of the lateral ventricle is cannulated through a precoronal burr hole (2 cm anterior to the coronal suture and 2 cm from the midline). The flexible endoscope, with a diameter of 3.9 mm is introduced and manipulated throughout the procedure using a free hand technique. At the third ventricle, the scope is guided backward toward the opening of the aqueduct to the midbrain. In case of tetraventricular hydrocephalus, the aqueduct is dilated and the scope passes quite easily into the fourth ventricle. At this phase, free irrigation is stopped, because the fourth ventricle is now completely trapped and additional liquid volumes can lead to life-threatening episodes of bradycardia.

The scope is postioned posteriorly, the median sulcus of the fourth ventricle is seen, it leads to the posterior triangle of the rhomboid fossa. The lateral recesses appear enlarged and both Luschka foramina are obstructed by thick membranes. A thick membrane is stretched from the borders of the calmus scriptorious to the pyramid of the vermis, occluding the foramen of Magendie. The membrane is perforated using monopolar coagulation or a "saline torch", and the opening is enlarged with the inflation of a Fogarty balloon. The endoscope is advanced to the cisterna magna inorder to assess its extent and confirm absence of adhesions. The endoscope is then carefully withdrawn with meticulous attention inorder not to injure the aqueductal tip or columns of the fornix.

4.4 Septum pellucidotomy

The endoscopic procedure for treatment of isolated lateral ventricle is fenestration of the septum pellucidum. The degree of difficulty of this procedure is grossly underestimated. This is because most patients requiring this procedure have one collapsed ventricle and one grossly dilated ventricle. It is so difficult to identify the septum in these patients that stereotactic assistance is recommended. In uncomplicated cases, the results of septum pellucidotomy are excellent, obviating the need for two shunts, and in some cases, the need for any shunting (Teo, 1998).

Surgical Technique

The patient is placed in the supine position with the head slightly flexed. The burr hole site is placed more laterally than the standard coronal burr hole used for shunt placement (5-6 cm from the midline), so that the endoscope approaches the target at an angle more perpendicular to the septum pellucidum. The surgeon is often faced with the dilemma of which ventricle to enter when performing a septostomy. Some authors (Teo, 1998) recommend working in the nondilated ventricle toward the dilated ventricle. Others (Abtin & Walker, 1998) recommend working in the larger ventricle toward the smaller one, where the surgeon can more easily maneuver the endoscope and instruments. The second procedure is more risky, because the opposite ventricle is small and caution is necessary inorder to avoid any direct or thermal injury to structures on the lateral wall of the contralateral ventricle.

The rigid endoscope is then introduced into the lateral ventricle, and the septum pellucidum is visualized. A safe target should be 1 cm above and 2 cm anterior to the foramen of Monro. An area of about 1.5 to 2 cm is then fenestrated with laser or other instrumentation. The site of fenestration is critical, if placed too high on the septum, the fenestration may open into the interhemispheric fissure, with potential injury of the anterior cerebral arteries. If the fenestration is made above the foramen of Monro, there is risk of injury to the fornix. If placed posterior to the foramen, there is risk of injury to the genu of the contralateral internal capsule, if the instrument used for fenestration penetrates too deeply. One should also pay attention to variants such as cavum septum pellucidum inorder to achieve a satisfactory septostomy (Abtin & Walker, 1998).

4.5 Endoscopic cyst fenestration

Multiloculated hydrocephalus is not uncommon in the hydrocephalic community, especially in those infants whose shunts have been complicated by infection or whose primary pathology was intraventricular hemorrhage. Both conditions cause fibrous septations as a result of chemical or bacterial ventriculitis. Infants with this condition usually require multiple shunts and therefore are subjected to the additive risk of complex shunts mainly malfunctioning (Teo, 1998). These patients are excellent candidates for the endoscopic procedure. The endoscope is used to communicate all the cysts and a shunt is then left in the largest ventricle, using the same burr hole through which the procedure was performed. Endoscopy offers a simple means of communicating isolated cerebrospinal fluid spaces and ventricles by membrane fenestration. In a recent report, endoscopy has led to avoiding, eliminating or simplifying the use of shunts, with a significant decrease in postoperative shunt revision rate (El-Ghandour, 2008).

Surgical Technique

The approach is individually designed in each case separately depending on location of the cysts, entry site of pre-existing ventricular catheter and the need for placement of a new shunt. Cysts located anteriorly are approached through a standard midpupillary coronal burr hole, whereas an occipital or posterior parietal route is used for posterior or temporal loculations. The burr holes are bevelled laterally to allow the endoscope to reach the contralateral ventricle and the trajectory is planned to fenestrate the maximum number of cysts. The ventricular system or cyst is cannulated with a # 14 french peel-away sheath and stylet. Care is taken to prevent the release of cerebrospinal fluid before the endoscope is introduced. After withdrawal of the stylet, a 2 mm diameter rigid lens (wide-angle, straight-forward, 0 degree) with angled eye piece and working channel diameter 3 mm is inserted.

Cyst fenestration is performed in a relatively avascular segment of the cyst wall sharply with bipolar electrocautery. The fenestration is widened to at least 1 cm in diameter to prevent early reclosure. This is achieved sharply by widening the initial hole or connecting multiple holes using the bipolar electrode. Devascularization of the cyst wall is done by coagulating its vascular supply to prevent or retard its regrowth. Pulsed irrigation with lactated Ringer's solution is used to prevent thermal injury and collapse of the ventricles. Any bleeding from the cyst wall usually stops with irrigation or coagulation. If there is significant intraventricular bleeding, it is better to put an external ventricular drain and postpone shunting procedure to a later date (El-Ghandour, 2008).

4.6 Aqueductoplasty

There are few indications for this high risk procedure. Most cases of noncommunicating hydrocephalus respond more favourably to third ventriculostomy. Some authors believe that it can be used as an adjunct to third ventriculostomy in patients with adult onset aqueductal stenosis (Oka et al., 1993). Patients who have an isolated fourth ventricle are also excellent candidates for this procedure. Endoscopic reopening of the aqueduct of Sylvius (aqueductoplasty) is considered to be the ideal treatment of isolated fourth ventricle, because it re-establishes communication between the fourth ventricle and the supratentorial ventricular system, equilibrating the transtentorial pressure and allowing a single supratentorial shunt to control the patient's hydrocephalus. However, endoscopic aqueductoplasty cannot be performed in all cases, it can be only performed if a membranous occlusion of the aqueduct is present in preoperative MR images. The standard precoronal approach can be used only in cases in which the supratentorial ventricular system is also dilated; in other cases a suboccipital approach should be used (Cinalli et al., 2006).

4.6.1 Precoronal approach

The patient is positioned supine with the head lying in a horseshoe-shaped head rest. The burr hole site is placed more anteriorly than the standard coronal burr hole used for shunt placement (just behind the hair line, 4-5 cm anterior to the coronal suture). The right lateral ventricle is cannulated with a peel-away sheath. A flexible endoscope is then inserted and careful inspection of the frontal horn usually allows easy identification of the foramen of Monro. The endoscope is then advanced through the foramen of Monro into the third ventricle, where the obstructed aqueduct inlet is identified.

The aqueduct should not be confused with suprapineal recess, which is located above the aqueduct and behind the posterior commisure. The membrane occluding the inlet of aqueduct is perforated simply by probing the aqueduct with the aid of the smooth tip of a Fogarty balloon catheter; this allows inspection of the cavity of the fourth ventricle. In short stenosis, the aqueduct is restored by gently inflating the balloon to a diameter of 3 mm. In long stenosis, a stent may be inserted into the aqueduct to prevent later occlusion by scarring (Schroeder & Gaab, 1999). However, implanting stents carries the risk of stent dislodgement and migration (Mohanty, 2005).

4.6.2 Suboccipital approach

The patient is placed prone with the head lying in a horseshoe-shaped head rest. The head is flexed as much as possible to create the best trajectory to the aqueduct. An infratentorial burr hole is drilled 2-3 cm from the midline over the right cerebellar hemisphere. The dilated fourth ventricle is cannulated with the aid of a peel-away sheath and then the endoscope is inserted. After the aqueduct has been identified, the obstructing membrane is perforated using a Fogarty balloon catheter while carefully avoiding any damage to the periaqueductal gray matter. Inspection of the aqueduct permits the operator to visualize the third ventricle. The limit of this approach is the lack of landmarks available for orientation in the unusual and distorted anatomy of a trapped fourth ventricle, where recognition of the inlet of aqueduct can be very difficult (Cinalli et al., 2006).

4.7 Endoscope-guided shunt placment

Although placement of a ventricular catheter using endoscopy has yet to be proven superior to other methods, the tip of the ventricular catheter can be properly placed in the desired position under direct visualization using small endoscope that passes through the shunt catheter. Endoscope-guided shunt placement can be done either using free hand method or by stereotactic assistance.

4.7.1 Free hand endoscopic shunt placment

Direct Placment

The ventricular catheter is "loaded" on an endoscope with the tip of the endoscope exposed for visualization. The shunt may then be placed directly into the ventricle via the appropriate trajectory. After placing the ventricular catheter into the ventricle, the operator can look through the endoscope to confirm the shunt catheter's position. If the ventricular catheter is not in a proper position, the shunt is withdrawn and modification of the trajectory can be done. The surgeon determines the preferred position of the shunt catheter, but the general consensus is that it should be as far as possible from the choroid plexus, a natural source of scar formation. Consequently, the frontal horn of the lateral ventricle has become a favored position for catheter placement by most of the neurosurgeons (Brockmeyer, 1998).

Peel-away Catheter

Another technique for endoscopic shunt placement, which applies to those neurosurgeons using a rod lens endoscope system, involves placing an appropriate-sized peel-away catheter into the ventricle, then inserting the endoscope through the peel-away catheter. In this way, the potential shunt position is confirmed and the length of the ventricular catheter can be estimated. Once the peel-away catheter is in an appropriate position, the endoscope is withdrawn and the ventricular catheter is passed through the peel-away sheath to the predetermined location. The sheath is then peeled away while the ventricular catheter is held gently with smooth forceps, leaving the ventricular catheter in place (Brockmeyer, 1998).

4.7.2 Stereotactic shunt placment

Applying stereotactic technology to endoscopic techniques has increased the safety and accuracy of such procedures. The available frameless stereotactic systems may be coupled to endoscopes and can be used to pass stereotactic probe to the target ventricle and then withdrawn. A fiberoptic endoscope already loaded with a shunt catheter is then passed down the probe tract under direct vision into the ventricle (Brockmeyer, 1998).

Endoscopic-assisted placement of a multiperforated shunt catheter into the fourth ventricle guided by frameless stereotaxy, has been recently advocated by some authors for the treatment of isolated fourth ventricle and multicompartmentalized hydrocephalus. The procedure is performed via a frontal transventricular approach using the flexible endoscope with dual-port intraventricular access for direct visualization and for mechanical manipulation of the catheter (Upchurch et al., 2007).

4.8 Ventricular catheter retrieval

Endoscopic retrieval of a retained intraventricular catheter is an excellent application of endoscopy in the management of hydrocephalus. The endoscope can be used to extract catheters from inside the ventricle either they are "free" or "adherent" in scar tissue. Adherent ventricular catheters are usually found in cases of multiloculated hydrocephalus. It has been reported that retained pre-existing malfunctioning ventricular catheters in multiloculated hydrocephalus could not be withdrawn safly without endoscopic assistance. Such catheters have to be dissected gently and dislodged under direct endoscopic visualization inorder to avoid the risk of hemorrhage and damage which can be induced if the catheter is pulled without being dissected (EL-Ghandour, 2008).

Surgical Technique

Any endoscope with a working channel can be used for such technique. If the ventricular catheter is "free" within the ventricle, a long grasping forceps is passed through the working channel and the endoscope is navigated into an appropriate position. Obviously, knowledge of the intraventricular anatomy is essential for navigating into correct position for catheter retrieval. The retained catheter is then grasped with the endoscopic forceps and withdrawn outside the ventricular system (Brockmeyer, 1998)

Endoscopy can be also used to remove adherent scarred-in ventricular catheters, and consequently it plays an important role in simplification of complex shunts in multiloculated hydrocephalus. One possible technique described by El-Ghandour, for shunts initially placed via occipital burr hole, involves placing a separate burr hole 2-3 cm above the old one, through which the endoscope is introduced parallel to the ventricular catheter with slight inclination toward its tip. Bipolar electrode is then used to coagulate the scarred-in choroid plexus and dislodge the shunt catheter, which can then be withdrawn gently and safely without risking intraventricular hemorrhage (El-Ghandour, 2008).

Alternatively, the Nd:YAG laser can be used to coagulate the choroid plexus and cut along the interface of the scar and silicone tubing inorder to dislodge the catheter. The adherent ventricular catheter is then removed under endoscopic visualization and a new ventricular catheter is placed in an appropriate position (Lewis et al., 1995).

4.9 Shunt revision

Intracranial neuroendoscopy can be very useful during routine shunt revision. It increases the surgeon's confidence that a ventricular catheter is placed in the appropriate position, and it is useful in repositioning previously inserted malfunctioning shunts under direct visualization.

Surgical Technique

After dislodging and removing the old ventricular catheter, a new ventricular catheter is loaded on a fiberoptic endoscope and passed down the same tract. The tract may be inspected for nests of scar tissue, membranes or webs. When the endoscope reaches an area in the ventricle free of scar, choroid plexus or membrane, it is withdrawn back through the ventricular catheter and cerebrospinal fluid flow is observed. The need for a longer or shorter ventricular catheter is easily confirmed by the endoscope and demonstrated by the presence or absence of cerebrospinal fluid flow. The flow of cerebrospinal fluid confirms the intraventricular position of a shunt catheter. This technique allows the operator to avoid the nest of scar tissue by direct visual confirmation inorder to place the new catheter in a more appropriate position (Brockmeyer, 1998).

4.10 Resection of intraventricular tumors

With increasing experience and improved endoscopic instruments (such as bipolar diathermy, laser instruments), an increasing number of tumors may be completely removed without microsurgical brain dissection. In certain cases, a neuroendoscopic approach to intraventricular tumors via a simple burr hole is as effective as microsurgery but less invasive. During endoscopic procedures, brain retraction can be completely avoided, and the tumor can be well visualized with the aid of endoscopy. The origin of the tumor and the amount of blood supply can be recognized prior to tumor biopsy or resection. Only a few publications in the neurosurgical literature address the endoscopic treatment of intraventricular tumors. Most authors have not reported details regarding endoscopic technique, complications or outcome (Gaab & Schroeder, 1998).

The ventricular enlargement provides sufficient space for manipulation with the endoscope and instruments. However, if the ventricles are small or the tumor is located in the posterior part of the third ventricle, it is advisable to use a guiding device to follow the ideal access route to the target, thus avoiding unnecessary brain traumatization. Frameless stereotaxy or neuronavigation has been used in conjunction with neuroendoscopy to increase the accuracy in determining the approach. For treatment of intraventricular tumors, rigid endoscopes are preferred because of the superior optical quality which maintains good vision even when small hemorrhages occur. The operating endoscope (wide-angle, straight-forward, 0 degree) with angled eye piece allows accurate guidance of the instruments in a straight line.

Using large operating sheath (approximately 6 mm in diameter) without separate working channels, makes effective piecemeal resection of the tumor possible. However, in most neuroendoscopes currently available, the working channel is no larger than 2.4 mm. It is obvious that removal of intraventricular tumors, even if small in size, is a tedious, time-consuming procedure with these scopes (Gaab & Schroeder, 1998). Some neurosurgeons recommend the insertion of a second working portal, enabling the use of larger instruments and thus accelerating tumor resection (Cohen, 1993; Jallo et al., 1996). Flexible endoscopes can be applied for final inspection. Various endoscopic instruments should be available inorder to make the procedure successful such as scissors, puncture needles, biopsy and grasping forceps, balloon catheters, laser fibers and monopolar electrodes.

Surgical Technique

Lateral Ventricular Tumors

Tumors of the frontal horn and ventricular body are approached via a standard midpupillary precoronal burr hole (3 cm paramedian and 2 cm precoronal). The tumor can be biopsied or resected, and septostomy can be performed if there is unilateral hydrocephalus. For tumors of the trigone, the burr hole is placed more anteriorly (4-6 cm precoronal) inorder to reach the tumor in a straight line through the ventricular body. A posterior approach can also be performed, it has the advantage that there is a shorter distance from the cortical surface to the tumor when entering the ventricle posteriorly than when entering it anteriorly. However, there is usually a very limited amount or almost no cerebrospinal fluid-filled working space in front of the tumor, which makes inspection of the lesion, orientation, and dissection extremely difficult or even impossible (Gaab & Schroeder, 1998).

Once the dura is opened, the operating sheath with trocar is inserted free hand or under navigational guidance into the lateral ventricle and fixed with two retractor arms. The trocar is then withdrawn and the rigid endoscope is introduced. The tumor is inspected and its relationship to the choroid plexus and the feeding arteries is visualized. After exploration of the tumor, the diagnostic scope is replaced by the operating scope. Before tumor dissection, capsule vessels are coagulated by bipolar diathermy or Nd:YAG laser. Depending on the tumor size, removal usually begins with intracapsular debulking or dissection in the plane between the tumor and the normal brain tissue. During this dissection, feeding arteries must be identified early and cauterized before bleeding obscures clear vision. If laser is used during resection, it requires vigorous irrigation to avoid thermal damage to adjacent brain tissue.

Hemostasis of small hemorrhages represents no problem as these usually stop spontaneously after a few minutes of irrigation. Larger vessels which are at risk of being torn during tumor resection, should be cauterized by the bipolar diathermy. After isolation of the lesion from the surrounding brain tissue, the tumor is resected in a piecemeal fashion with the aid of grasping and biopsy forceps. In general, the foramen of Monro is usually patent after tumor resection. If the foramen is obstructed, a septostomy through the septum pellucidum may be performed to release cerebrospinal fluid circulation. After successful tumor removal, the region of resection is inspected again with the diagnostic scope to ensure good hemostasis. The ventricles are vigorously rinsed to remove any clots and the operating sheath is then withdrawn and the wound is closed.

Third Ventricular Tumors

For tumors located in the anterior part of the third ventricle such as colloid cysts, the lesion can be approached via a transcoronal burr hole. The burr hole should be placed (about 1 cm) infront of the coronal suture and far laterally (5-7cm from the midline) in order to directly visualize the cyst wall. Placing the burr hole too close to the midline will decrease visualization of the cyst significantly. Also widening of the outer edges of the burr hole provides a more conical opening which allows greater freedom in maneuvering the endoscope with enough angulation to reach the contralateral ventricle. Laser is usually essential to open the cyst wall and bipolar cautery is usually unsuccessful in opening the tough cyst wall. Monopolar electrode was found to be equally effective like laser and it is less cumbersome (El-Ghandour, 2009).

Devascularizing the outer layer of the colloid cyst is a crucial step that should be done in all the cases. It shrinks the capsule to open the foramen of Monro, cuts off the nutrients to the inner layer that secretes the colloid and prevents regrowth (Fig 1). Residual parts of the capsule firmly attached to the roof of the ventricle should be coagulated rather than vigorously removed, because pulling may cause severe venous bleeding. Re-establishing cerebrospinal fluid pathways is an important step that should be performed in all the cases. The aqueduct of Sylvius is visualized to ensure a clear pathway between the lateral, third and fourth ventricles. The septum pellucidum is often fenestrated to ensure a balanced flow of cerebrospinal fluid between the lateral ventricles. An external ventricular drain is not required, unless uncontrolled bleeding has occurred. Most bleeding will stop with direct irrigation at the bleeding site. Some neurosurgeons prefer inserting an external ventricular catheter routinely to prevent aseptic ventriculitis that may be caused by free-floating colloid material within the ventricular system (Hellwig et al., 2008).

For tumors located in the posterior third ventricle, such as pineal body tumors, an endoscopic supracerebellar infratentorial approach has been used by some authors (Gore et al., 2008). Nevertheless, this approach has considerable risks for many reasons; 1) A simple burr hole is not sufficient to identify the transverse sinus and therefore a small craniotomy has to be performed. 2) Thick arachnoid membranes often cover the pineal region, hindering accurate orientation. 3) The superior cerebellar bridging veins and deep incisural veins are at risk when inserting the endoscope (Gaab & Schroeder, 1998). Other neurosurgeons recommend performing endoscopic third ventriculostomy for the management of the associated obstructive hydrocephalus and obtaining tissue samples sufficient for pathological diagnosis which can be taken endoscopically through the same transcoronal burr hole (Chernov et al., 2006; Al-Tamimi et al., 2008).

5. Complications

The complications of endoscopic procedures can be grouped into three groups: general, neurological, and vascular

5.1 General complications

This group includes wound infection, ventriculitis, cerebrospinal fluid leaks, and subgaleal fluid collections. It is worth noting that the use of normal saline for irrigation is contraindicated due to the fact that it is strongly acidic and it can lead to chemical

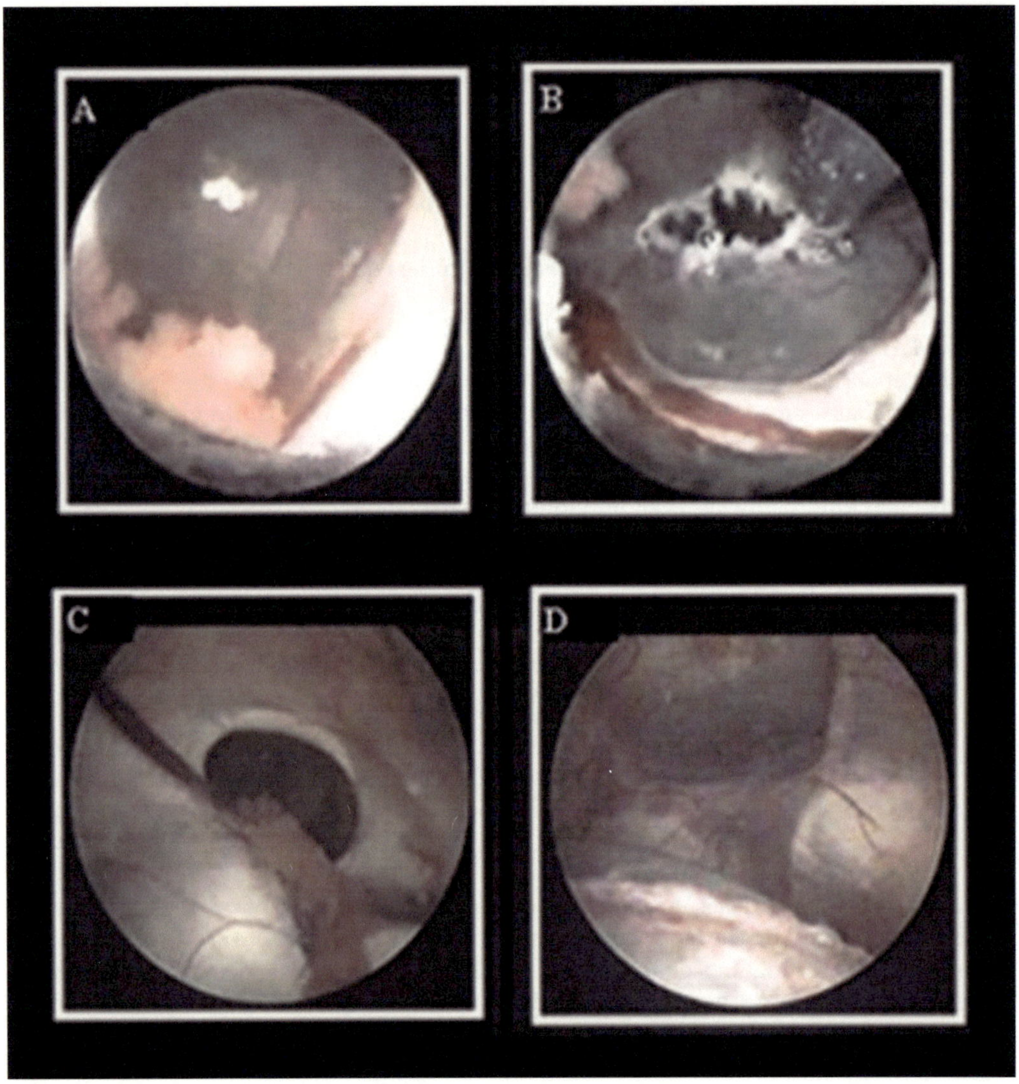

Fig. 1. Intraoperative neuroendoscopic views. A, Photograph showing anterior colloid cyst bulging through and obstructing the formen of Monro. B, Photograph of the same case where monopolar electrode is used to open the cyst wall and shrink it to a tiny nonvascular remnant. C, Photograph showing posterior colloid cyst causing a bulge in the floor of the lateral ventricle. Note the formen of Monro is open in this case. D, Photograph of the same case where the endoscope is introduced inside the third ventricle through the formen of Monro. Note both mammillary bodies. The colloid cyst is seen at 7 o'clock. Endoscopic third ventriculostomy was done in this case. [Reprinted with permission from El-Ghandour NM (2009). Endoscopic treatment of third ventricular colloid cysts: a review including ten personal cases. *Neurosurg Rev*,Vol. 32, No. 4, (October 2009), pp. 395-402, ISSN 0344-5607].

ventriculitis. Lactated Ringer's solution is considered to be the perfusate of choice because its chemical composition is closest to cerebrospinal fluid. The irrigation rate should be controlled inorder to prevent dangerous acute intracranial hypertension which may result in significant postoperative neurological sequelae. Inorder to avoid such complication, care is taken to maintain sufficient outflow of irrigating fluid (Jimenez, 1998).

5.2 Neurological complications

During the procedure of endoscopic third ventriculostomy or any other intraventricular endoscopic surgery, injury to the fornix can occur, and it leads to transient deficit in short-term memory. Oculomotor and other cranial nerve palsies can also occur due to incorrect placement of the fenestration off the midline, in a lateral position. The oculomotor nerve can be injured by laterally directing the endoscope while perforating the tuber cinereum. Oculomotor palsy may be transient or permanent depending on the degree of damage that occur during the endoscopic procedure.

Damage to the hypothalamus can occur due to traction injury associated with the use of the tip of a large endoscope to create the fenestration on the floor of the third ventricle. This can lead to hyponatremia, lethargy, diabetes insipidus, transient syndrome of inappropriate antidiuretic hormone secretion and permanent or temporary weight gain. Midbrain injury and hemiparesis have also been reported. Although seizures can occur following insertion of a large peel-away or rigid introducers through the cortical mantle, this complication has not been found to occur clinically after endoscopic procedures (Jimenez, 1998).

5.3 Vascular complications

The most dangerous complication during endoscopic surgery is injury to the superior basilar artery complex, which is manifested intraoperatively by massive intraventricular hemorrhage with complete obscuration of the endoscopic field. Although reported previously (Schroeder et al., 2002), it is considered to be a rare complication. The bleeding is usually profuse, however, it usually stops following persistent and vigorous irrigation. Inorder to avoid this vascular injury, perforation of the floor of the third ventricle should be performed in the midline, halfway between the infundibular recess and the mammillary bodies, just behind the dorsum sellae.

Less serious although equally bothersome is damage to the ventricular veins, such as thalamostriate, caudate, septal or internal cerebral veins. Bleeding associated with these low pressure venous systems usually stops after few minutes of continuous irrigation. Intraventricular clots can be easily removed with the use of grasping forceps and suction (Jimenez, 1998).

6. Outcome and prognosis

A successful outcome following endoscopic third ventriculostomy is defined as resolution of symptoms associated with increased intracranial pressure secondary to cerebrospinal fluid flow obstruction. It should be highlighted that if there is no decrease in ventricular size in postoperative imaging, it should not be taken as a nonsuccessful outcome, because a large number of patients continue to demonstrate ventriculomegaly following successful endoscopic third ventriculostomy. This is particularly true in patients with long standing hydrocephalus (Jimenez, 1998).

Postoperative MR imaging may show a decrease in ventricular size and/or improvement of transependymal edema especially in acutely or subacutely developing hydrocephalus. It should also demonstrate a flow void in the floor of the third ventricle, otherwise a cine MR imaging is obtained for a better demonstration of systolic/diastolic cerebrospinal fluid flow through the created fenestration (Jallo et al., 2005).

Reported success rates for endoscopic third ventriculostomy vary between 15% and 80%. Several factors appear to be related to poor results and those include younger patients (< 2 years), a history of meningitis, intraventricular or subarachnoid hemorrhage, infants with myelodysplasia, and a history of previous radiation therapy (Jimenez, 1998).

Endoscopic third ventriculostomy plays a crucial role in the treatment of obstructive hydrocephalus secondary to tumors obstructing cerebrospinal fluid pathways. Excellent results were obtained in a series of 32 pediatric patients with obstructive hydrocephalus secondary to midline posterior fossa tumors (20 medulloblastomas, 12 ependymomas). Intracranial hypertension symotoms improved postoperatively in 31 out of 32 cases (96.9%). Ataxia improved in 4 out of 10 cases (40%), sixth nerve palsy improved in 6 out of 9 cases (66.7%). All the 4 cases presented with deteriorated conscious level became fully conscious (100%), immediately postoperatively. Improvement of hydrocephalus in postoperative imaging occurred in 28 out of 32 cases (87.5%) (Fig 2) (El-Ghandour, 2011)

Endoscopy plays an important role in the treatment of complex hydrocephalus. Among 24 pediatric patients with multiloculated hydrocephalus operated by endoscopic cyst fenestration, improvement of hyrocephalus occurred in 18 cases (75%), the need for shunt insertion was avoided in 3 cases (12.5%), shunt revision rate was reduced from 2.9 per year before fenestration to 0.2 per year after fenestration. During the overall mean follow-up period (30 months), repeated endoscopic procedure was necessary in 8 cases (33%). Six out of these 8 patients (75%) had already undergone shunt placement before endoscopy (El-Ghandour, 2008).

Suprasellar arachnoid cysts, which cause hydrocephalus by obstructing the foramen of Monro, can be marsupialized to the ventricular system endoscopically (Fig 3). Excellent results have been obtained in a recent study including 25 pediatric patients operated by endoscopy. In this study, patients were divided into 2 groups. Patients in group A (11 patients) underwent ventriculocystostomy with a mean follow-up 55 months, and those in group B (14 patients) underwent ventriculocystocisternostomy with a mean follow-up of 64.7 months. Both procedures proved to be almost equally effective clinically and radiologically.

The incidence of improvement of hydrocephalus-related symptoms was 63.6% in group A, compared with 85.7% in group B. Improvement in cyst size and hydrocephalus after ventriculocystostomy was 81.8% and 63.6% respectively, compared with 100% and 85.7% respectively after ventriculocystocisternostomy (Fig 4). However because of the statistically significant difference between the incidence of recurrence after ventriculocystostomy and ventriculocystocisternostomy during the long-term follow-up (27.3% versus 0%, $p < 0.05$), the author concluded that ventriculocystocisternostomy should be considered as the procedure of choice in the treatment of these cases (El-Ghandour, 2011).

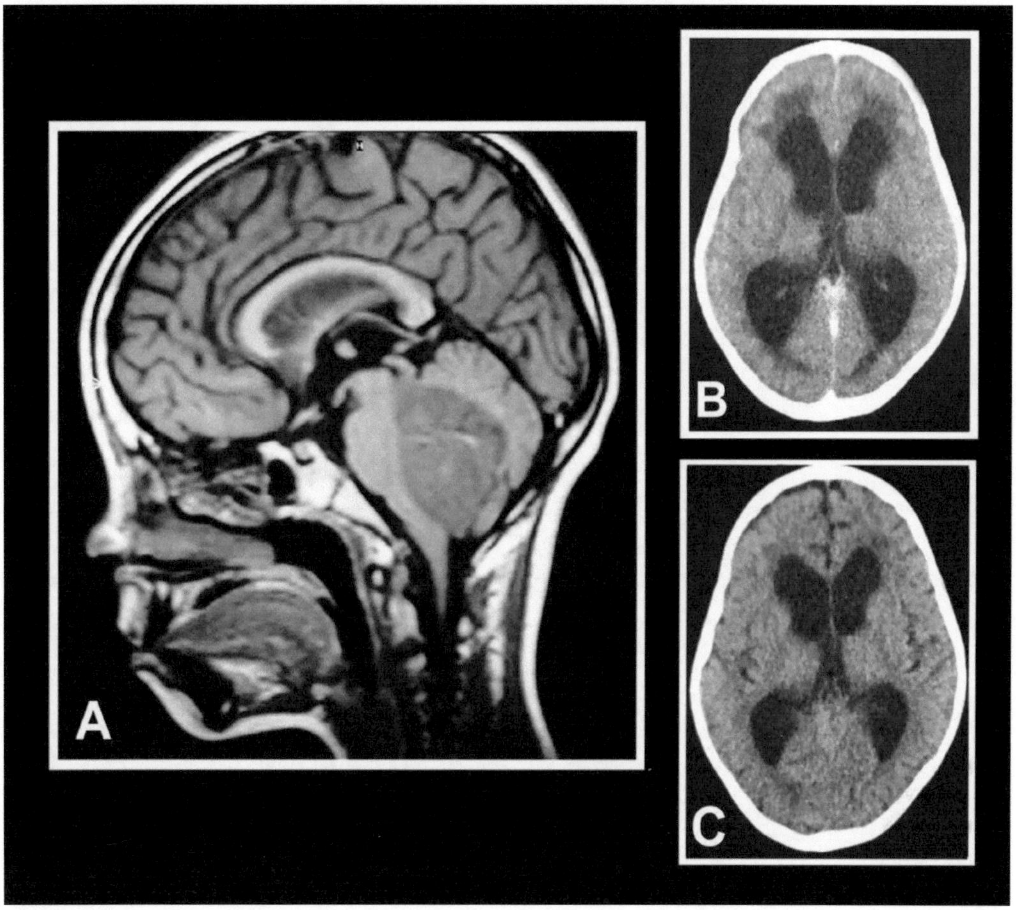

Fig. 2. A: Magnetic resonance imaging T1 weighted sagittal view of a case of posterior fossa tumor (medulloblastoma), demonstrating communication between third ventricle and prepontine cistern after endoscopic third ventriculostomy . B: Preoperative axial CT scan image showing severe obstructive hydroceophalus due to posterior fossa tumor. The presence of massive periventricular edema signifies acutely occurring hydrocephalus. C: Postoperative axial CT scan image obtained 3 days after endoscopic third ventriculostomy showing mild reduction in ventricular size, resolution of periventricular edema, and opening of subarachnoid space. [Reprinted with permission from El-Ghandour NM (2011). Endoscopic third ventriculostomy versus ventriculoperitoneal shunt in the treatment of obstructive hydrocephalus due to posterior fossa tumors in children. *Childs Nerv Syst*, Vol. 27, No. 1, (January 2011), pp. 117-126, ISSN 0256-7040].

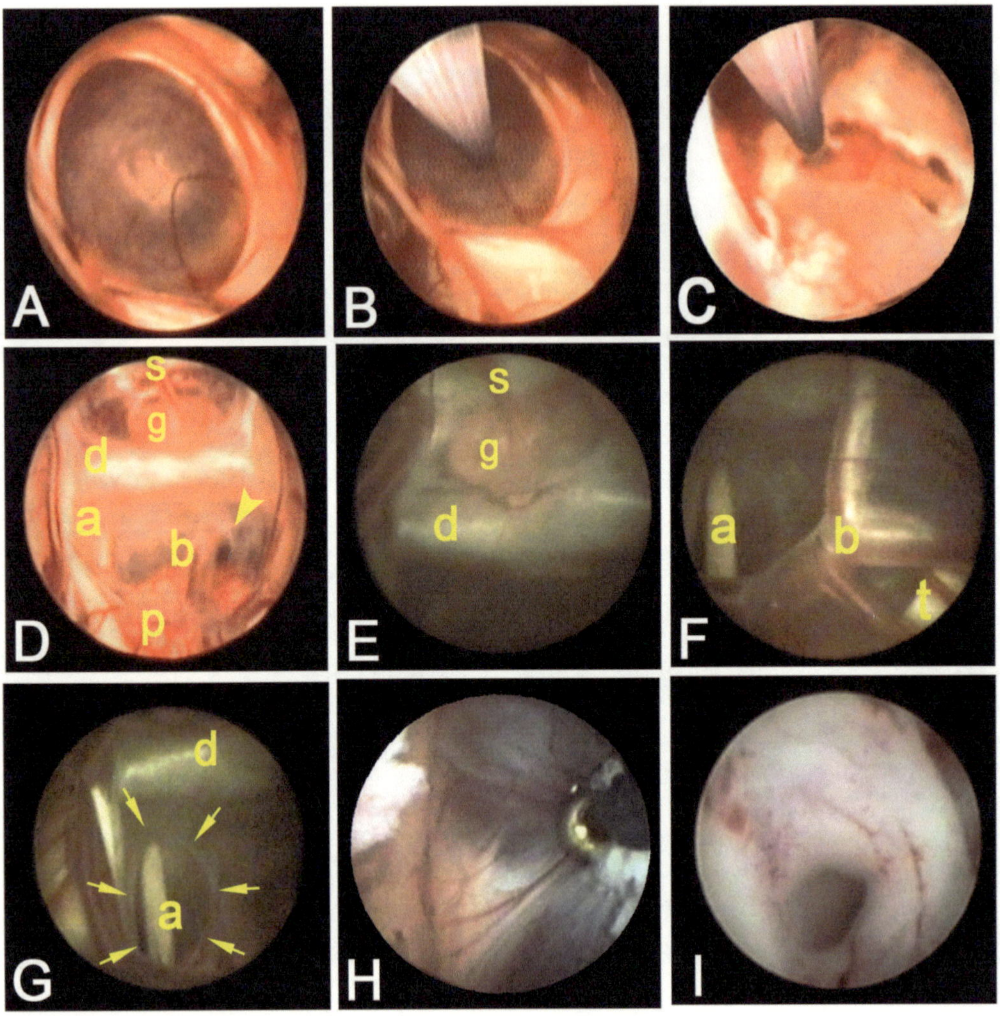

Fig. 3. Intraoperative neuroendoscopic views. A: Bluish-colored apical dome of surasellar arachnoid cyst bulging through and obstructing the foramen of Monro. B: Opening of upper cyst wall using bipolar electrode. C: Ventriculocystostomy, widening of the fenestration is done by bipolar diathermy. D: Anatomical landmarks as seen through the cyst membrane; a = abducent nerve; b = basilar artery; d = dorsum sellae; g = pituitary gland; p = pons; s = pituitary stalk; arrow head = valve like structure. E: Suprasellar compartment showing pituitary gland (g), pituitary stalk (s), dorsum sellae (d). F: Prepontine compartment as seen through the cyst membrane, a = abducent nerve; b = basilar artery apex; t = trigeminal nerve. G: Cystocisternostomy, a = abducent nerve; d = dorsum sellae; arrows = fenestration. H: Shrinking of the cyst membrane by bipolar diathermy. **I:** At end of the procedure, the aqueduct of Sylvius is patent [Reprinted with permission from El-Ghandour NM (2011). Endoscopic treatment of suprasellar arachnoid cysts in children. *J Neurosurg Pediat* Vol. 8, No. 1, (July 2011), pp. 6-14, ISSN 1933-0707].

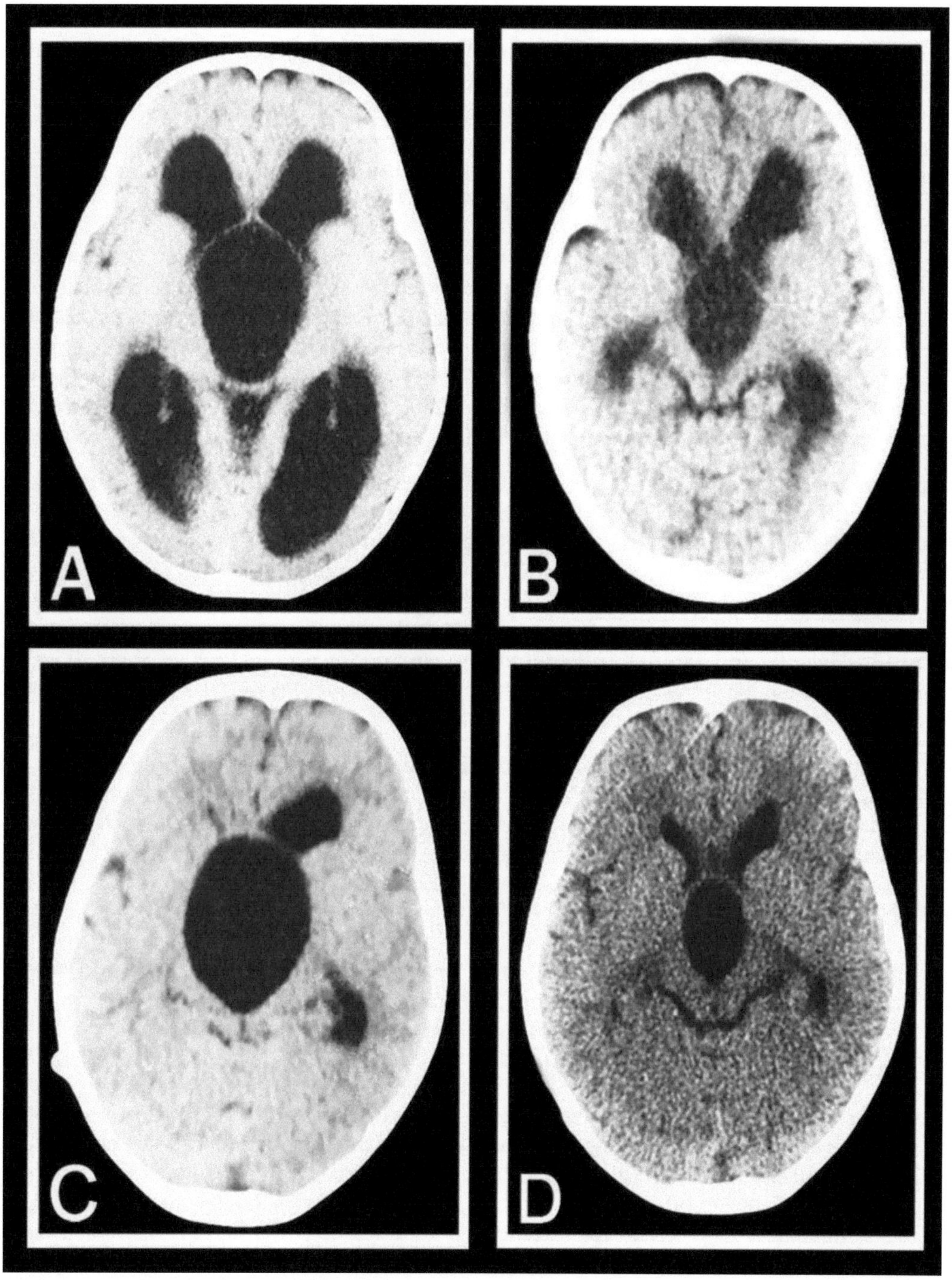

Fig. 4. A: Axial T1 weighted MR imaging showing a huge suprasellar arachnoid cyst with marked obstructive hydrocephalic changes. B: Axial CT scan performed 3 months after endoscopic ventriculocystocisternostomy showing apparent decrease in size of both the cyst and hydrocephalus with opening of the subarachnoid space. C: Axial CT scan showing

a huge suprasellar arachnoid cyst. A right sided ventriculoperitoneal shunt is seen, which was inserted in an outside institution due to a misdiagnosis of aqueduct stenosis. D: Axial CT scan performed 6 months after endoscopic ventriculocystocisternostomy and shunt removal showing apparent decrease in size of both the cyst and hydrocephalus with opening of the subarachnoid space [Reprinted with permission from El-Ghandour NM (2011). Endoscopic treatment of suprasellar arachnoid cysts in children. *J Neurosurg Pediat* Vol. 8, No. 1, (July 2011), pp. 6-14, ISSN 1933-0707].

Although there is an arguement about the role of endoscopy in the management of normal pressure hydrocephalus, some studies have reported good outcome. In a series including 110 patients with idiopathic normal pressure hydrocephalus operated by endoscopic third ventriculostomy, postoperative clinical improvement occurred in 76 cases (69.1%). Among the 34 patients who did not improve, 24 (21.8%) were unchanged and stable on the postoperative follow-up examination, whereas 10 (9%) showed clinical progression despite the endoscopic treatment (Gangemi et al., 2008).

Neuroendoscopic management of third ventricular colloid cysts is emerging as a safe, effective alternative to microsurgery. Among 10 cases operated endoscopically in a recent study, near-total excision of the cyst was achieved in 8 cases (80%), all of them were anteriorly located within the third ventricle. In the remaining 2 cases (20%), excision was subtotal, and remnants of the cyst wall were left obstructing the aqueduct of Sylvius. These 2 cases were located in the posterior part of the third ventricle, endoscopic third ventridculostomy and septum pellucidotomy were performed in both of them (Fig 5). Restoration of the foramina of Monro was achieved in all the patients (100%) (El-Ghandour, 2009).

Endoscopic third ventriculostomy and concomitant endoscopic biopsy has been reported by many authors as the procedure of choice in the treatment of pineal region tumors. In cases such as germinomas, establishing pathological diagnosis is quite sufficient, and it obviates the need for open surgery, since these tumors are radiosenstive. In a series of 23 patients with pineal tumors operated by such strategy, the obtained tissue sample was sufficient for pathological diagnosis in all the cases (100%) (Chernov et al., 2006). Endoscopic biopsy has the advantage of being combined with endoscopic third ventriculostomy to treat hydrocephalus and obtain cerebrospinal fluid for tumor markers and cytology, and allows tissue bites to be taken under direct vision (Al-Tamimi et al., 2008).

7. Ventriculostomy versus shunting

There are many studies which discuss the role of endoscopic third ventriculostomy in the management of noncommunicating hydrocephalus, but the comparison between endoscopic third ventriculostomy and ventriculoperitoneal shunting has rarely been addressed in the literature. A recent study compares both procedures in the management of obstructive hydrocephalus due to posterior fossa tumors. It included 53 pediatric patients which were divided into 2 groups: group A (32 cases) operated by endoscopic third ventriculostomy and group B (21 cases) operated by ventriculoperitoneal shunting. Both procedures proved to be almost equally effective clinically and radiologically.

Intracranial hypertension symptoms improved in 31 out of 32 patients (96.9%) included in group A, and in all the patients (100%) included in group B. Improvement of hydrocephalus

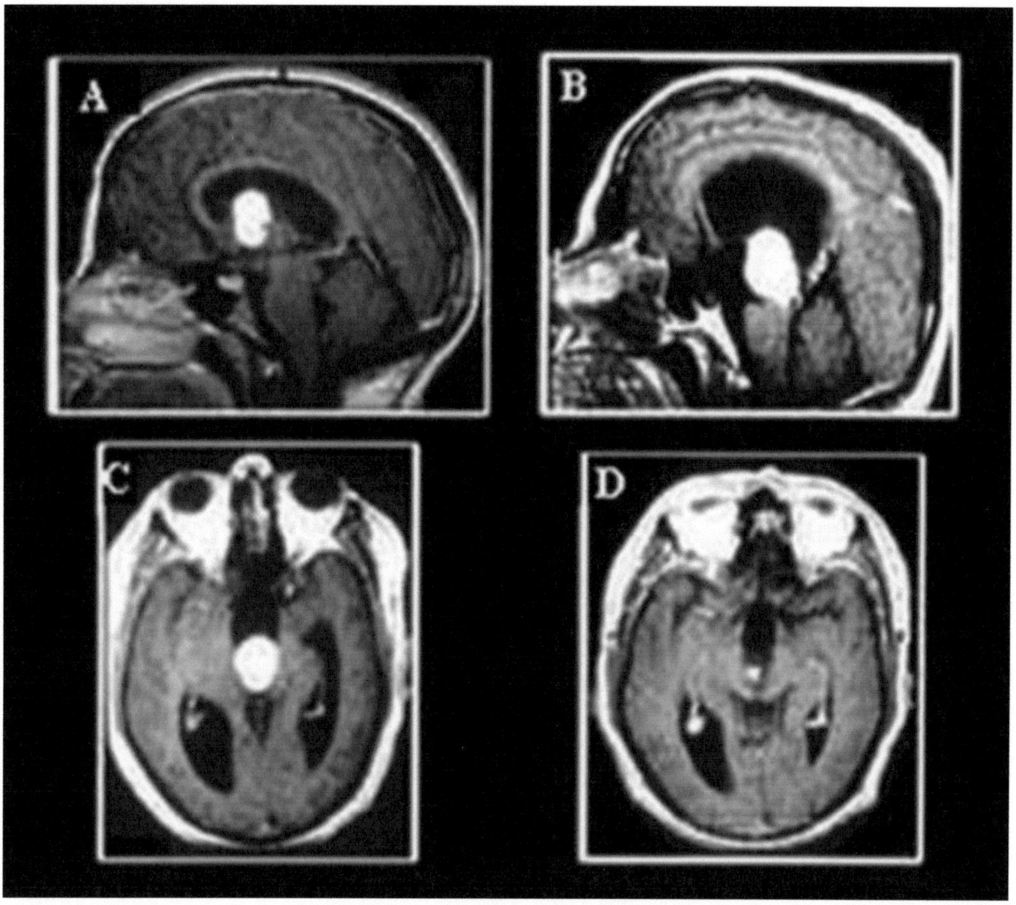

Fig. 5. A, Preoperative midsagittal MR imaging brain showing colloid cyst within the anterior aspect of the third ventricle. B, Preoperative midsagittal MR imaging brain showing colloid cyst within the posterior aspect of the third ventricle. C, Preoperative axial MR imaging brain of the same patient with posteriorly located colloid cyst. D, Postoperative axial MR imaging brain with gadolinium performed 1 year after endoscopic removal of the colloid cyst. Improvement of hydrocephalus and remnant of the cyst wall are noted. [Reprinted with permission from El-Ghandour NM (2009). Endoscopic treatment of third ventricular colloid cysts: a review including ten personal cases. *Neurosurg Rev*, Vol. 32, No. 4, (October 2009), pp. 395-402, ISSN 0344-5607].

in postoperative CT scan occurred in 28 out of 32 patients (81.3%) included in group A (Fig 2) and in all the 21 patients (100%) included in group B. The mean duration of surgery in group A was 15 minutes compared to 35 minutes in group B ($p<0.01$, highly significant).

The incidence of complications after ventriculostomy was 9.3% (3 out of 32 cases) and after ventriculoperitoneal shunting was 38% (8 out of 21 cases). The difference in the incidence of complications between both groups is statistically significant ($p<0.05$). In group A, intraoperative bleeding occurred in 2 patients (it was minor and stopped spontaneously within few minutes with irrigation), and cerebrospinal fluid leakage occured in 1 patient. In group B, shunt infection occurred in 2 patients, one of these 2 patients died 4.5 months postoperatively from ventriculitis. Subdural collection occurred in 2 patients, and upward brain herniation in 1 patient (Table 1).

Morbidity and mortality	ETV group (32 cases)	VPS group (21 cases)	P value
Morbidity (Total)	3 (9.3%)	8 (38%)	0.03
Bleeding	2 (6.2%)	0	--
CSF leak	1 (3.1%)	0	--
Infection	0	2 (9.4%)	--
Subdural collection	0	2 (9.4%)	--
Epidural hematoma	0	1 (4.7%)	--
Upward herniation	0	1 (4.7%)	--
Pseudomeningocele	0	2 (9.4%)	--
Mortality (Total)	0	1 (4.7%)	0.8
Hydrocephalus-related	0	1 (4.7%)	0.8
Nonhydrocephalus-related	0	0	--

Table 1. Morbidity and mortality in 53 pediatric patients with obstructive hydrocephalus due to posterior fossa tumors
ETV = endoscopic third ventriculostomy; VPS = ventriculoperitoneal shunt. [Reprinted with permission from El-Ghandour NM (2011). Endoscopic third ventriculostomy versus ventriculoperitoneal shunt in the treatment of obstructive hydrocephalus due to posterior fossa tumors in children. *Childs Nerv Syst*, Vol. 27, No. 1, (January 2011), pp. 117-126, ISSN 0256-7040].

Recurrence of hydrocephalus occurred in 2 out of 32 patients (6.2%) operated by endoscopic third ventriculostomy, at 6.5 and 14 months postoperatively respectively (both patients had intraoperative bleeding at initial surgery). Among 21 patients operated by ventriculoperitoneal shunting, shunt revision was performed 15 times in 8 patients. The incidence of recurrence of hydrocephalus was 6.2% among ventriculostomy patients, compared to 38% among shunt patients ($p < 0.01$, highly significant) (Table 2). All the 32 patients included in group A were shunt free among the mean follow-up duration of 27.4 months, whereas all the 21 patients included in group B were shunt dependent among the mean follow-up duration of 25 months.

The number of revisions per patient (among the 8 patients with postoperative failure included in group B) was 1.8, and the mean duration which lapsed between the shunting procedure and the first revision procedure was 5.6 months. Kaplan-Meier survival curve for both groups shows a more progressive decrease of the cumulative survival in the ventriculoperitoneal shunt group. The mean survival time in group A is higher than in group B (logrank test is highly significant, $p < 0.01$) (Fig 6).

The author concluded that endoscopic third ventriculostomy is superior than ventriculoperitoneal shunting because of the shorter duration of surgery, the lower incidence of morbidity, absence of mortality and the lower incidence of procedure failure. It renders the patient independent from a failure-prone shunt system, and offers a good opportunity to become shunt free. It is a preliminary, simple, safe, effective, minimally invasive and physiological method of bypassing obstruction in cerebrospinal fluid circulation in cases of obstructive hydrocephalus (El-Ghandour, 2011).

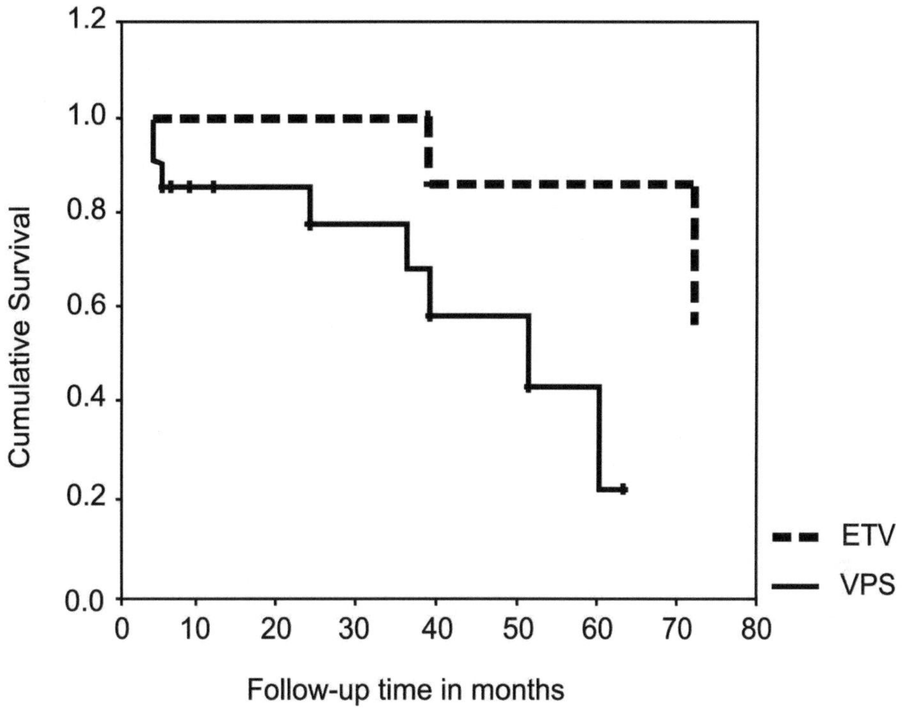

Fig. 6. Kaplan-Meier survival curve plotted for endoscopic third ventriculostomy (group A) and ventriculoperitoneal shunt (group B) showing a more progressive decrease of the cumulative survival in the ventriculoperitoneal shunt group. There is a higher mean survival time for endoscopic third ventriculostomy as compared to ventriculoperitoneal shunt (the logrank test is highly significant, $p<0.01$) [Reprinted with permission from El-Ghandour NM (2011). Endoscopic third ventriculostomy versus ventriculoperitoneal shunt in the treatment of obstructive hydrocephalus due to posterior fossa tumors in children. *Childs Nerv Syst*, Vol. 27, No. 1, (January 2011), pp. 117-126, ISSN 0256-7040].

Results of outcome	ETV group (32 cases)	VPS group (21 cases)	P value
Improvement of symptoms			
Intracranial hypertension	31/32(96.9%)	21/21(100%)	0.2
Gait ataxia	4/10(40%)	2/8(25%)	0.8
Sixth nerve palsy	6/9(66.7%)	3/6(50%)	0.9
Conscious level	4/4(100%)	2/2(100%)	--
Bulbar symptoms	0/2(0%)	0/3(0%)	--
Improvement of hydrocephalus (in postoperative C.T. scan)	28/32 (87.5%)	21/21(100%)	0.2
Duration of follow-up in months (mean $\pm$ SD)	27.4 ($\pm$ 20.5)	25 ($\pm$ 19.7)	0.6
Postoperative failure	2 (6.2%)	8 (38%)	0.003
Time to first failure in months (mean $\pm$ SD)	10.3($\pm$ 5.3)	5.6($\pm$ 4.6)	0.2
Shunt free patients	32 (100%)	0	--
Shunt dependent patients	0	21 (100%)	--
Number of revisions in postoperative failure patients (mean $\pm$ SD)	1	1.8($\pm$ 0.8)	0.2

Table 2. Results of outcome in 53 pediatric patients with obstructive hydrocephalus due to posterior fossa tumors.
ETV = endoscopic third ventriculostomy; VPS = ventriculoperitoneal shunt.; SD = standard deviation [Reprinted with permission from El-Ghandour NM (2011). Endoscopic third ventriculostomy versus ventriculoperitoneal shunt in the treatment of obstructive hydrocephalus due to posterior fossa tumors in children. *Childs Nerv Syst*, Vol. 27, No. 1, (January 2011), pp. 117-126, ISSN 0256-7040].

8. Conclusions

A significant advance in the treatment of hydrocephalus has been the evolution of endoscopy. Hydrocephalus represents the classic indication for a neuroendoscopic approach. Currently, hydrocephalus remains the most frequent intracranial disease treated endoscopically. The success of neuroendoscopy in recent years has relied heavily on the success of endoscopic third ventriculosromy in the treatment of obstructive hydrocephalus.

Endoscopic third ventriculostomy has become a well established procedure for the treatment of noncommunicationg hydrocephalus. In our experience, third ventriculostomy has been successful in controlling obstructive hydrocephalus caused by posterior fossa tumors, and it was much more superior than shunting in terms of morbidity and incidence of procedure failure.

The role of endoscopy in the treatment of complex hydrocephalus is indispensable. Our results of using endoscopy in the treatment of these cases are encouraging. Endoscopic cyst fenestration has led to avoiding or eliminating the need for shunts in some cases, simplification of complex shunts and reduction of shunt revision rate. It can be also used as an adjunct to shunting. It improves the results of shunting, and it plays a crucial role in shunt revision and retrieval of malfunctioning ventricular catheters.

In addition to tumor biopsy sampling, the endoscope has been used for the resection of colloid cysts and other intraventricular lesions. Our results of using endoscopy in the treatment of these cases are excellent. The use of the neuroendoscope provides the unique ability to perform tumor resection, tumor biopsy sampling, restoration of obstructed cerebrospinal fluid pathways (e.g. foramen of Monro and aqueduct of Sylvius), performing endoscopic third ventriculostomy, and cerebrospinal fluid sampling, all can be done in a single procedure.

Over the last few years, the field of neuroendoscopy has been expanded to treat a wide array of neurosurgically managed conditions. A seemingly limitless number of neurosurgical applications await the endoscope. In the future, one can expect routine use of the endoscope in the management of hydrocephalus, either as the primary surgery or as an adjunct. The continued evolution of this modality will rely on new technological advances, improved understanding of endoscopically demonstrated neurosurgical anatomy, discovery of new applications, and the training of neurosurgeons. Endoscopy is expected to become a routine procedure in modern neurosurgical practice and training. Pediatric neurosurgeons should acquire the needed skill in using endoscopy inorder to manage one of the most common neurosurgical problems in children, which is hydrocephalus.

9. References

Abdou MS, Cohen AR (1998). Endoscopic treatment of colloid cysts of the third ventricle. Technical note and review of the literature. *J Neurosurg,* Vol. 89, No. 6, pp. 1062-1068, (December 1998), ISSN 0022- 3085

Abtin K, Walker ML (1998): Endoscopic management of complex hydrocephalus. In: *Intracranial Endoscopic Neurosurgery,* Jimenez DF, pp. 135-145, AANS publication committee, ISBN 0-9624246-6-8, Illinois.

Albright AL, Reigel DH (1977). Management of hydrocephalus secondary to posterior fossa tumors. *J Neurosurg,* Vol. 46, No. 1, (January 1977), pp. 52-55, ISSN 0022-3085

Al-Tamimi YZ, Bhargava D, Surash S, Ramirez RE, Novegno F, Crimmins DW, Tyagi AK, Chumas PD (2008). Endoscopic biopsy during third ventriculostomy in pediatric pineal region tumors. *Childs Nerv Syst,* Vol. 24, No.11, (November 2008), pp. 1323-1326, ISSN 0256-7040

Bradley WG Jr, Whittemore AR, Watanabe AS, Davis SJ, Teresi LM, Homyak M (1991). Association of deep white matter infarction with chronic communicating hydrocephalus: implications regarding the possible origin of normal-pressure hydrocephalus. *AJNR Am J Neuroradiol*, Vol.12, No. 1 (January- February 1991), pp. 31-39, ISSN 0195-6108

Brockmeyer DL (1998). The use of endoscopes for shunt placement. In *Endoscopy of the central and peripheral nervous system*, King W, Frazee J & De Salles A, pp. 91-99, Thieme, ISBN 0- 86577-690-3, New York

Chernov MF, Kamikawa S, Yamane F, Ishihara S, Kubo O, Hori T (2006). Neuroendoscopic biopsy of tumors of the pineal region and posterior third ventricle: indications, technique, complications and results. *Neurosurgery*, Vol. 59, No. 2, (August 2006), pp. 267-277, ISSN 0148-396x

Cinalli G, Spennato P, Savarese L, Ruggiero C, Aliberti F, Cuomo L, Cianciulli E, Maggi G (2006). Endoscopic aqueductoplasty and placement of a stent in the cerebral aqueduct in the management of isolated fourth ventricle in children. *J Neurosurg* Vol. 104, No. 1 (Suppl Pediatrics), (January 2006), pp. 21-27, ISSN 0022-3085

Cohen AR (1993). Endoscopic ventricular surgery. *Pediatr Neurosurg*, Vol. 19, No. 3, (May-June 1993), pp. 127-134, ISSN 1016-2291

Culley DJ, Berger MS, Shaw D, Geyer R (1994). An analysis of factors determining the need for ventriculoperitoneal shunts after posterior fossa tumor surgery in children. *Neurosurgery*, Vol. 34, No. 3, (March 1994), pp. 402-408, ISSN 0148-396x

Dandy WE (1918). Extirpation of the choroid plexus of the lateral ventricle in communicating hydrocephalus. *Ann Surg*, Vol. 70, No. 6, (December 1918), pp. 569-579, ISSN 0003-4932

El-Ghandour NM (2006). Multiloculated hydrocephalus: A study of 24 patients operated by endoscopic cyst fenestration. *Neurosurgery*, Vol. 59, No. 2, (August 2006), p 477, ISSN 0148-396x (Abstr).

El-Ghandour NM (2008). Endoscopic cyst fenestration in the treatment of multiloculated hydrocephalus in children. *J Neurosurg Pediatr*, Vol.1, No. 3, (March 2008), pp. 217-222, ISSN 1933-0707

El-Ghandour NM (2009). Endoscopic treatment of third ventricular colloid cysts: a review including ten personal cases. *Neurosurg Rev*, Vol. 32, No. 4, (October 2009), pp. 395-402, ISSN 0344-5607

El-Ghandour NM (2011). Endoscopic third ventriculostomy versus ventriculoperitoneal shunt in the treatment of obstructive hydrocephalus due to posterior fossa tumors in children. *Childs Nerv Syst*, Vol. 27, No. 1, (January 2011), pp. 117-126, ISSN 0256-7040

El-Ghandour NM (2011). Endoscopic treatment of suprasellar arachnoid cysts in children. *J Neurosurg Pediat*, Vol. 8, No. 1, (July 2011), pp. 6-14, ISSN 1933-0707

Epstein FJ (1993). Medulloblastoma: indications for shunt placement. *Pediatr Neurosurg*, Vol.19, No. 6, (June 1993), pp. 300-302, ISSN 1016-2291

Farwell JR, Dohrmann GJ, Flannery JT (1977). Central nervous system tumors in children. *Cancer*, Vol. 40, No. 6, (December 1977), pp 3123-3132, ISSN 1097-0142

Fiorindi A, Longatti PL, Martinuzzi A (2004). Failure of endoscopic third ventriculostomy in treatment of idiopathic normal pressure hydrocephalus. *Minim Invasive Neurosurg*, Vol. 47, No. 6, (December 2004), pp. 342-345, ISSN 0946-7211

Gaab MR, Schroeder HW (1998). Neuroendoscopic treatment of intraventricular tumors. In: *Intracranial Endoscopic Neurosurgery*, Jimenez DF, pp. 171-183, AANS publication committee, ISBN 0-9624246-6-8, Illinois.

Gangemi M, Maiuri F, Naddeo M, Godano U, Mascari C, Broggi G, Ferroli P (2008). Endoscopic third ventriculostomy in idiopathic normal pressure hydrocephalus: an Italian multicenter study. *Neurosurgery*, Vol. 63, No. 1, (July 2008), pp. 62-69. ISSN 0148-396x

Gore PA, Gonzalez LF, Rekate HL, Nakaji P (2008). Endoscopic supracerebellar infratentorial approach for pineal cyst resection : technical case report. *Neurosurgery*, Vol. 62, No. 3 (Suppl 1) (March 2008), pp. 108-109, ISSN 0148-396x

Greitz D (2004). Radiological assessment of hydrocephalus : new theories and implications for therapy. *Neurosurg Rev*, Vol. 27, No. 3, (July 2004), pp. 145-167, ISSN 0344-5607

Hellwig D, Bauer BL, Schulte M, Gatscher S, Riegel T, Bertalanffy H (2008). Neuroendoscopic treatment for colloid cysts of the third ventricle : the experience of a decade. *Neurosurgery* Vol. 62, No. 6, (Suppl 3) (June 2008), pp. 1101-1109, ISSN 0148-396x

Jallo GI, Abbott R (1996). Introduction of a second working portal for neuroendoscopy. A technical note. *Pediatr Neurosurg*, Vol. 24, No.2, (February 1996), pp. 56-60, ISSN 1016-2291

Jallo GI, Kothbauer KF, Abbott IR (2005). Endoscopic third ventriculostomy. *Neurosurg Focus*, Vol. 19, No. 6, (December 2005), E11, ISSN 1092- 0684

Jeeves MA, Simpson DA, Geffen G (1979). Functional consequences of the transcallosal removal of intraventricular tumors. *J Neurol Neurosurg Psychiatry*, Vol. 42, No. 2, (February 1979), pp. 134- 142, ISSN 0022-3050

Jimenez DF (1998). Third ventriculostomy. In: *Intracranial Endoscopic Neurosurgery*, Jimenez DF, pp. 101-110, AANS publication committee, ISBN 0-9624246-6-8, Illinois.

Jones RFC, Stening WA, Brydon M (1990). Endoscopic third ventriculostomy. *Neurosurgery*, Vol. 26, No. 1,(January 1990), pp. 86-92, ISSN 0148-396x

Lee M, Wisoff JH, Abbott R (1994). Management of hydrocephalus in children with medulloblastoma: prognostic factors for shunting. *Pediatric Neurosurg*, Vol.20, No. 4 (April 1994), pp. 240 -247, ISSN 1016-2291

Lewis AI, Keiper GL, Crone KR (1995). Endoscopic treatment of loculated hydrocephalus. *J Neurosurg*, Vol.82, No.5, (May 1995), pp. 780-785, ISSN 0022- 3085

Lewis AI, Crone KR (1998). Endoscopic removal of colloid cysts. In: *Intracranial Endoscopic Neurosurgery*, Jimenez DF, pp. 125-133, AANS publication committee, ISBN 0-9624246-6-8, Illinois.

Li KW, Nelson C, Suk I, Jallo GI (2005). Neuroendoscopy : past, present, and future. *Neurosurg Focus*, Vol.19, No.6, (December 2005), E1, ISSN 1092- 0684

Longatti P, Fiorindi A, Feletti A, Baratto V (2006). Endoscopic opening of the foramen of Magendie using transaqueductal navigation for membrane obstruction of the fourth ventricle outlets. Technical note. *J Neurosurg*, Vol. 105, No. 6, (December 2006), pp. 924-927, ISSN 0022-3085

Mathiesen T, Grane P, Lindquist C, von Holst H (1993). High recurrence rate following aspiration of colloid cysts in the third ventricle. J *Neurosurg, Vol.* 78, No. 5, (May 1993), pp. 748-752,. ISSN 0022- 3085

McNickle HF (1947). The surgical treatment of hydrocephalus. A simple method of performing third ventriculostomy. *Br J Neurosurg*, Vol. 34, No. 135, (January 1947), pp. 302-307, ISSN 0268-8697

Meier U, Zeilinger FS, Schonherr B (2000). Endoscopic third ventriculostomy versus shunt operation in normal pressure hydrocephalus: diagnostics and indication. *Minim Invasive Neurosurg*, Vol. 42, No. 2, (June 2000), pp. 87-90, ISSN 0946-7211

Mitchell P, Mathew B (1999). Third ventriculostomy in normal pressure hydrocephalus. *Br J Neurosurg*, Vol. 13, No. 4 (August 1999), pp. 382-385, ISSN 0268-8697

Mixter WJ (1923). Ventriculoscopy and puncture of the floor of the third ventricle. *Boston Med Surg*. Vol. 188, (1923), pp. 277-278, ISSN 0003-4819

Mohanty A (2005). Endoscopic options in the management of isolated fourth ventricles. Case report. *J Neurosurg: Pediatrics*, Vol. 103, No. 1, (July 2005), pp. 73-78, ISSN 0022-3085

Mohanty A, Biswas A, Satish S, Vollmer DG (2008). Efficacy of endoscopic third ventriculostomy in fourth ventricular outlet obstruction. *Neurosurgery*, Vol. 63, No. 5 (November 2008), pp. 905-914, ISSN 0148-396x

Nulsen FE, Spitz EB (1951). Treatment of hydrocephalus by direct shunt from ventricle to jugular vein. *Surgical Forum*, Vol. 2, (1951), pp. 399-403, ISSN 00718041

Oi S, Matsumoto S (1986). Pathophysiology of aqueductal obstruction in isolated IV ventricle after shunting. *Childs Nerv Syst*, Vol. 2, No. 6, (June 1986), pp. 282-286, ISSN 0256-7040

Oka K, Yamamoto M, Ikeda K (1993). Flexible endoneurosurgical therapy for aqueductal stenosis. *Neurosurgery*, Vol. 33, No. 2, (August 1993), pp. 236-243, ISSN 0148-396x

Papo I, Caruselli G, Luongo A (1982). External ventricular drainage in the management of posterior fossa tumors in children and adolescents. *Neurosurgery*, Vol. 10, No. 1, (January 1982), pp. 13-15, ISSN 0148-396x

Polednak AP, Flannery JT (1995). Brain, other central nervous system, and eye cancer. *Cancer*, Vol. 75, No.1 (Suppl 1) (January 1995), pp. 330-337, ISSN 1097-0142

Pudenz RH (1981). The surgical treatment of hydrocephalus: a historical review. *Surg Neurol*, Vol. 15, No. 1, (January 1981), pp. 15-26, ISSN 0090-3019

Raimondi AJ, Tomita T (1981). Hydrocephalus and infratentorial tumors. Incidence, clinical picture, and treatment. *J Neurosurg*, Vol. 55, No. 2, (August 1981), pp. 174-182, ISSN 0022-3085

Ray P, Jallo GI, Kim RY, Kim BS, Wilson S, Kothbauer K, Abbott R (2005). Endoscopic third ventriculostomy for tumor-related hydrocephalus in a pediatric population. *Neurosurg Focus*, Vol. 19, No. 6, (December 2005), E8, ISSN 1092-0684

Scarff JE (1935) Third ventriculostomy as the rational treatment of obstructive hydrocephalus. *J Pediatr*, Vol. 6, (1935), pp. 870-871, ISSN 0022-3476

Shin M, Morita A, Asano S, Ueki K, Kirino T (2000). Neuroendoscopic aqueductal stent placement procedure for isolated fourth ventricle after ventricular shunt placement. *J Neurosurg*, Vol. 92, No. 6, (June 2000), pp. 1036-1039, ISSN 0022-3085

Schroeder HW, Gaab MR (1999). Endoscopic aqueductoplasty: technique and results. *Neurosurgery*, Vol. 45, No. 3, (September 1999), pp. 508-518, ISSN 0148-396x

Schroeder HW, Gaab MR (1999). Intracranial endoscopy. *Neurosurg Focus*, Vol. 6, No. 4 (April 1999), E1, ISSN 1092-0684

Schroeder HW, Niendorf WR, Gaab MR (2002). Complications of endoscopic third ventriculostomy. *J Neurosurg*, Vol. 69, No. 6, (June 2002), pp. 1032-1040, ISSN 0022-3085

Teo C (1998). Endoscopy for the treatment of hydrocephalus. In *Endoscopy of the central and peripheral nervous system*, King W, Frazee J & De Salles A, pp. 59-67, Thieme, ISBN 0- 86577-690-3, New York

Upchurch K, Raifu M, Bergsneider M (2007). Endoscope-assisted placement of a multiperforated shunt catheter into the fourth ventricle via a frontal transventricular approach. *Neurosug. Focus*, Vol. 22, No. 4 (April 2007), E8, ISSN 1092-0684

Walker ML (2001). History of ventriculostomy. *Neurosurg Clin N Am*, Vol. 12, No.1 (January 2001), pp. 101-110, ISSN 1042-3680

Yamini B, Refai B, Rubin CM, Frim DM (2004). Initial endoscopic management of pineal region tumors and associated hydrocephalus: clinical series and literature review. *J Neurosurg*, Vol. 100, No. 5 (Suppl Pediatrics), (May 2004), pp. 437-441, ISSN 0022-3085

9

Transcranial Doppler Ultrasonography in the Management of Neonatal Hydrocephalus

Branislav Kolarovszki and Mirko Zibolen
Jessenius Faculty of Medicine, Comenius University
Slovakia

1. Introduction

Neonatal hydrocephalus is characterised by an excessive accumulation of cerebrospinal fluid with enlargement of cerebral ventricles, that occurs as a result of disturbance of production, flow or resorption of cerebrospinal fluid.

The pathophysiological changes of progressive neonatal hydrocephalus include: increased intracranial volume of cerebrospinal fluid, progressive dilatation of cerebral ventricles, decreased intracranial compliance, raised intracranial pressure, alteration of cerebral circulation and subsequent secondary brain tissue damage (decreased cerebral blood flow, hypoperfusion, ischaemia), alteration of energy metabolism (tissue acidosis, higher lactate concentration), changes in neurotransmiter systems, damage of white matter, associative tracts and cerebral cortex. The primary target of injury are periventricular axons and myelin. Secondary changes in neurons reflect the compensation to the stress or ultimately the disconnection (De Riggo et al., 2007).

Transcranial color coded Doppler sonography provides a bedside noninvasive and repeatable method of monitoring of the cerebral circulation with good clinical applications. Progressive hydrocephalus leads to the stretching, displacement and compression of cerebral vessels with increased vascular resistance. Doppler parameters reflect good the changes of cerebral circulation. In generall, there is a good corelation between the increase of intracranial pressure and changes in Doppler curve parameters, mainly decreased end-diastolic blood flow velocity and increased resistive index and pulsatility index. The mean cerebral blood flow velocity is mainly determined by diastolic blood flow. In the cases of intracranial hypertension, the arterial blood flow is more affected during diastole than during systole, resulting in an increase of resistive index and pulsatility index. Transcranial Doppler ultrasonography can be used as a noninvasive method for the indirect monitoring of intracranial pressure and dynamics in newborns with hydrocephalus.

2. Transcranial Doppler ultrasonography

The introduction of transcranial Doppler ultrasonography by Aaslid et al., in 1982 offered a noninvasive method for the assessment of cerebral blood flow velocity in the major intracranial arteries (Aaslid et al., 1982). This new method was used also in the examination of children with hydrocephalus. Neonatal Doppler studies date from 1979 (Bada et al., 1979).

2.1 Transcranial color coded Doppler ultrasonography

Transcranial color coded Doppler ultrasonography, first performed by Schoning et al. in 1989, allows direct visualization at basal cerebral arteries and demostrates cerebral blood flow easily because of the color coding (Schoning et al., 1989).

During the examination of newborn by transcranial Doppler ultrasonography is important to comply with precise method of examination. The examiner should not to upset the child. The newborn has to lie calm, the vessel cross-sectional area and the position of sample volume in the vessel should be constant. Also an inadequate rotation of head could decrease the venous outflow and change the real Doppler parameters of cerebral vessels. Color coding enables visualization of the selected segment of cerebral vessels and detection of blood flow direction. The measurement of the blood flow velocity depends upon the angle between the Doppler beam and the longitudinal axis of the vessel. The angle of insonation should be kept as close to zero as posssible. The measurement of Doppler curve parameters is made by the software equipment.

In neonatal transcranial Doppler studies are used following acoustic windows:

- transfontanellar - through the anterior fontanelle, mainly for the visualization of anterior cerebral artery, internal carotid artery and basilar artery (Fig. 1)
- transtemporal - through the temporal bone, for the visualization of middle cerebral artery and posterior cerebral artery (Fig. 2)
- suboccipital - through the foramen magnum, visualization of distal segments of vertebral arteries and basilar artery
- transorbital and submandibular - are used only occasionally

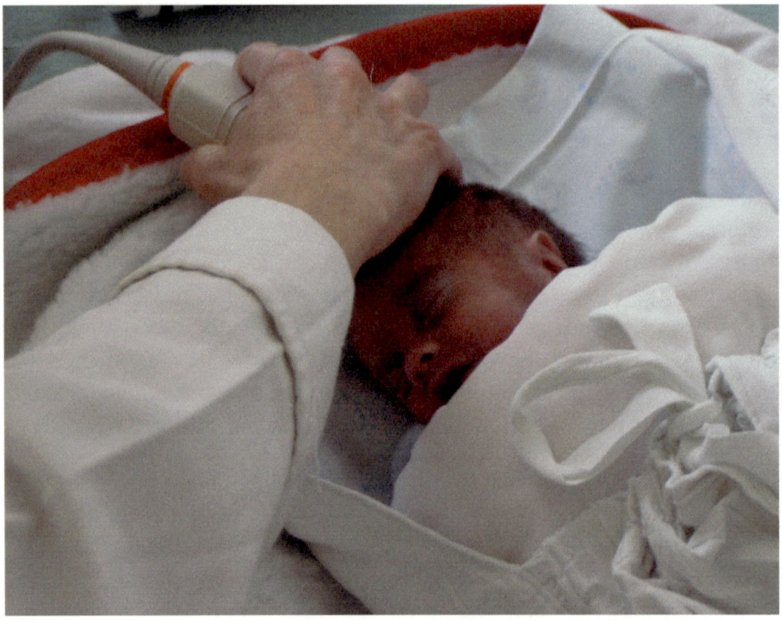

Fig. 1. Transcranial Doppler ultrasonography - examination of the newborn, transfontanellar acoustic window (photo - authors)

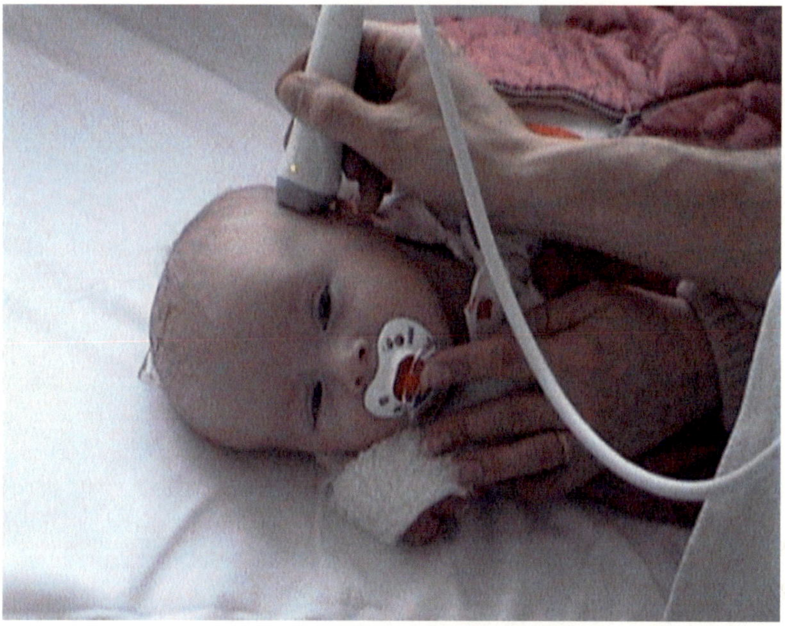

Fig. 2. Transcranial Doppler ultrasonography - examination of the infant, transtemporal acoustic window (photo - authors)

2.2 Doppler curve and parameters

The cerebral circulation is a low-resistive vascular system, which is typicall for organs with the need of constant high minute blood flow. Therefore Doppler curve of cerebral vessels has the positive blood flow during systole and also during diastole (Fig. 3).

Several factors influence the shape and parameters of Doppler curve. The pressure gradient in arteries is produced by myocardial contractility. The systolic peak of Doppler curve is related to the pressure gradient, arterial elasticity and blood viscosity. The shape of diastole is determined mainly by distal vessels resistance, but can be influenced also by systematic arterial, venous and intrathoracic pressure. In the cases of increased peripheral vessels resistance, the diastolic blood flow velocity is decreased. The zero or reverse end-diastolic blood flow is always pathological.

The mainly used Doppler curve parameters are:

- peak systolic blood flow velocity (Vsyst) - the maximal velocity during systole (m/s, cm/s)
- end-diastolic blood flow velocity (Ved) - the blood flow velocity at the end of diastole (m/s, cm/s)
- mean flow velocity (Vmean) - the mean value of blood flow velocity between the begining of systole and the end of diastole.

Analysis of Doppler curve enables the calculation of qualitative Doppler parameters, which are less influenced by the angle of insonation and local turbulent flow in arterial lumen. The mainly used qualitative Doppler curve indices are:

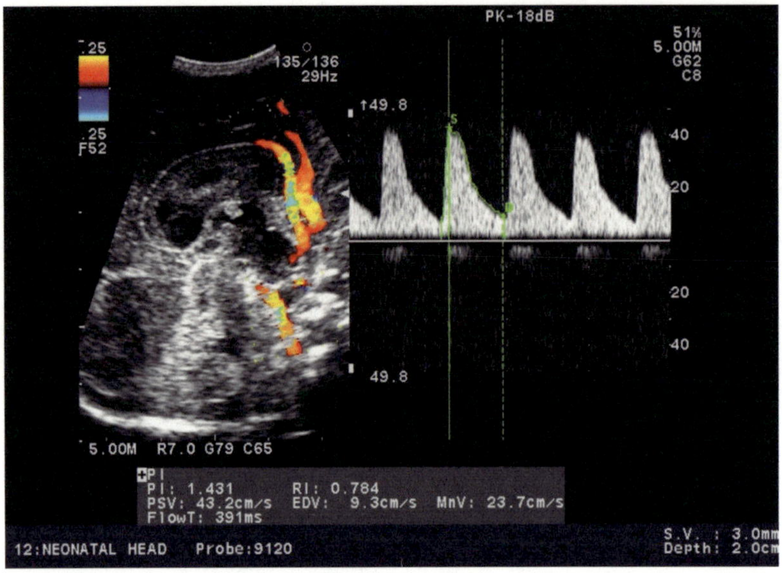

Fig. 3. Doppler curve of pericallosal artery: PI - pulsatility index, RI - resistive index, PSV - peak systolic blood flow velocity, EDV - end-diastolic blod flow velocity, MnV - mean blood flow velocity, FlowT - flow time (figure - authors)

- resistive index (RI, Pourcelot, 1975) - reflects the blood vessel resistance. Is defined as:

$$RI = Vsyst - Ved / Vsyst$$

- pulsatility index (PI, Gösling et al., 1974) - the value of pulsatility index is higher than resistive index. The assessment of pulsatility index is helpfull in the situation of zero or reverse diastolic blood flow, when the calculation of resistive index or S/D ratio is impossible. Pulsatility index is defined as:

$$PI = Vsyst - Ved / Vmean$$

- S/D ratio (S/D index, Stuart et al., 1980) - is defined as:

$$S/D = Vsyst / Ved$$

- trans-systolic time - reflects the time-related changes of the cerebral blood flow velocities (Hanlo et al., 1995a)

The basal Doppler parameters are measured at first. There is only a light contact between sonographic probe and the surface of anterior fontanelle through the layer of gel. Than anterior fontanelle compressive test is performed - the Doppler parameters are measured during the compression of anterior fontanelle using sonographic probe. The compression of anterior fontanelle by means of ophtalmodynamometer allows exact determination of applied pressure (g/cm2). The Doppler parameters could be measured through transtemporal acoustic window (Taylor et al., 1994; Taylor et al., 1996; Westra et al., 1998). If the value of basal resistive index increased more than 25% or the value of compressive resistive index is more than 0,90, the compressive test is considered to be positive (Westra et al., 1998).

2.3 Reference values of Doppler parameters

There were published several studies with the analysis of reference values of Doppler parameters of cerebral vessels in newborns and children (Babikian & Wechsler, 1993; Bode, 1988; Bode & Wais, 1988; Brouwers, 1990; Deeg & Rupprecht, 1989; Hayashi et al., 1992; Horgan et al., 1989; Ozek et al., 1995; Schöning et al.,1996).

The determination of generally accepted normal Doppler parameters of the cerebral circulation have some limitations:

- use of different sonographic technique
- the changes in the quality of sonographic equipment
- sometimes unclear method of examination
- ununiformity of documentation and results presentation.

Therefore the presented data can not be generally used for each institution. In our institution, the reference values of Doppler parameters of selected cerebral vessels were determined by Minarik (2000) using transcranial color coded Doppler ultrasonography: ultrasonographic equipment Aloka Color Doppler SSD-830, probes 3,5 and 5 MHz for B-picture, 2 MHz for CW (continuous wave Doppler) and PW (pulsed wave Doppler). The analysis of Doppler signal was performed using Fourier transformation with the spectrum visualization. The sample volume was 1 mm3 and low frequency filter 100 kHz was used. The adjustment of alliasing and the angle of insonation was performed. The reference values of Doppler parameters of selected cerebral vessels in the first year of life determined by Minarik (2000) are presented in the Table 1, Table 2 and Table 3.

There is a linear corelation between the gestational age and the blood flow velocity of all cerebral arteries during the first 21 days of life. The cerebral blood flow velocity is increased by increasing gestational age. In generally, the preterm newborns have decreased cerebral blood flow velocity and increased value of resistive index (Table 4). The main changes of cerebral blood flow velocity occur during first hours and days after delivery, when the increase of blood flow velocity and decrease of resistive index is most rapid. The prematurity and low birth weight is associated with the changes of end-diastolic blood flow velocity (Minarik, 2000).

	1. month	1. month	3. month	3. month	6. month	6. month	12. month	12. month
	A1	A3	A1	A3	A1	A3	A1	A3
Vsyst (cm/s)	67-82	56-69	74-87	64-77	81-90	68-85	95-104	87-96
Ved (cm/s)	19-28	18-27	21-34	20-31	26-34	25-33	25-44	33-40
Vmean (cm/s)	36-46	29-42	36-54	30-50	46-58	38-54	57-67	51-63
RI	0,65-0,73	0,60-0,69	0,59-0,71	0,59-0,69	0,62-0,68	0,58-0,65	0,57-0,63	0,58-0,62

Table 1. The reference values of Doppler parameters of A1 and A3 segment of anterior cerebral artery during the first year of life (Minarik, 2000). Published with author´s permission.

	1. month	1. month	3. month	3. month	6. month	6. month	12. month	12. month
	M1	M3	M1	M3	M1	M3	M1	M3
Vsyst (cm/s)	75-86	65-80	80-90	70-79	91-100	83-92	104-115	95-106
Ved (cm/s)	20-30	19-28	24-35	22-32	32-40	28-36	41-49	36-45
Vmean (cm/s)	39-51	35-49	46-60	41-55	56-68	51-65	64-80	61-74
RI	0,65-0,74	0,63-0,73	0,61-0,70	0,60-0,70	0,60-0,65	0,59-0,66	0,55-0,61	0,56-0,62

Table 2. The reference values of Doppler parameters of M1 and M3 segment of right middle cerebral artery during the first year of life (Minarik, 2000). Published with author´s permission.

	1. month	1. month	3. month	3. month	6. month	6. month	12. month	12. month
	M1	M3	M1	M3	M1	M3	M1	M3
Vsyst (cm/s)	75-85	64-79	80-90	70-82	91-99	81-90	103-112	96-106
Ved (cm/s)	20-29	19-28	23-34	22-30	32-40	29-37	41-48	38-45
Vmean (cm/s)	39-51	35-49	48-62	40-56	57-68	50-66	64-80	57-72
RI	0,65-0,73	0,62-0,71	0,63-0,68	0,60-0,68	0,59-0,65	0,56-0,68	0,56-0,61	0,57-0,64

Table 3. The reference values of Doppler parameters of M1 and M3 segment of left middle cerebral artery during the first year of life (Minarik, 2000). Published with author´s permission.

< 33. gestational week	$0{,}77 \pm 0{,}09$
> 34. gestational week	$0{,}70 \pm 0{,}07$

Table 4. The reference values of resistive index of Doppler curve in the vertical segment of pericallosal artery before the genu corporis callosi in preterm newborns (Bode, 1988; Chadduck & Seibert, 1989; Westra et al., 1998) (table - authors)

2.4 Factors that influence Doppler parameters of cerebral circulation

The values of Doppler parameters are influenced by several factors that change mainly diastolic, but also systolic part of Doppler curve. The significant fluctuation of qualitative indices during the examination is the sign of alteration of cerebral autoregulation.

The crying and restlessness of newborn, unequale and unadequate compression of anterior fontanelle by the sonographic probe, influence the Doppler parameters of cerebral circulation (Hadač, 2000).

Interindividual changes - the method of examination and technical parameters of sonographic equipment have to be taken in the consideration. When the conclusion of sonographic examination is not unambiguous, it is better to assess the dynamic intraindividual trends (Myers et al., 1987).

The studies of several authors showed the influence of physical and mental activity on the cerebral blood flow (Diehl et al., 1998; Roberts & McKinney, 1998; Owega et al., 1998). There is a significant increase of systolic, diastolic and mean blood flow velocity in proximal and distal segments of cerebral vessels during the period of increased mental activity of child. The value od resistive index is not significantly changed (Minarik, 2000).

The manipulation and suction from orotracheal tube can influence the cerebral blood flow velocity (Perlman & Vople, 1983). The cerebral circulation is affected also by bradycardia and apnoic pauses (Perlman & Volpe, 1985).

The review of extracranial and intracranial factors that influence Doppler parameters of the cerebral circulation is presented in Table 5.

2.4.1 Pathologic conditions with increased resistive index

- hypocapnia – decreased value of paCO2 leads to the vasoconstriction of cerebral arteries with subsequently decreased cerebral blood flow. The loss of CO2 vasoreactivity corelates with the severity and prognosis of clinical status of infant (Klingelheofer & Sander, 1992; Miller et al., 1992). The decrease of paCO2 leads to the decrease of end-diastolic blood flow velocity and increase of resistive index. Sometimes the end-diastolic blood flow velocity can be zero. During the extreme decrease of paCO2, also the decrease of systolic blood flow velocity occurs (Macko et al., 1993; Menke et al., 1993; Vergesslich et al., 1989; Wyatt et al., 1991).

- hyperoxia – increased value of paO2 leads to mild cerebral vasoconstriction and decreased cerebral blood flow. The paO2 cerebral vasoreactivity is more uniform than paCO2 vasoreactivity.

- acute intracranial hypertension – in brain injury, cerebral oedema or active hydrocephalus negatively affects the cerebral blood flow. End-diastolic blood flow velocity is decreased and resistive index increased. The systolic blood flow velocity is changed in relationship to the systemic arterial blood pressure adaptation response. Blood flow during the diastole is affected first. When the value of intracranial pressure is the same than diastolic blood pressure, the end-diastolic block occurs (Barzo et al., 1991; Czernicki, 1992; Hanlo et al., 1995b; Kopniczky et al., 1995).

- intraventricular haemorrhage – in the brain tissue near intracerebral or intraventricular haemorrhage is resistive index increased because of cerebral vasoconstriction. In the cases of severe intraventricular haemorrhage, the vasoconstriction could occur also in all main cerebral arteries (Bada et al., 1979).

- brain infarction – typically there is no detectable blood flow in the occluded segment of cerebral artery, in proximal part of the artery is detected decreased end-diastolic blood flow velocity and increased resistive index (Babikian & Wechsler, 1993).

- congenital heart disease with left-right shunt – for example persistent arterial duct or truncus arteriosus, affects cerebral blood flow. Typically, the persistent arterial duct leads to the decrease or reverse diastolic blood flow with increased resistive index. The extent of the cerebrovascular changes is related to the hemodynamic severity of left-right cardiac shunt (Bissonnette & Benson, 1998; Wright, 1988). When the compensation mechanisms are sufficient, there is no decrease of cerebral blood flow under the ischaemic border. In the case of the combination with another pathological findings, the status of achieved hemodynamic equilibrium could be lost with the potential ischaemic damage of brain tissue (Shortland et al., 1990).

- blood hyperviscosity - polyglobulia is associated with the decrease of absolute values of cerebral blood flow velocity, the value of resistive index is increased only slightly. The vascular changes are seen in proximal and distal segments of cerebral arteries. The changes of haematocrit, blood viscosity and rheological properties of blood lead to the alteration of Doppler parameters.

- indomethacin - the administration of indomethacin leads to the cerebral vasoconstriction with the increase of resistive index. Inadequate use of indomethacin can cause ischaemic damage of brain tissue (Lundel et al., 1986).

- critically ill newborns - in severe arterial hypotension with decreased cardiac output the diastolic blood flow is more affected than systolic blood flow and therefore resistive index of cerebral vessels is increased.

- brain death - the Doppler curve demonstrates diastolic block or reverse diastolic blood flow at cerebral arteries.

2.4.2 Pathologic conditions with decreased resistive index

- hypercapnia - leads to the vasodilatation of cerebral vessels and increased cerebral blood flow. End-diastolic blood flow velocity is increased and resistive index is decreased. When the value of $paCO2$ is more increased, also the systolic blood flow velocity increases (Fisher & Truemper, 1993; Menke et al., 1993).

- hypoxemia, hypoxia - decrease of $paO2$ causes the cerebral vasodilatation (Ausina et al., 1998; Curz et al., 1998; Dings et al., 1996).

- seizures - increased brain metabolism leads to the cerebral vasodilatation

- inflammation - inflammatory brain congestion and the cerebral vasodilatation cause decrease of resistive index.

- asphyxia - hypercapnia, hypoxia, tissue hypoperfusion and acidosis have negative influence on the cerebral circulation. The alteration of cerebral autoregulation is presented. The Doppler curve parameters changes include decrease of resistive index and increase of end-diastolic blood flow velocity.

- idiopathic respiratory distress syndrom - the combination of hypoxia, hypercapnia and arterial hypotension decreases the resistance of cerebral arteries, resistive index is decreased

- increased cardiac output, hypervolemia

- increased central venous pressure - for example pnemothorax and right sided cardiac failure can decrease resistive index of cerebral arteries

- cerebral arteriovenous malformation – the cerebral blood flow is ussualy bidirected with increased end-diastolic blood flow velocity and decreased resistive index.

	EXTRACRANIAL FACTORS	INTRACRANIAL FACTORS
INCREASED RESISTIVE INDEX	hypocapnia, hyperoxia, congenital heart disease with left-right shunt (persistent arterial duct, truncus arteriosus), blood hyperviscosity, increased hematocrit, polyglobulia, indomethacin, severe arterial hypotension, decreased cardiac output, brain death	acute intracranial hypertension (brain injury, cerebral oedema, active hydrocephalus), brain infarction, intraventricular and intracerebral haemorrhage
DECREASED RESISTIVE INDEX	hypercapnia, hypoxemia, hypoxia, seizures, asphyxia, idiopathic respiratory distress syndrom, increased cardiac output, hypervolemia, increased central venous pressure (pnemothorax , right sided cardiac failure)	inflammatory brain tissue congestion, cerebral arteriovenous malformation, seizures

Table 5. Extracranial and intracranial factors that influence Doppler parameters of the cerebral circulation (table – authors)

3. The assessment of cerebral circulation by means of transcranial Doppler ultrasonography in neonatal hydrocephalus

The analysis of Doppler parameters of the cerebral circulation in neonatal and pediatric hydrocephalus remains still disputable. In recent years, the main interest is focused on the monitoring of intracranial biomechanics, analysis of pressure-volume relationship, intracranial compliance, intracranial pressure and changes of cerebral circulation in hydrocephalus. The knowledge and clinical application of pathophysiological mechanisms of hydrocephalus is the base for the improvement of treatment of newborns and children with hydrocephalus.

In generally, there is a good corelation between resistive index, pulsatility index of cerebral vessels and intracranial pressure. The population of newborns is heterogenous. Because of different gestational age and biomechanical properties of head the analysis of relationship between resistive index and intracranial pressure in different subgroups is needed. Imporant is the fact, that during the progression of hydrocephalus occur not only the enlargement of cerebral ventricles and increase of intracranial pressure, but also the main cerebral arteries are stretched, compressed or distorsed (Finn et al., 1990).

The relationship between intracranial pressure and Doppler parameters of cerebral arteries is of a complex nature. Many extracranial and intracranial factors may influence the cerebral blood flow.

The relationship between increased resistive index and increased intracranial pressure in preterm infants with posthaemorrhagic hydrocephalus was first described by Bada et al. (Bada et al., 1982).

The changes of resistive index of anterior cerebral artery in newborns with hydrocephalus was assessed by Hill & Volpe (1982). In 9 from 11 cases with raised intracranial pressure, the dilatation of cerebral ventricles was presented. In all cases the resistive index was increased. The significant decrease of resistive index after the successful drainage procedure was detected.

The study of Fisher & Livingstone (1989) showed increased pulsatility index, significantly decreased end-diastolic blood flow velocity and slight decrease of peak systolic blood flow velocity in anterior cerebral circulation (anterior cerebral artery, middle cerebral artery, internal carotid artery) in pediatric hydrocephalus. The values of Doppler parameters after the drainage procedure with functional internal drainage system were normal. The dilatation of cerebral ventricles (except the width of third ventricle) persisted also after the drainage procedure. There was found no corelation between the size of cerebral ventricles and peak systolic blood flow velocity. The relationship between end-diastolic blood flow velocity and the size of cerebral ventricles was intraindividual. Pulsatility index showed the highest level of corelation with the size of cerebral ventricles. The width of third ventricle seems to be the most sensitive morphological parameter of intracranial volume changes. Anterior cerebral artery and middle cerebral artery are the most sensitive cerebral vessels to the intracranial dynamics (Aaslid, 1984; Fisher & Livingstone, 1989). Also the studies of another authors confirmed the significant increase of pulsatility index of cerebral vessels before the drainage operation and significant decrease of pulsatility index after the drainage procedure (Jindal & Mahapatra, 1998; Nadvi et al., 1994).

Nishimaki et al. (1990) were interested in the changes of resistive index of anterior cerebral artery and basilar artery in children with hydrocephalus. There was increased resistive index of both arteries before the drainage procedure. The successful drainage operation led to the significant decrease of resistive index of anterior cerebral artery and basilar artery. The decrease of resistive index of anterior cerebral artery was significantly higher than decrease of resistive index of basilar artery. Normal values of resistive index of anterior cerebral artery in children are lower than the values of resistive index of basilar artery. The difference between the haemodynamic changes of anterior cerebral artery and basilar artery can be caused by the anatomical localisation of vessels. The anterior cerebral artery has close relationship to the lateral cerebral ventricles and third ventricle, basilar artery is localised in pontine cistern. In most cases of pediatric hydrocephalus, the progressive dilatation of lateral cerebral ventricles and third ventricle is greater than the dilatation of fourth ventricle. Therefore authors suggest, that the enlargement of cerebral ventricles in hydrocephalus affects more haemodynamic parameters of the anterior cerebral artery than basilar artery.

Quinn & Pople (1992) in their study confirmed increased pulsatility index in the cases of malfunction of ventriculoperitoneal shunt in children with hydrocephalus. After revision surgery the pulsatility index decreased. The change of the dilatation of cerebral ventricles was detected only in 10 from 32 patients with malfunction of ventriculoperitoneal shunt. In spite of stable dilatation of cerebral ventricles, there were presented clinical signs of intracranial hypertension and an increase of pulsatility index before the revision surgery.

Goh et al. (1991) studied the corelation between resistive index of cerebral arteries and intracranial pressure in newborns and children with hydrocephalus. There was found good intraindividual corelation between the resistive index and intracranial pressure in newborns, whereas in older children the corelation between resistive index and intracranial pressure was good in generally. The differences between age groups are probably caused by highly individual volume-pressure compensation mechanisms in newborns in different stages of hydrocephalus and different compliance of neonatal head (biomechanical and fibroelastic properties of bones, sutures and soft tissue of head). The intracranial dynamics in older children is more uniform, therefore the corelation of resistive index of cerebral arteries and intracranial pressure is generally good. There was found significant decrease of resistive index and increase of end-diastolic blood flow velocity after the drainage procedure in all age groups, but only in newborns was detected moderate increase of peak systolic blood flow velocity and mean blood flow velocity. The same haemodynamic Doppler changes of cerebral vessels were found in the cases of shunt malfunction and after the successful revision surgery.

Goh et al. (1995) in their study confirmed, that there was no increase of resistive index of cerebral vessels in newborns with hydrocephalus in the cases of stable dilatation of cerebral ventricles. The results of the study suggest, that the increase of resistive index of cerebral arteries is caused by raised intracranial pressure and not by enlargement of cerebral ventricles alone.

In spite of detection of increased values of resistive index of cerebral vessels there was found also altered CO2 cerebral vasoreactivity in children with hydrocephalus with the need of drainage procedure. After the insertion of shunt or revision surgery for shunt malfunction, the improvement of CO2 cerebral vasoreactivity was confirmed (De Oliveira & Machado, 2003).

Vajda et al. (1999) found the significant decrease of pulsatility index of middle cerebral artery in children with obstructive hydrocephalus after successful endoscopic third ventriculostomy in relationship to the preoperative value. The function of ventriculostomy was confirmed by the detection of cerebrospinal fluid flow by means of magnetic resonance imaging. The clinical symptomatology improved in 17 from 22 patients. There was found no corelation between the pulsatility index and the age and sex of children. The results of this study show the role of transcranial Doppler sonography in the indirect assessment of the function of endoscopic third ventriculostomy in the early postoperative period.

Cosan et al. (2000) analysed the haemodynamic changes of cerebral circulation in neonatal rats with progressive communicating hydrocephalus by means of transcranial Doppler ultrasonography. There was confirmed, than in the acute phase of hydrocephalus, the dilatation of cerebral ventricles was not accompanied by the alteration of Doppler parameters of cerebral vessels (the value of pulsatility index was normal). During the progression of communicating hydrocephalus an increase of the size of cerebral ventricles and an increase of pulsatility index occured. The enlargement of cerebral ventricles alone in the initial phase of communicating neonatal hydrocephalus did not lead to the changes of pulsatility index of cerebral vessels. The alteration of Doppler parameters of cerebral vessels (increased pulsatility index, decreased end-diastolic blood flow velocity) occured in the phase of progression with increased intracranial pressure. In this phase, the cerebral circulation is more affected by increased intracranial pressure than by the dilatation of cerebral ventricles. The raised intracranial pressure leads to the compression of brain capillaries and increase of vascular resistance of cerebral arteries with increased pulsatility index (Cosan et al., 2000; Seibert et al., 1989). In the chronic phase of hydrocephalus, the enlargement of cerebral ventricles and haemodynamic changes of cerebral circulation are accompanied by several pathologic changes (Del Bigio, 1993).

Taylor et al. (1994) analysed the anterior fontanelle compressive test as a part of the examination of newborns with altered intracranial compliance by means of transcranial Doppler sonography. Basal and compressive values of resistive index of middle cerebral artery were measured. The basal resistive index in the preterm newborns and term newborns with altered intracranial compliance was significantly higher than in healthy term newborns. There was only a minimal change of basal resistive index during the anterior compressive test in healthy preterm and term newborns. In newborns with altered intracranial compliance, the value of resistive index during the compressive test was increased. In newborns with hydrocephalus with increased intracranial pressure, increased values of basal resistive index were detected. After the drainage procedure, the haemodynamic response on anterior fontanelle compression was improved.

In another study Taylor et al. (1996) assessed the haemodynamic response of anterior cerebral artery on anterior fontanelle compression in newborns with hydrocephalus. The results suggest, that the significant increase of resistive index was found in newborns with increased intracranial pressure with the need of drainage procedure.

Also the study of another authors confirmed increased basal and compressive values of resistive index of anterior cerebral artery in children with hydrocephalus in the cases of increased intracranial pressure. After the successful drainage procedure, the significant decrease of basal and compressive values of resistive index was found. The borderline value of basal resistive index of anterior cerebral artery was defined as 0,70, for positive anterior compressive test as 0,90 or increase of basal resistive index more than 25% (Westra et al., 1998).

Gera et al. (2002) were interested in the assessment of Doppler parameters of anterior cerebral artery in newborns and children with hydrocephalus in relationship to the need of drainage procedure. There was found a significant increase of basal and compressive resistive index in patients with the need of drainage operation. After the drainage procedure, the significant decrease of basal and compressive resistive index was detected. The results of the study suggest significant increase of intracranial compliance after the drainage procedure. There was no significant change of head circumference after surgery. The importance of the assessment of resistive index of anterior cerebral artery in newborns and children with hydrocephalus in relationship to the need of drainage procedure was defined: basal resistive index - sensitivity 72,5%, specificity 80%, diagnostic accuracy 75%, false negativity 25%, compressive resistive index - sensitivity 75%, specificity 100%, diagnostic accuracy 83,3%, false negativity 25%.

The asessment of Doppler parameters of cerebral vessels in premature newborns with hydrocephalus is still disputable. The results of published studies are sometimes different and incoherent. The reason for this discrepancy can be the use of different type of sonographic equipment, method of sonographic examination, heterogenity of the group of premature newborns (gestational age, weight, extracranial factors, medication, number of patients) and different indication for drainage procedure.

Perlman & Volpe (1982) analysed the Doppler parameters of anterior cerebral artery in 32 premature newborns with intraventricular haemorrhage. The gestational age of premature newborns was in the range from 26 to 34 weeks. There was found no corelation between intraventricular haemorrhage and resistive index of anterior cerebral artery. In 29 cases, the intraventricular haemorrhage was not accompanied by the decrease of cerebral blood flow velocity. There was no corelation betwen the time of the onset of intraventricular haemorrhage and the value of resistive index. In 9 cases with pneumothorax, the significant decrease of resistive index was detected. Another authors described increased value of resistive index (more than 0,90) of cerebral arteries in premature newborns with intraventricular haemorrhage.

Van Bel et al. (1988) analysed the Doppler parameters of anterior cerebral artery in 10 premature newborns with posthaemorrhagic hydrocephalus. There was found a significantly increased pulsatility index and peak systolic blood flow velocity before the drainage procedure. After the drainage procedure, a significant decrease of pulsatility index and peak systolic blood flow velocity was detected. The values of postoperative pulsatility index were normal. There were found no significant changes of end-diastolic blood flow velocity and mean blood flow velocity before and after the drainage procedure. The increase of pulsatility index before the surgery was caused by an increase of peak systolic blood flow velocity. The reason for the earliest indication of drainage procedure was the reduction of the damage of cerebral circulation. The indication criterion included the progressive dilatation of cerebral ventricles with increased size more than 97th percentil. The same results were published by Alvisi et al. (1985). Authors suggest, that the increase of peak systolic blood flow velocity before the drainage procedure is caused by the dislocation and compression of anterior cerebral artery by enlarged cerebral ventricles. The transport of cerebrospinal fluid into the white matter also causes the loss of transmural pressure gradient (Alvisi et al., 1985; Weller & Shulman, 1972; Wozniak et al., 1975).

The frequency and timing of intermitent drainage of cerebrospinal fluid in newborns with posthaemorrhagic hydrocephalus is still the topic of discussion. One of the aims of intermitent drainage of cerebrospinal fluid is the prevention of negative influence of raised intracranial pressure on cerebral circulation.

Kempley & Gamsu (1993) assessed the changes of intracranial pressure and Doppler parameters of anterior cerebral artery in the group of 6 newborns with posthaemorrhagic hydrocephalus before and after the drainage of cerebrospinal fluid (23 drainage procedures). There was found significant decrease of intracranial pressure after the derivation of cerebrospinal fluid. The decrease of intracranial pressure was accompanied by an increase of mean blood flow velocity and decrease of pulsatility index. The results of the study suggest, that the derivation of cerebrospinal fluid in newborns with posthaemorrhagic hydrocephalus leads to the significant improvement of haemodynamic parameters of cerebral circulation. Authors recommend, that the alteration of Doppler parameters of cerebral vessels should be taken in the consideration in the indication and timing of drainage procedure in newborns with posthaemorrhagic hydrocephalus.

Also the results of the study by Nishimaki et al. (2004) confirmed an increase of resistive index of anterior cerebral artery before the drainage procedure in newborns with posthaemorrhagic hydrocephalus. The drainage procedure, lumbar punction or punction of subcutaneous reservoir, with the aspiration of cerebrospinal fluid (5-10 ml/kg) led to the significant decrease of resistive index.

Maertzdorf et al. (2002) analysed the Doppler parameters of anterior cerebral artery and middle cerebral artery in premature newborns with posthaemorrhagic hydrocephalus. The authors performed repeated aspiration of cerebrospinal fluid from the subcutaneous reservoir. The increased resistive index and decreased end-diastolic blood flow velocity was confirmed in the cases of increased intracranial pressure (≥ 6cm H2O) before the aspiration of cerebrospinal fluid. After the derivation of cerebrospinal fluid with a decrease of intracranial pressure (≤ 6cm H2O), a significant increase of end-diastolic blood flow velocity and decrease of resistive index was found. There was no significant change of peak systolic blood flow velocity after the drainage procedure. The results of the study suggest a good intraindividual corelation between the resistive index of anterior cerebral artery and middle cerebral artery and intracranial pressure in premature newborns with posthaemorrhagic hydrocephalus.

The qualitative indices of Doppler waveform (resistive index, pulsatility index) have certain disadvantages. Both indices are influenced by the heart rate and have a broad range of reference values, especially in children. Hanlo et al. (1995a) presented a hydrodynamic model, which showed the effects of raised intracranial pressure on the cerebral circulation. The authors defined a new Doppler index, the trans-systolic time, reflecting specific changes in the Doppler waveform induced by changes in the intracranial pressure.

Leliefeld et al. (2009) analysed the relationship between the trans-systolic time of Doppler waveform of middle cerebral artery and intracranial pressure in infants with hydrocephalus.

There was found significant decrease of the intracranial pressure after the drainage procedure ($p<0.005$), accompanied by the significant increase of trans-systolic time ($p<0.005$), significant decrease of pulsatility index ($p<0.05$) and significant decrease of resistive index ($p<0.05$). Trans-systolic time has a strong correlation with the intracranial pressure ($p<0.005$). Trans-systolic time reflects the relative changes in the cerebral blood flow velocity caused by intracranial dynamics changes. The results of the study suggest, that the trans-systolic time has a closer relation to intracranial pressure than the pulsatility index and the resistive index.

The changes of Doppler parameters of pericallosal artery before and after the drainage procedure in preterm newborn with posthaemorrhagic hydrocephalus are shown in Figures 4-7.

Transcranial Doppler ultrasonography plays an important role in the management of newborn with hydrocephalus. Is widely used because of it´s noninvasivity, repeatability and the possibility of bedside examination. The clinical applications of transcranial Doppler ultrasonography in the management of neonatal hydrocephalus include:

- the indication and timing of drainage procedure
- monitoring of the efficacy of the drainage procedure – shunts, external ventricular drainage, derivation of cerebrospinal fluid from subcutaneous reservoir in

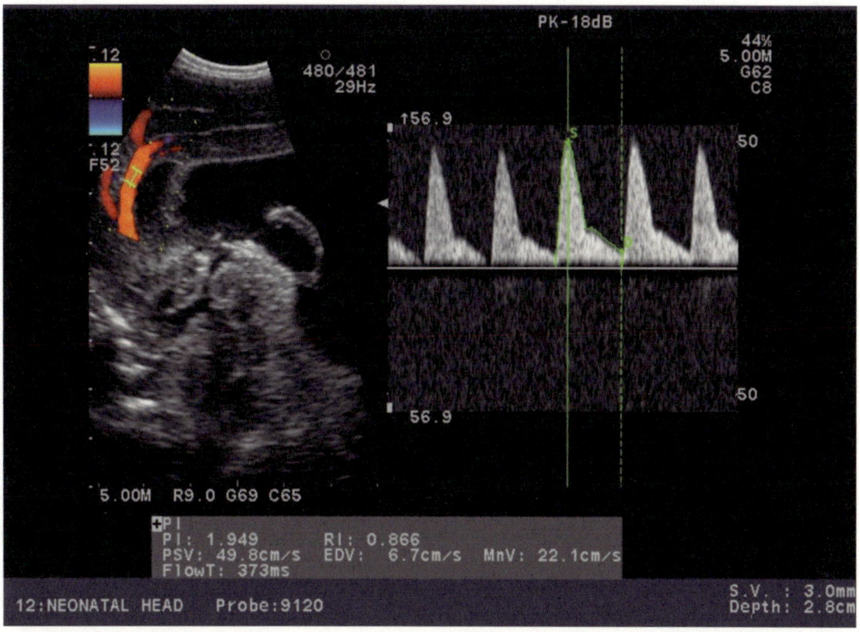

Fig. 4. Basal Doppler parameters of pericallosal artery in preterm newborn with posthaemorrhagic hydrocephalus before the drainage procedure: decreased end-diastolic blood flow velocity, increased resistive index, increased pulsatility index (figure - authors)

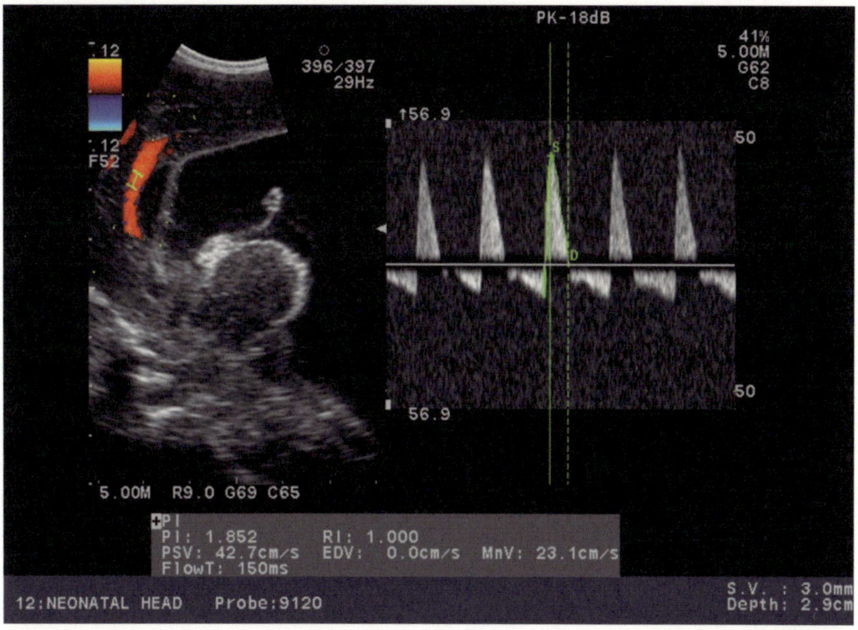

Fig. 5. Positive anterior fontanelle compressive test, compressive Doppler parameters of pericallosal artery in preterm newborn with posthaemorrhagic hydrocephalus before the drainage procedure -reverse end-diastolic blood flow (figure - authors)

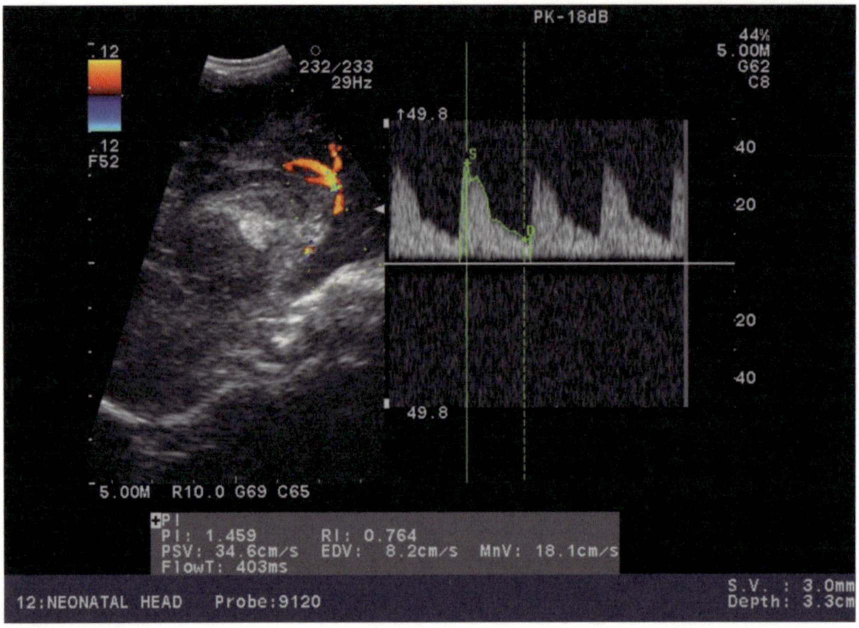

Fig. 6. Basal Doppler parameters of pericallosal artery in preterm newborn with posthaemorrhagic hydrocephalus after the drainage procedure: increased end-diastolic blood flow velocity, decreased resistive index, decreased pulsatility index (figure - authors)

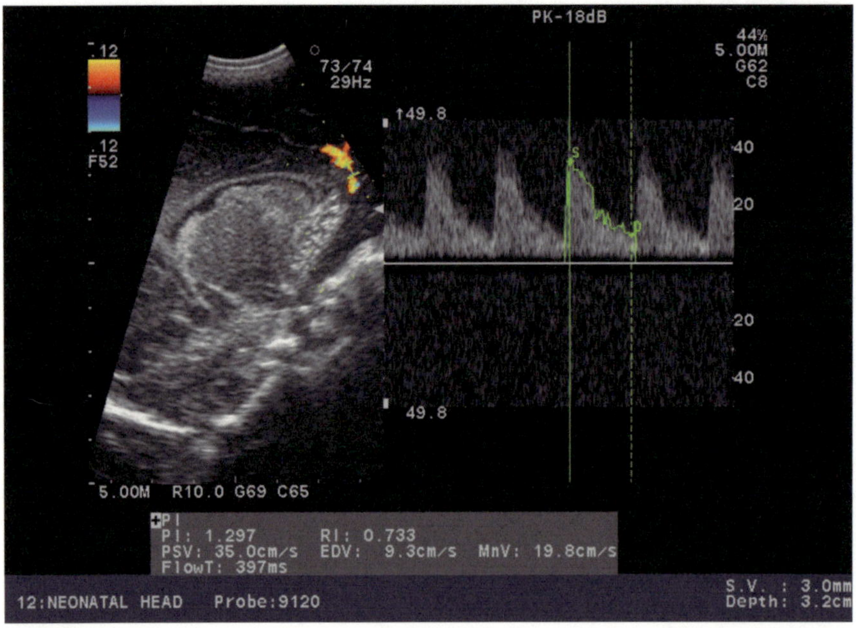

Fig. 7. Negative anterior fontanelle compressive test, compressive Doppler parameters of pericallosal artery in preterm newborn with posthaemorrhagic hydrocephalus after the drainage procedure (figure - authors)

posthaemorrhagic hydrocephalus (frequency and the volume of derivated cerebrospinal fluid), endoscopic third ventriculostomy
- monitoring of the function and the detection of malfunction of internal (shunts) and external drainage systems (external ventricular drainage) and endoscopic third ventriculostomy
- detection of shunt-dependency of newborn with hydrocephalus - the change of external ventricular drainage or subcutaneous reservoir to the shunt, the need of revision surgery of the shunt with malfunction

4. Conclusion

Increased intracranial pressure in progressive neonatal hydrocephalus leads to the alteration of cerebral circulation (decreased cerebral blood flow, hypoperfusion and ischaemia). Transcranial color coded Doppler sonography provides a noninvasive method of monitoring of the blood flow velocities in cerebral vessels. In generall, there is a good corelation between the increase of intracranial pressure and changes in Doppler curve parameters. Before the drainage procedure there was confirmed increased basal and compressive values of resistive index and pulsatility index of cerebral arteries. After the successful drainage procedure, the significant decrease of basal and compressive values of resistive index and pulsatility index was found.

The published studies and clinical experiences confirm, that transcranial Doppler ultrasonography can be routinely used as a noninvasive method for the monitoring of cerebral circulation, indirect monitoring of intracranial pressure and compliance with good clinical applications in the indication of drainage procedure or the monitoring of the function of drainage systems and endoscopic third ventriculostomy in newborns with hydrocephalus.

5. Acknowledgment

This work was supported by project „Center of Excellence of Perinatology Research (CEPV II)", ITMS code: 26220120036, which is co-financed by EU sources.

6. References

Aaslid, R., Hubert, P., & Nornes, H. (1984). Evaluation of cerebrovascular spasm with transcranial Doppler ultrasound. *J Neurosurg*, Vol. 60, No. 1, (January 1984), pp. 37-41

Aaslid, R., Markwalder, TM., & Nornes, H. (1982). Noninvasive transcranial Doppler ultrasound recording of flow velocity in basal cerebral arteries. *J Neurosurg*,Vol. 57, No. 6, (December 1982), pp. 769-774

Alvisi C., Cerisoli M., Giulioni M., Monari P., Salvioli GP., Sandri F., Lippi C., Bovicelli L., & Pilu G. (1985). Evaluation of cerebral blood flow changes by transfontanelle Doppler ultrasound in infantile hydrocephalus. *Childs Nerv Syst*, Vol. 1, No. 5, (November 1985), pp. 244-247

Ausina, A., Baquena, M., Nadal, M., Manrique, S., Ferrer, A., Sahuquillo, J., & Garnacho, A. (1998). Cerebral haemodynamic changes during sustained hypocapnia in severe head injury: can hyperventilation cause cerebral ischemia? *Acta Neurochir Suppl,* Vol. 71, (1998), pp. 1-4

Babikian, VL. & Wechsler, LR. (1993). *Transcranial doppler ultrasonography* (1st edition), Mosby-Year Book Inc., St. Louis, USA

Bada, HS., Hajjar, W., Chua, C., & Summer, DS. (1979). Noninvasive diagnosisof neonatal asphyxia and intraventricular hemorrhage by Doppler ultrasound. *J Pediat,* Vol. 95, No. 5, (November 1979), pp. 775-779

Bada, HS., Miller, JE., Menke, JA., Menten, TG., Bashiru, MSM., Binstadt, D., Sumnera, DS., & Khanna, NN. (1982). Intracranial pressure and cerebral arterial pulsatile flow measurements in neonatal intraventricular haemorrhage. *J Pediatr,* Vol. 100, No. 2, (February 1982), pp. 291-296

Barzo, P., Doczi, T., Csete, K., Buza, Z., & Bodosi, M. (1991). Measurements of regional cerebral blood flow and blood flow velocity in experimental intracranial hypertension: infusion via the cisterna magna in rabbits, *Neurosurgery,* Vol. 28, No. 6, (June 1991), pp. 821-825

Bissonnette, B. & Benson, LN. (1998). Closure of persistently patent arterial duct and its impact on cerebral circulatory haemodynamics in children, *Can J Anaesth,* Vol. 45, No. 3, (March 1998), pp. 199-205

Bode, H. & Wais, U. (1988). Age dependence of flow velocities in basal cerebral arteries, *Arch Dis Child,* Vol. 63, No. 6, (June 1988), pp. 606-611

Bode, H. (1988). *Pediatric applications of transcranial Doppler sonography* (1st edition), Springer-Verlag, Vienna, Austria

Brouwers, PJAM., Vriens, EM., Musbach, M., Wieneke, GH., & Van Huffelen, AC. (1990). Transcranial pulsed Doppler measurements of blood flow velocity in the middle cerebral artery: reference values at rest and during hyperventilation in healthy children and adolescents in relation to age and sex. *Ultrasound Med Biol,* Vol. 16, No. 1, (January 1990), pp. 1-8

Chadduck, WM. & Seibert, JJ. (1989). Intracranial duplex Doppler: practical uses in pediatric neurology and neurosurgery. *J Child Neurol,* Vol. 4, Suppl, (January 1989), pp. S77-86

Cosan, TE., Gucuyener, D., Dundar, E., Arslantas, A., Vural, M., Uzuner, K., & Tel, E. (2001).Cerebral blood flow alterations in progressive communicating hydrocephalus: transcranial Doppler assessment in an experimental model. *Journal of Neurosurgery,* Vol. 94, No. 2, (February 2001), pp. 265-269

Cruz, J. (1998). The first decade of continuous monitoring of jugular bulb oxyhemoglobinsaturation: management strategies and clinical outcome. *Crit Care Med,* Vol. 26, No. 2, (February 1998), pp. 344-351

Czernicki, Z. (1992). Use of transcranial Doppler ultrasonography for evaluation of intracranial pressure. *Neurol Neurochir Pol,* Vol. 26, No. 3, (May-June 1992), pp. 375-382

De Oliveira, RS. & Machado, HR. (2003). Transcranial color-coded Doppler ultrasonography for evaluation of children with hydrocephalus. *Neurosurg Focus,* Vol. 15, No. 4, (October 2003), ECP3

De Riggo, J., Kolarovszki, B., Richterova, R., Kolarovszka, H., Sutovsky, J., & Durdik P. (2007). Measurement of the blood flow velocity in the pericallosal artery of children with hydrocephalus by transcranial Doppler ultrasonography-preliminary results.

Biomed Pap Med Fac Univ Palacky Olomouc Czech Repub., Vol. 151, No. 2, (December 2007), pp. 285-289

Deeg, KK. & Rupprecht, TH. (1989). Pulsed Doppler sonographic measurement of normal values for the flow velocities in the intracranial arteries of healthy newborns. *Pediatric Radiology*, Vol. 19, No. 2, (January 1989), pp. 71-78

Del Bigio, MR. (1993). Neuropathological changes caused by hydrocephalus. *Acta Neuropathol*, Vol. 85, No. 6, (May 1993), pp. 573-585

Diehl, B., Stodieck, SR., Diehl, RR., & Ringelstein, EB. (1998). The photic driving EEG response and photoreactive cerebral blood flow in the posterior cerebral artery in controls and patients with epilepsy. *Electroencephalogr Clin Neurophysiol*, Vol. 107, No. 1, (July 1998), pp. 8-12

Dings, J., Meixensberger, J., Amschler, J., Hamelbeck, B., & Roosen, K. (1996). Brain tissue pO2 in relation to cerebral perfusion pressure, TCD findings and TCD-CO2 reactivity after severe head injury. *Acta Neurochir (Wien)*,Vol. 138, No. 4, (April 1996), pp. 425-434

Finn, JP., Quinn, MW., Hall-Craggs, MA., & Kendall BE. Impact of vessel distortion on transcranial Doppler velocity measurements: correlation with magnetic resonance imaging. *J Neurosurg*, Vol. 73, No. 4, (October 1990), pp. 572-575

Fisher, AQ. & Livingstone II, JN. Transcranial Doppler and real-time cranial sonography in neonatal hydrocephalus. *J Child Neurol*, Vol. 4, No. 1, (January 1989), pp. 64-69

Gera, P., Gupta, R., Sailukar, M., Agarwal, P., Parelkar, S., & Oak, S. (2002). Role of transcranial Doppler sonography and pressure provacation test to evaluate the need for cerebrospinal fluid drainage in hydrocephalic children, *Annual Conference of IAPS*, Ahmedabad, 2002

Goh, D., Minns, RA., & Pye, SD. (1991). Transcranial Doppler (TCD) ultrasound as a noninvasive means of monitoring cerebrohaemodynamic change in hydrocephalus. *Eur J Pediatr Surg*, Vol. 1, Suppl I, (December 1991), pp. 14-17

Goh, D. & Minns, RA. (1995). Intracranial pressure and cerebral arterial flow velocity indices in childhood hydrocephalus: current review. *Childs Nerv Syst*, Vol. 11, No. 7, (July 1995), pp. 392-396

Gösling, RG. & King, DH. (1974). Continuous wave ultrasound as an alternative and complement to X-ray in vascular examinations, In: *Cardiovascular applications of ultrasound*, Reneman, RE., pp. 266-282, North-Holland, Amsterdam

Hadač, J. (2000). *Ultrazvukové vyšetření mozku přes velkou fontanelu* (1st edition), Triton, ISBN 80-7254-110-2, Prague, Czech Republic

Hanlo, PW., Peters, RJ., Gooskens, RH., Heethaar, RM., Keunen, RW., van Huffelen, AC., Tulleken, CA., & Willemse J. (1995a). Monitoring intracranial dynamics by transcranial Doppler-a new Doppler index: trans systolic time. *Ultrasound Med Biol*, Vol. 21, No. 5, (1995), pp. 613-621

Hanlo, PW., Gooskens, RH., Nijhuis, IJ., Faber, JA., Peters, RJ., van Huffelen, AC., Tulleken, CA., & Willemse, J. (1995b). Value of transcranial Doppler indices in predicting raised ICP in infantile hydrocephalus. A study with review of literature. *Childs Nerv Syst*, Vol. 11, No. 10, (October 1995), pp. 595-603

Hayashi, T., Ichiyama, T., Uchida, M., Tashiro, N., & Tanaka, H. (1992). Evaluation by colour Doppler and pulsed Doppler sonography of blood flow velocities in intracranial arteries during the early neonatal period. *Eur J Pediatr,* Vol. 151, No. 6, (June 1992), pp. 461-465

Hill, A. & Volpe, JJ. (1982). Decrease in pulsatile flow in anterior cerebral arteries in infantile hydrocephalus. *Pediatrics,* Vol. 69, No. 1, (January 1982), pp. 4-7

Horgan, JG., Rumack, CM., Hay, T., Manco-Johnson, ML., Merenstein, GB., & Esola, Ch. (1989). Absolute intracranial blood flow velocities evaluated by duplex Doppler sonography in asymptomatic preterm and term neonates. *Am J Roentgenol,* Vol. 152, No. 5, (May 1989), pp. 1059-1064

Jindal, A. & Mahapatra, AK. (1998). Correlation of ventricular size and transcranial Doppler findings before and after ventricular peritoneal shunt in patients with hydrocephalus: prospective study of 35 patients. *J Neurol Neurosurg Psychiatry,* Vol. 65, No. 2, (August 1998), pp. 269-271

Kempley, ST. & Gamsu, HR. (1993). Changes in cerebral artery blood flow velocity after intermittent cerebrospinal fluid drainage. *Arch Dis Child,* Vol. 69, 1 Spec No., (July 1993), pp. 74-76

Kingelhofer, J. & Sander, D. (1992). Doppler CO2 test as an indicator of cerebral vasoreactivity and prognosis in severe intracranial hemorrhages. *Stroke,* Vol. 23, No. 7, (July 1992), pp. 962-966

Kopniczky, Z., Barzo, P., Pavics, L., Doczi, T., Bodosi, M., & Csernay, L. (1995). Our policy in diagnosis and treatment of hydrocephalus. *Childs Nerv Syst,* Vol. 11, No. 2, (February 1995), pp. 102-106

Leliefeld PH., Gooskens RH., Peters RJ., Tulleken CA., Kappelle LJ., Han KS., Regli L., & Hanlo PW. (2009). New transcranial Doppler index in infants with hydrocephalus: transsystolic time in clinical practice. *Ultrasound Med Biol,* Vol. 35, No 10, (October 2009), pp. 1601-1606

Lundell BP., Sonesson SE., & Cotton RB. (1986). Ductus closure in preterm infants. Effects on cerebral hemodynamics. *Acta Paediatr Scand,* Vol. 329, Suppl., (1986), pp. 140-147

Macko, RF., Ameriso, SF., Akmal, M., Hill., AP., Mohler, JG., Massry, SG., Meiselman, HJ., & Fisher, M. (1993). Arterial oxygen content and age are determinants of middle cerebral artery blood flow velocity. *Stroke,* Vol. 24, No. 7, (July 1993), pp. 1025-1028

Maertzdorf, WJ., Vles, JS., Beuls, E., Mulder, ALM, & Blanco, CE. (2002). Intracranial pressure and cerebral blood flow velocity in preterm infants with posthaemorrhagic ventricular dilatation. *Arch Dis Child Fetal Neonatal Ed,* Vol. 87, No. 3, (November 2002), pp. 185-188

Menke, J., Michel, E., Rabe, H., Bresser, W., Grohs, B., Schidtt, M., & Jorch, G. (1993). Simultaneous influence of blood flow pressure, pCO2, pO2 on cerebral blood flow velocity in preterm infants of less than 33 weeks gestatio. *Pediat Res,* Vol. 34, No. 2, (August 1993), pp. 173-177

Miller, JD., Smith, RR., & Holaday, HR. (1992). Carbon dioxide reactivity in the evaluation of cerebral ischemia. *Neurosurgery,* Vol. 30, No. 4, (April 1992), pp. 518-521

Minarik, M. (2000). *Transkraniálna farebná duplexná sonografia dojčiat* (1st edition), Osveta, ISBN 80-8063-041-0, Martin, Slovak Republic

Myers, TF., Patrinos, ME., Muraskas, J., Caldwell, CC., Lambert, GH., & Anderson, CL. (1987). Dynamic trend monitoring of cerebral blood flow velocity in newborn infants. *J Pediatr,* Vol. 110, No. 4, (April 1987), pp. 611-616

Nadvi, SS., Du Trevou, MD., Vandelen, JR., & Gouws E. (1994). The use of TCD ultrasonography as a method of assessing ICP in hydrocephalic children. *Br J Neurosurg,* Vol. 8, No. 5, (January 1994), pp. 573-577

Nishimaki, S., Iwasaki, Y., & Akamatsu, H. (2004). Cerebral blood flow velocity before and after cerebrospinal fluid drainage in infants with posthemorrhagic hydrocephalus. *J Ultrasound Med,* Vol. 23, No. 10, (October 2004), pp. 1315-1319

Nishimaki, S., Yoda, H., Seki, K., Kawakami, T., Akamatsu, H., & Iwasaki, Y. (1990). Cerebral blood flow velocities in the anterior cerebral arteries and basilar artery in hydrocephalus before and after treatment. *Surg Neurol,* Vol. 34, No. 6, (December 1990), pp. 373-377

Owega, A., Klingelhofer, J., Sabri, O., Kunert, HJ., Albers, M., & Sass, H. (1998). Cerebral blood flow velocity in acute schizophrenic patients. A transcranial Doppler ultrasonography study. *Stroke,* Vol. 29, No. 6, (June 1998), pp. 1149-1154

Ozek, E., Koroglu, TF., & Karakoc, F. (1995). Transcranial Doppler assessment of cerebral blood flow velocity in term newborns. *Eur J Pediatr,* Vol. 154, No. 1, (January 1995), pp. 60-63

Perlman, JM. & Volpe, JJ. (1982). Cerebral blood flow velocity in relation to intraventricular hemorrhage in the premature newborn infant. *J Pediatr,* Vol. 100, No. 6, (June 1982), pp. 956-959

Perlman, JM. & Volpe, JJ. (1985). Episodes of apnea and bradycardia in preterm newborn: impact on cerebral circulatio. *Pediatrics,* Vol. 76, No. 3, (September 1985), pp. 333-338

Perlman, JM. & Volpe, JJ. (1983). Suctioning in the preterm infant: Effects on cerebral blood flow velocity and arterial blood pressure. *Pediatrics,* Vol. 72, No. 3, (September 1983), pp. 329-334

Pourcelot, L. (1975). Applications cliniques de l'examen Doppler transcutané, In: *Vélocimétrie ultrasonore Doppler,* Peronneau, P., pp. 213-240, INSERM, Paris, France

Quinn, MV. & Pople, JK. (1992). MCA pulsatility in children with blocked CSF shunt. *J Neurol Neurosurg Psychiatry,* Vol. 55, No. 4, (April 1992), pp. 325-327

Roberts, AE. & McKinney, WM. (1998). Blood flow velocities in three cerebral arteries in the same subject modulate during thinking. *J Neuroimaging,* Vol. 8, No. 4, (October 1998), pp. 191-196

Seibert, JJ., McCowan, TC., Chadduck, WM., Adametz, JR., Glasier, ChM., Williamson, SL., Taylor, BJ., Leithiser, RE., Jr., McConnell, JR., Stansell, CA., Rodgers, AB., & Corbitt, SL. (1989). Duplex pulsed Doppler US versus intracranial pressure in the neonate: clinical and experimetal studies. *Radiology,* Vol. 171, No. 1, (April 1989), pp. 155-159

Shortland, DB., Gibson, NA., Levene, MI., Archer, LNJ., Evans, DH., & Shaw, DE. (1990). Patent ductus arteriosus and cerebral circulation in preterm infants. *Development Med Child Neurol,* Vol. 32, No. 5, (May 1990), pp. 386-393

Schöning, M. & Hartig, B. (1996). Age dependence of total cerebral blood flow volume from childhood to adulthood. *J Cereb Blood Flow Metab,* Vol. 16, No. 5, (September 1996), pp. 827-833

Stuart, B., Drumm, J., Fitzgerald, DE., & Duignan, NM. (1980). Fetal blood velocity waveforms in normal pregnancy. *Br J Obstet Gynaecol,* Vol. 87, No.9 (September 1980), pp. 780-785

Taylor, GA. & Madsen, JR. (1996). Neonatal hydrocephalus: hemodynamic response to fontanelle compression - correlation with intracranial pressure and need for shunt placement. *Radiology,* Vol. 201, No. 3, (December 1996), pp. 685-689

Taylor, GA., Phillips, MD., Ichord, RN., Carson, BS., Gates, JA., & James, CS. (1994). Intracranial compliance in infants: evaluation with Doppler US. *Radiology,* Vol. 191, No. 3, (June 1994), pp. 787-791

Vajda, Z., Büki, A., Vető, F., Horváth, Z., Sándor, J., & Dóczi, T. (1999). Transcranial Doppler-determined pulsatility index in the evaluation of endoscopic third ventriculostomy (preliminary data). *Acta Neurochir (Wien),* Vol. 141, No. 3, (March 1999), pp. 247-250

Van Bel, F., van de Bor, M., Baan, J., Stijnen, T., & Ruys, JH. (1988). Blood flow velocity pattern of the anterior cerebral arteries. *J Ultrasound Med,* Vol. 7, No. 10, (October 1988), pp. 553-559

Vergesslich, KA., Weninger, M., Ponhold, W., & Simbruner, G. (1989). Cerebral blood flow in newborn infants with and without mechanical ventilation. *Pediatr Radiol,* Vol. 19, No. 8, (September 1989), pp.509-512

Weller, RO, & Shulman, K. (1972). Infantile hydrocephalus: Clinical, histological and ultrastructural study of brain damage. *J Neurosurg,* Vol. 36, No. 3, (March 1972), pp. 255-265

Westra, SJ., Lazareff, J., Curran, JG., Sayere, JW., & Kawamoto, H., Jr. (1998). Transcranial Doppler ultrasonography to evaluate need for cerebrospinal fluid drainage in hydrocephalic children. *J Ultrasound Med,* Vol. 17, No. 9, (September 1998), pp. 561-569

Wozniak, M., McLone, DG., & Raimondi, AJ. (1975). Micro- and macrovascular changes as a direct cause of parenchymal destruction in congenital murine hydrocephalus. *J Neurosurg,* Vol. 43, No. 5, (November 1975), pp. 535-545

Wright, LL., Baker, KR., Hollander, DI., Wright, JN., & Nagey DA. (1988). Cerebral blood flow velocity in term newborn infants: changes associated with ductal flow. *J Pediatr,* Vol. 112, No. 5, (May 1988), pp. 768-773

Wyatt, JS., Edwards, AD., Cope, M., Delpy, DT., McCormick, DC., Potter, A., & Reynolds, EO. (1991). Response of cerebral blood volume to change in arterial carbon dioxide tension in preterm and term infants. *Pediatr Res,* Vol. 29, No. 6, (June 1991), pp. 553-557

10

Novel Method for Controlling Cerebrospinal Fluid Flow and Intracranial Pressure by Use of a Tandem Shunt-Valve System

Yasuo Aihara
Department of Neurosurgery, Tokyo Women's Medical University, Tokyo, Japan

1. Introduction

In general, cerebrospinal fluid (CSF) shunt valves control the intracranial pressure rather than fluid flow or other aspects. [1-4] There are various kinds of shunt valves including fixed pressure and programmable valves. Fixed pressure valves usually have low, medium or high pressure settings. The choice of valve pressure is based on preoperative intracranial pressure, clinical course, cerebral ventricle size, age, and the lifestyle of the patient.[5-8]

Programmable valves with or without anti-siphon devices were subsequently developed. [9-16] CSF flow is regulated by adjusting the pressure via a magnetically-controlled valve. However, CSF dynamics are complicated because production and absorption rates of CSF may vary in any given patient. Consequently, the existing shunt systems cannot correspond to each of these situations. With regard to intracranial pressure; treatment *in vivo* involves not only setting the shunt's valve pressure but also taking into consideration the CSF flow rate; which is a very important parameter.[17, 18]. Even with anti-siphon devices attached to some valves, despite their advantages, there is still no perfect valve system in neurosurgery as devices with these attachments still fail to adequately control pressure requirements as well as CSF flow rates at the same time. Practically, we sometimes experience a patient with over-drainage problem even using an anti-siphon device.

To overcome the difficulties of the existing shunt valve systems in achieving adequate CSF pressure and flow control, we contrived a novel tandem shunt valve system. We performed *in vitro* experiments using a manometer, and report the first clinical application of the novel tandem shunt system in humans.

2. Material and methods

An *in vitro* system with a manometer was built to measure pressure and flow rates of water in open and closed systems using the Codman (Codman; Johnson & Johnson Co., Raynham) Hakim programmable valve (CHPV) and the STRATA programmable valve (Medtronic, Inc, Minneapolis) as shown in figures 1 and 2, respectively. Single (Fig. 1a and Fig. 2a) and two single shunt valves (Fig. 1b and Fig. 2b) connected in series (the tandem shunt system) were connected to the manometer to check the pressure.

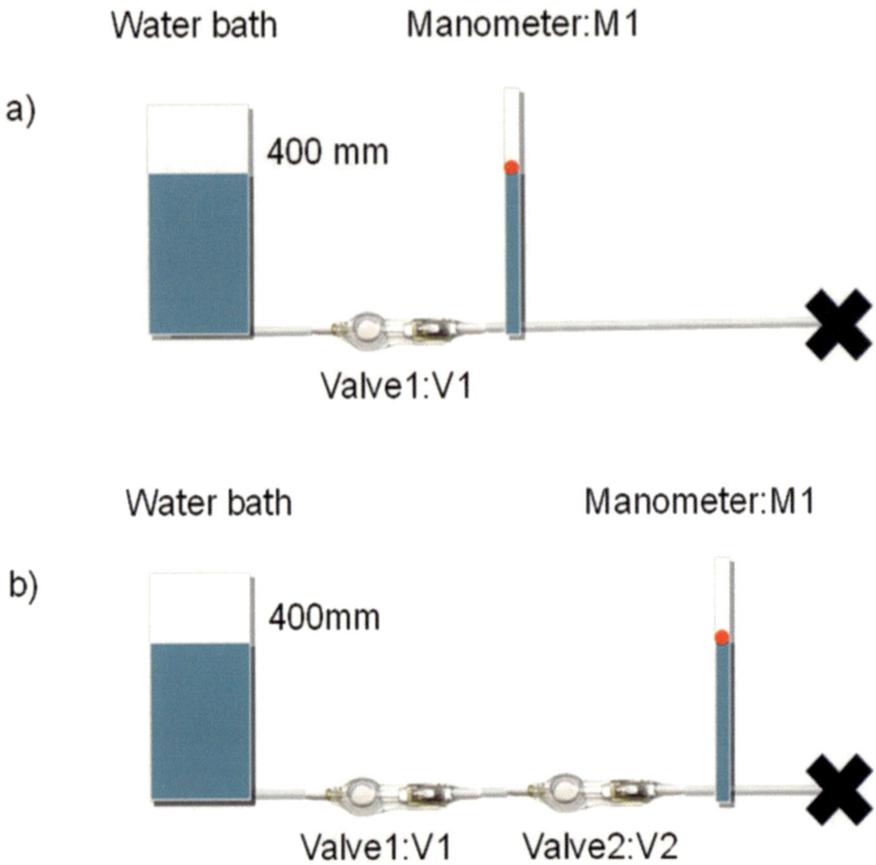

Top (1a): single shunt valve setup with clamp to close the system.
Bottom (2b): closed setup with two shunt valves connected in series (tandem shunt valve system) with clamp to close the system.

Fig. 1. *In Vitro* closed system with Codman (Codman; Johnson & Johnson Co., Raynham) Hakim programmable valves (CHPV)

2.1 In vitro closed system with water bath (Fig. 1)

In the closed single shunt valve system experiment, as shown in figure 1a, we measured the pressure in the original bath to be 400 mmH_2O with a closed valve (V1). We conducted 3 changes to V1, the valve pressure of the CHPV, and took 5 measurements each at V1=50, V1=100 and V1=200. Figure 1b shows the setup in a closed tandem shunt valve system. If we set V1=50 and V2=50, the total pressure setting of the valves (V) is V1 + V2 = 100. Other combinations of V1 and V2 were taken and six are reported below.

2.2 In vitro open system with manometer (Fig. 2)

An open system represents the real world environment. Unlike figure 1a and figure 1b, figure 2 does not have a clamp at the endpoint to keep the system closed. In our experiment we have the STRATA valve directly connected to the manometer and a scale at the other

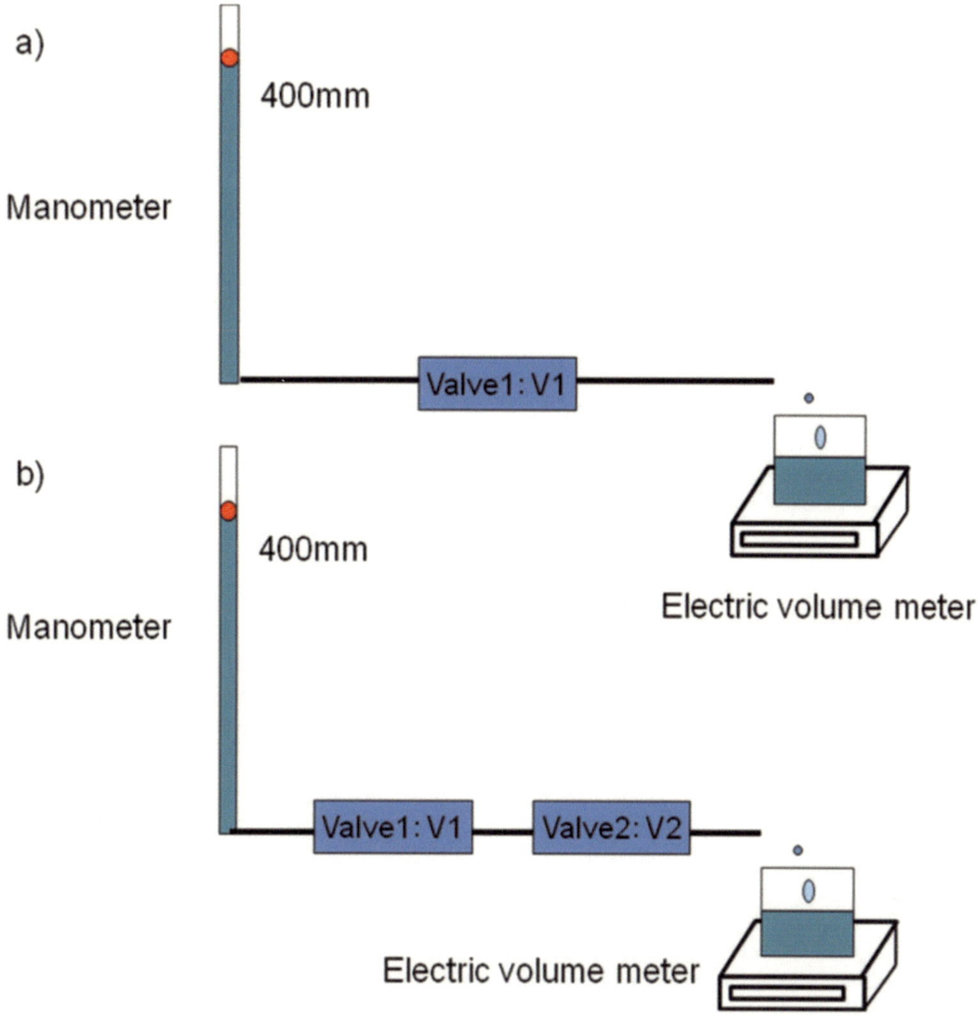

Top (2a): Manometer connected to the single shunt valve with a scale on the opposite end to measure volume of water over time.
Bottom (2b): the inclusion of another STRATA shunt valve connected in series was the only change made to the system.

Fig. 2. *In Vitro* Open system with STRATA programmable valves (Medtronic, Inc, Minneapolis)

end to measure the volume of water as seen in figure 2. In our single valve open system experiment the manometer was set to 400 mmH_2O and the STRATA valve used had 5 programmable settings (0.5, 1.0, 1.5, 2.0, and 2.5). These are referred to as performance levels (PL) by STRATA and we took manometer readings at each PL. An electric flow meter was also used to measure the volume of water every 30 seconds for each PL. The same measurements for the open tandem shunt valve system (Fig. 2b) were also taken but for different combinations of PLs. This experiment helped us illustrate the effects of a tandem shunt valve system in hydrocephalus cases.

3. Results

3.1 In vitro closed system with water bath

In the single shunt valve system experiment, when V1 was adjusted to 50, the final measurement in the manometer equaled around 350 mmH_2O (Fig. 3a). When V1=100, the final manometer reading was around 300 mmH_2O. Subsequently a V1 adjustment of 200 resulted in a final manometer reading of around 200 mmH_2O. Based on these results, we can conclude that the original water bath pressure = V1 pressure value + final manometer value (M1) as shown in figure 3a, where the average results of 5 measurements at (V1=50, 100 and 200) were taken. In the closed tandem shunt valve system experiment, when the final manometer reading was 300 mmH_2O, the sum of V1 + V2 always equaled around 100. We conducted further experiments that measured five manometer readings at different combinations of V1 and V2 such that (V1 + V2 = 100, 150, 200, 250, 300 and 400) and averaged the results as summarized in figure 3b. Based on our experiment, the final manometer pressure is the original water bath pressure minus (V1+V2). This principal holds for any value of V1 and V2. In conclusion, when two valves (Fig. 1b) are connected in series, regardless of whether one is higher than the other, their sum will always behave in the same way as the one valve in the closed system as shown in figure 1a.

3.2 In vitro open system with manometer

In an open system, at any value of V1, the manometer represents the same value as V1. At PL of 0.5 on the STRATA valve the final manometer reading was approximately 30mmH_2O after we had allowed the system to run for some time. Subsequent PL settings were measured and their final pressure manometer readings are as follow: 1.0≅40 mmH_2O; 1.5≅100 mmH_2O, 2.0≅170 mmH_2O, and 2.5≅200 mmH_2O as seen in the legend of figure 4. Figure 4 also shows the calculated flow rate (ml/min) curve over time. At the highest PL setting of 2.5 we achieved a lower flow rate as expected.

Figure 2b shows two valves connected in series in an open system (tandem system). In our tandem valve open system experiment we varied V1 and V2 and measured the final manometer readings for each combination and a summarized table of results is shown in Table 1. Interestingly, in the tandem system, the final pressure was almost equal to the highest pressure setting of one of the valves in the system. In a single valve system the flow rate changed depending on the valve pressure (Fig. 4). On the other hand, the flow rate in the tandem system depends on the total pressure of each shunt valve setting (Fig. 5). Furthermore, based on our experiments, we concluded that in an open system, along with reducing the flow rate, we discovered that we could control pressure because the final pressure reading on the manometer was always equal to the highest pressure value of either V1 or V2.

We assessed all combinations of tandem shunt valve pressures. The result was that the flow rate depended on the total valve pressure in the system (Fig. 5). Of considerable significance in table 1 is the experiment with STRATA performance level (1.0 + 1.0) and STRATA performance level (2.0). We would expect the final manometer pressure to be the same for these two experiments (because the PL totals are the same) but they are actually 50 mmH_20 and 170 mmH_20, respectively. There are two significant points here 1) flow rate and 2) final

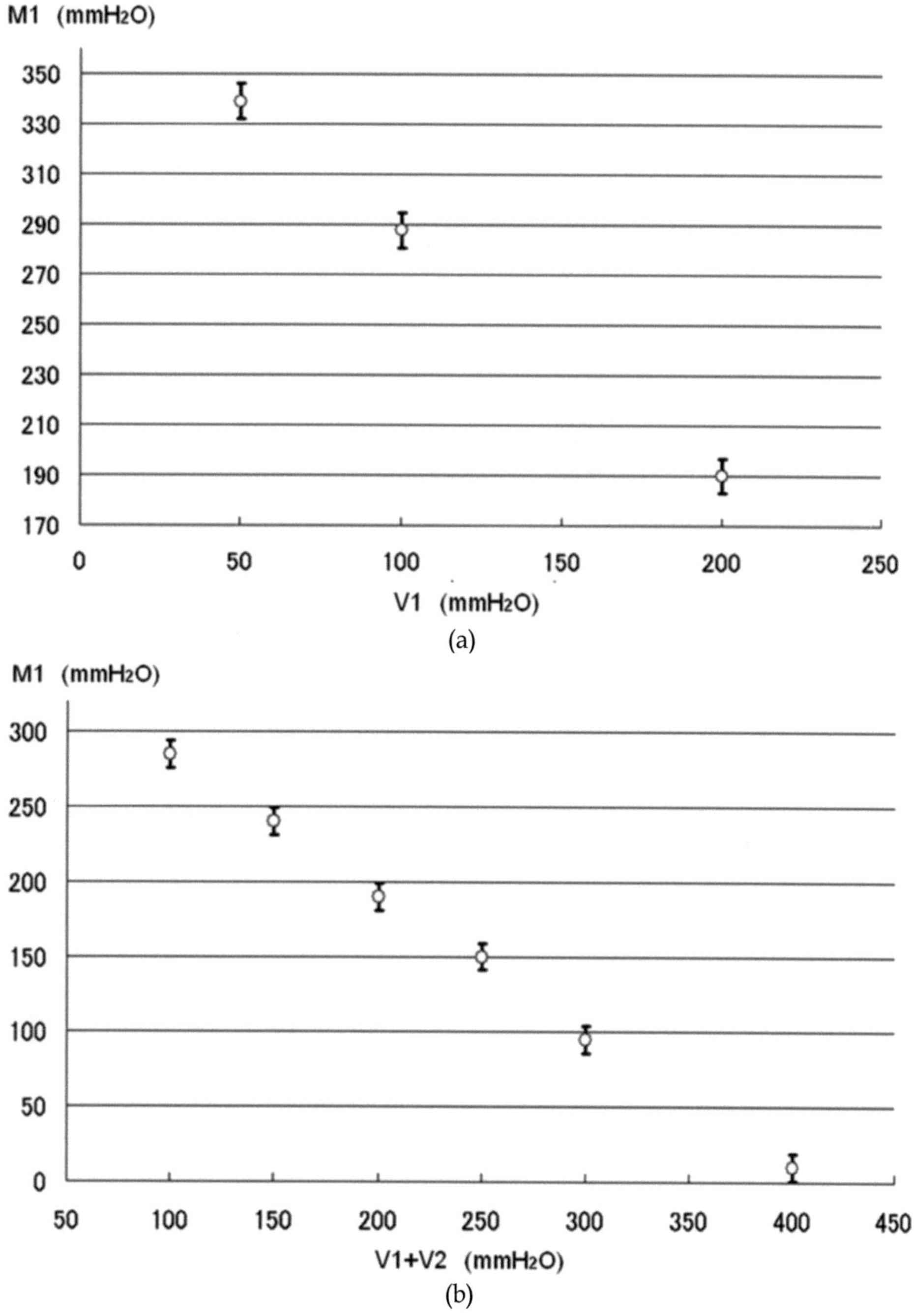

Demonstrating that the original water bath pressure = V1 pressure + final manometer reading (M1). With two valves connected in series, the following relationship continues to exist: original water bath pressure = (V1 pressure + V2 pressure) + final manometer reading (M1).

Fig. 3. (a) Single shunt valve experiment results for the closed system (b) Tandem shunt valve experiment results for the closed system

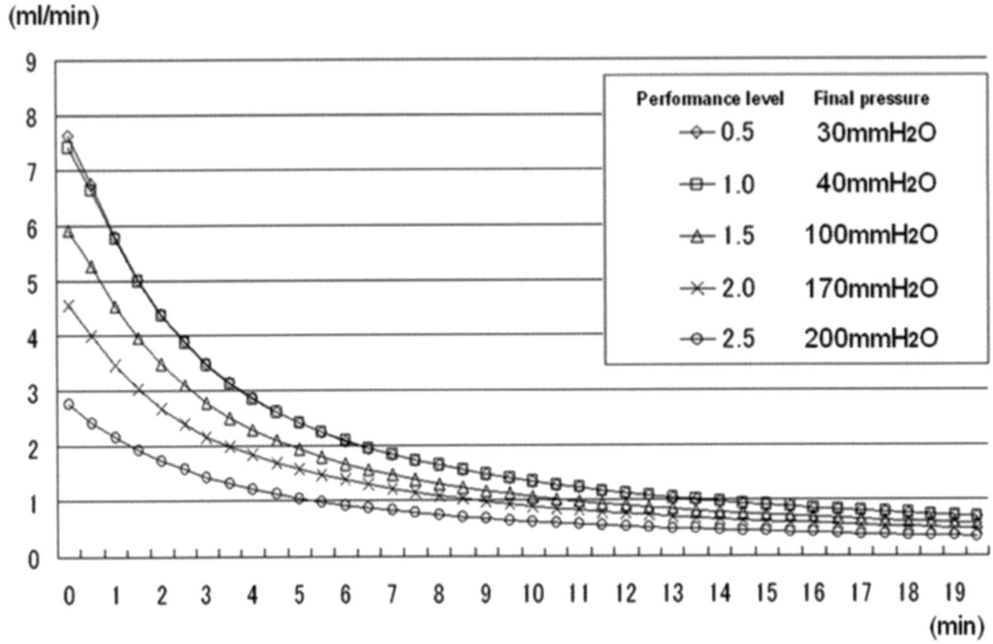

Each performance level setting on the STRATA valve corresponds to a final pressure reading as shown in the legend. Flow rate depends on shunt valve pressure setting.

Fig. 4. Single shunt valve experiment results for the open system

Single Valve	Tandem Valve System	
V1 (STRATA PL)	V2 (STRATA PL)	Final pressure
0.5	-	30mmH2O
1.0	-	40mmH2O
1.0	1.0	50mmH2O
1.5	-	100mmH2O
2.0	-	170mmH2O
2.0	0.5	180mmH2O
2.5	-	200mmH2O

PL : performance level

Table 1. Results comparing the Single shunt valve with Tandem shunt valve in the Open system. In the tandem system, with V1 at 1.0 and V2 at 1.0 the final pressure (50 mmH2O) is always close to the final pressure (40 mmH2O) when V1 is at 1.0 in a single valve system.

pressure. From figure 5, if we compare the rate of decrease between the two experiments we find that the curves follow similar flow rates, which indicates that even at different pressures we can control the flow rate. In fact, at PL (1.0 + 1.0), the final pressure of 50 mmH_20 is quite similar to that of a single valve with PL (1.0), where pressure is 40 mmH_20 as shown in table 1, but exhibits flow rates similar to PL (2.0). Similarly compare the experiments where performance level (2.0 + 0.5) with performance level (2.5) and the same property exist.

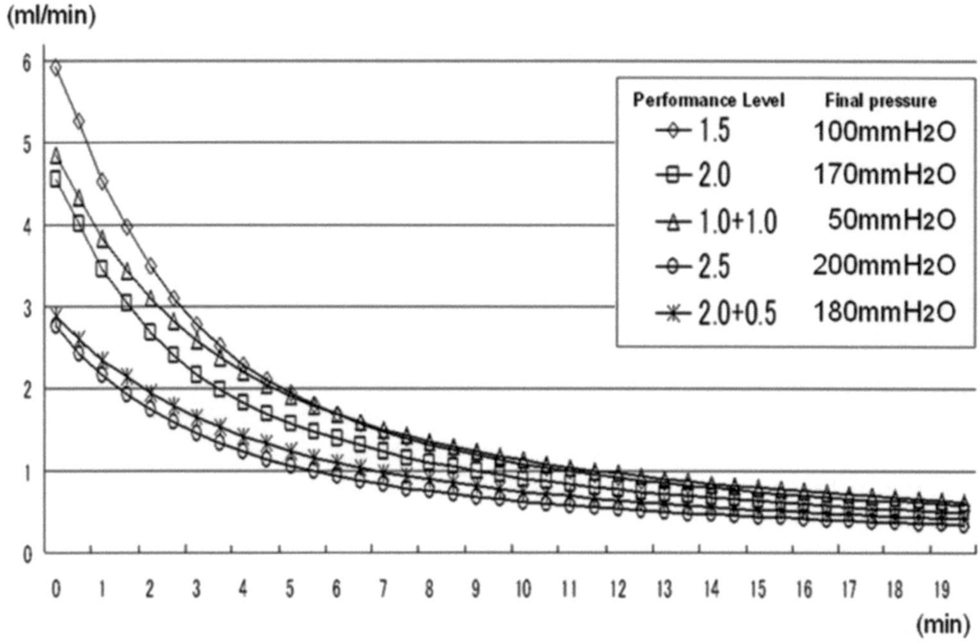

When the total performance levels are the same, the flow rates are similar. However, flow rates can decrease while maintaining final pressures.

Fig. 5. Tandem shunt valve experiment results for the open system

In conclusion, we can decrease flow rate without a major change in pressure using a tandem shunt valve system. After obtaining these *in vitro* results, we implemented tandem shunt valve systems in two shunt cases where problems associated with shunt implants such as slit like ventricle and or intractable hydrocephalus were present.

Case 1

A 6-year-old girl with a malignant glioma underwent bilateral ventricle-peritoneal (V-P) shunt (CHPV) for obstructive hydrocephalus. Although the patient's intracranial pressure was controlled by the shunt system (valve pressure was 150 mmH_2O), hydrocephalus developed during chemotherapy and radiotherapy. The lateral ventricle size and abdominal circumference increased due to a peritoneal fluid collection caused by tumor tissue dissemination through the V-P shunt tract. The shunt valve pressure was adjusted from 150 to 180 mmH_2O to solve this over-drainage problem. However this caused acute hydrocephalus with deteriorating consciousness. The shunt valve pressure was decreased from 180 to 140 mmH_2O. Although the ventricular size decreased and her consciousness improved, the fluid collection in the peritoneal cavity rapidly increased, which caused dyspnea due to high peritoneal pressure. We informed her parents about the two paradoxical problems that needed to be solved simultaneously, 1) finding the best V-P shunt valve pressure to prevent the hydrocephalus, and 2) reducing the amount of peritoneal fluid collection containing the brain tumor tissue and debris. To solve the opposing problems of obtaining sufficient CSF drainage to treat the hydrocephalus but not so much that it would cause peritoneal fluid collection, we tested the therapeutic possibility of the tandem shunt system by adding another adjustable valve (CHPV) with anti-siphon to the current setup. The new tandem shunt system was a connection from the lateral ventricle CHPV (1st valve) connected to the CHPV (2nd valve) with siphon guard to the peritoneal cavity. The performance level of the new tandem shunt system was adjusted to 140 mmH_2O for the 1st valve and 100 mmH_2O for 2nd valve. Hydrocephalus remarkably improved without peritoneal fluid collection and the patient was able to walk soon after the implant.

Case 2

A one and a half-year-old boy infected with Group B Streptococcus during pregnancy, born prematurely in July, 2007 at the gestational age of 28 weeks and weighing 1230g presented with progressive enlargement of head circumference as compared with his body size. Ultrasonography and CT scans revealed hydrocephalus caused by subependymal hemorrhage and periventricular leukomalacia. After controlling intracranial pressure using the Ommaya reservoir, a V-P shunt (Programmable STRATA non siphon control (NSC) Valve) was implanted at the age of 98 days (42 weeks gestation). The intracranial pressure was well controlled at the programmable performance valve level of 1.5. However, the performance level was changed to 2.5 (maximum pressure), because a CT scan showed slit lateral ventricles 6 months after the first shunt placement. After a temporary slight increase in size of the lateral ventricle, the patient was unable to keep a head-up position, which was judged to be a symptom of slit ventricles. Although an anti-siphon device (Delta chamber, Medtronic, Inc., Minneapolis) was added to the shunt system, which resulted in improvement of his symptoms for a month, he continued to suffer from depressed mood and loss of appetite in the head-up position. Moreover, he presented with acute hydrocephalus one day after the transient ligation of the shunt system to check the shunt system dependency. His parents were informed about the details of CSF over-drainage symptoms and the therapeutic possibility of tandem shunt valve system connection surgery. An extra adjustable STRATA NSC valve was connected to the previous shunt system. The final whole view of the tandem shunt valve system was a connection from the lateral ventricle to the STRATA NSC programmable valve (1st valve) connected to the STRATA NSC programmable valve (2nd valve) with anti-siphon system (Delta chamber) to the peritoneal cavity. The performance level of the new tandem shunt system was adjusted to 2.5 (1st valve) and 0.5 (2nd valve) but there was no remarkable change in his condition. After a few days, his second shunt valve performance level was adjusted from 0.5 to 1.0 and his general condition improved dramatically and he was able to keep head-up position over several hours.

4. Discussion

Intra-ventricular cerebrospinal fluid, shunt valve opening pressure, and intra-abdominal pressure are, through common use in neurosurgery and convention, called ICP, valve pressure and abdominal pressure, respectively. If we also consider the tube connecting the head to the abdominal, a difference of water pressure is present, conventionally referred to as hydrostatic pressure. If we assume (ICP + hydrostatic pressure) - (valve pressure + abdominal pressure) = 0, then this simplifies to ICP = (valve pressure + abdominal pressure) - hydrostatic pressure.

The difference in pressure causes fluid flow, however, other parameters to consider include the coefficient of viscosity caused by protein in the CSF, resistance between inner wall shunt tube and CSF flow (tube diameter), the positioning of the shunt valve (forehead or back of the head) and the intra-abdominal tube length and so on. All these parameters contribute to complicated flow dynamics, but a simpler approach is to only use pressures to help us describe fluid flow in a shunt system. In our *in vitro* experiment, we kept all other parameters the same and only changed pressure via valve settings and in the tandem shunt valve system, an additional shunt valve. This tandem system allowed us to precisely control the pressure and flow rate. Until now, CSF flow rate was always the result of the shunt's valve pressure but there has been no study to control the CSF flow rate and ICP individually. Our *in vitro* experiment showed that the tandem system was able to control CSF flow rate and ICP independently of each other.

Intracranial pressure automatically changes when the position of the head and abdominal changes (e.g. compare heights of standing versus sleeping person); these changes cause a siphon effect, which makes it extremely difficult to control ICP with only a single shunt system. [19-21]

Even with an anti-siphon system in place, controlling CSF flow is still difficult. However, with the tandem shunt valve system in place we were able to create a low CSF flow rate environment without increasing the intracranial pressure. In a single valve shunt system it was impossible to create such an environment while maintaining a constant ICP even with an anti-siphon system installed, because, as shown in our experiments, CSF flow is always directly related to the pressure setting at the valve. However, in the tandem valve shunt system, the most significant finding was that the final pressure was equal to the highest valve pressure of the two valves (Fig. 6). This means that in practice, this system has the possibility to control the intracranial pressure without increasing the pressure that is required by the patient.

Figure 6 demonstrates the mechanism behind the tandem shunt valves. It is used to show that the final pressure is equal to the highest valve pressure of the two tandem valves. M, V1 and V2 represent ICP in the human body, and the pressure settings at the shunt valve respectively. In M1 and M2 we add two walls V1 and V2 as shown in figure 6. It shows that regardless of where the highest wall is placed, the final water level at the highest wall will always be the same as the water level in column M. This demonstrates that the final pressure always equals the final pressures setting of either V1 or V2 (Fig 6a, b).

In terms of pressure management in the brain, when there are two valves present in a tandem shunt valve system, ICP pressure is controlled at the highest valve setting at the

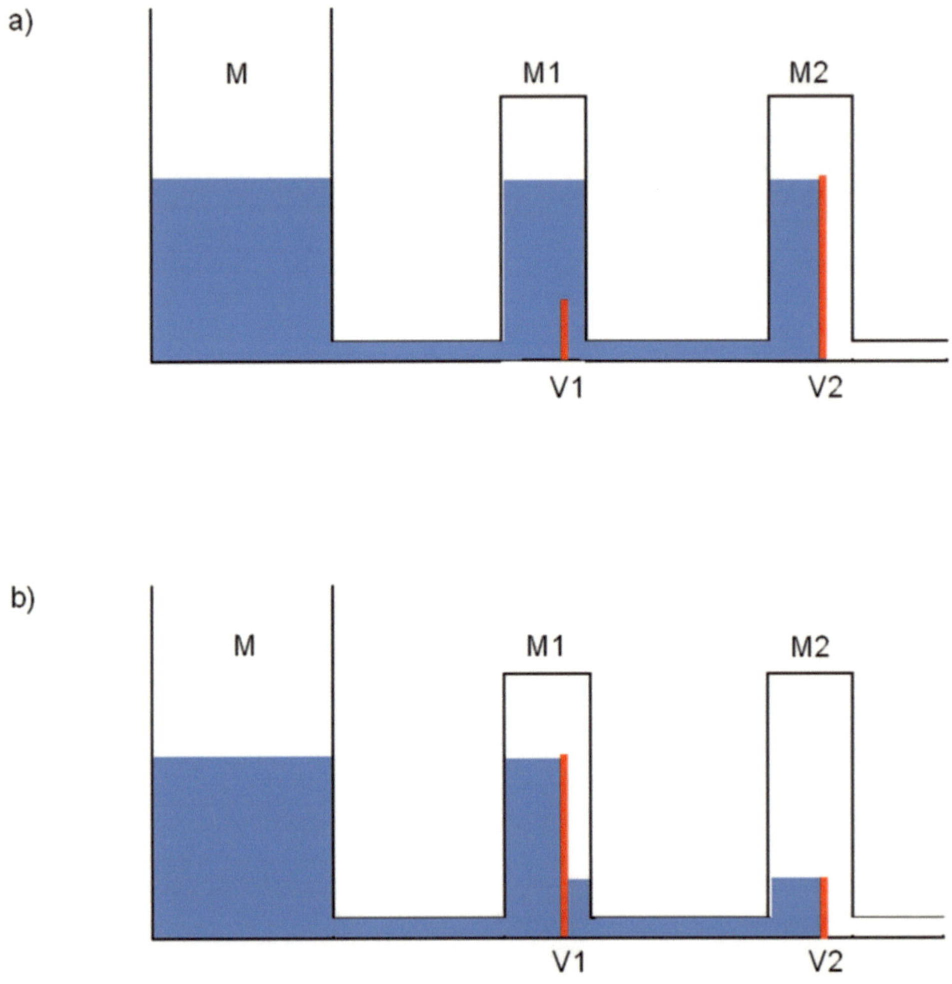

Top (6a): Liquid filled column system with two walls V1 and V2. Water level at M equals water level of V2 demonstrating that final pressure equals the pressure setting at the shunt, or in this case, height of the wall. M gauges pressure in this system, and represents ICP in the body.
Bottom (6b): Liquid filled column system with two walls V1 and V2 heights reversed. Water height at the highest wall is the same as the water height at M. Regardless of the ordering of V1 or V2, the final pressure will always equal to the highest pressure setting of either V1 and or V2. In real life ICP is controlled by the height of the highest setting of the two shunts.

Fig. 6. Controlling ICP - a special mechanism of tandem shunt valves shunt, while CSF flow rate is controlled by adjusting the valve settings. Until now, shunted patients in a single valve system have always been treated with respect to pressure. That is, we do not attempt to control the flow rate but attempt to control the pressure setting at the valve and flow rate is just a consequence of the pressure setting at the valve; that is higher pressure, lower CSF flow and vice versa. We have shown here that we can control CSF rate and ICP independently in the tandem shunt valve system.

Assume a performance level of 3.0 was required of a patient in a single shunt valve system using the STRATA valve. We could only do this by using 2 STRATA valves; the first (V1) connected to another STRATA (V2) shunt valve with the following V1 + V2 patterns available: (2.5 + 0.5, 2.0 + 1.0, 1.5 + 1.5). Each of these patterns result in 1) achieve the performance level of 3.0 and 2) set up the final ICP so that it would be controlled at 2.5, 2.0, and 1.5 (the highest valve pressure of the two valves). With only a single valve, the performance level of 3.0 would not be possible because the maximum performance level is 2.5. Furthermore, we were able to control the pressure while changing the flow rate with the tandem shunt valve system using the STRATA valves.

While the STRATA valve has only 5 settings, the CHPV has settings from 30 to 200 at increments of 10. If we try to create a 250 environment with the CHPV, as required by the patient, it would be impossible to do so with only one valve. In a tandem system there are eight patterns available: (200 +50, 190 +60, 180 +70, 170 +80, 160 +90, 150+100, 140 +110, and 130 +120) with the CHPV shunt valve connected to another CHPV directly; creating a tandem shunt valve system. Each pattern could set up the final ICP controlled at 200, 190, 180, 170, 160, 150, 140, and 130, respectively. These results would be the same condition as the STRATA example, that is, flow rate would be adjustable while keeping ICP controlled to the highest pressure setting of either V1 or V2. Because of the different combinations available we could select the best shunt valve pressure pair depending on the condition of the patient.

With the above mechanism, the tandem shunt valve systems (performance level (2.5+1.0)) prevent intracranial pressure to increase thereby decreasing cerebrospinal fluid flow as opposed to the single valve system performance level (2.5); which is extremely significant for treating slit-like ventricle. We can prevent an increasing ICP and limit flow rate at the same time, which is especially substantial for treating cases of over drainage. Our case studies have demonstrated that this control is only possible with a tandem shunt valve system in place and not a single valve system.

Given the associated problems that come with the usage of a single shunt, there will be a firm requirement for a shunt with tandem shunt valve properties in the future. Our mission is to assist development in this area is through the establishment of a new tandem shunt valve which contains two programmable valves in one device/chassis allowing for the best CSF flow and final ICP combination condition (Figure 7) in hydrocephalus patients. Since there have already been two successful clinical cases further studies to investigate clinical performance will only benefit hydrocephalus cases. The new tandem shunt valve system described here will provide future opportunities to achieve ICP pressure and CSF flow control in hydrocephalus and other related conditions requiring the prevention of pressure fall and fluid flow management at the same time.

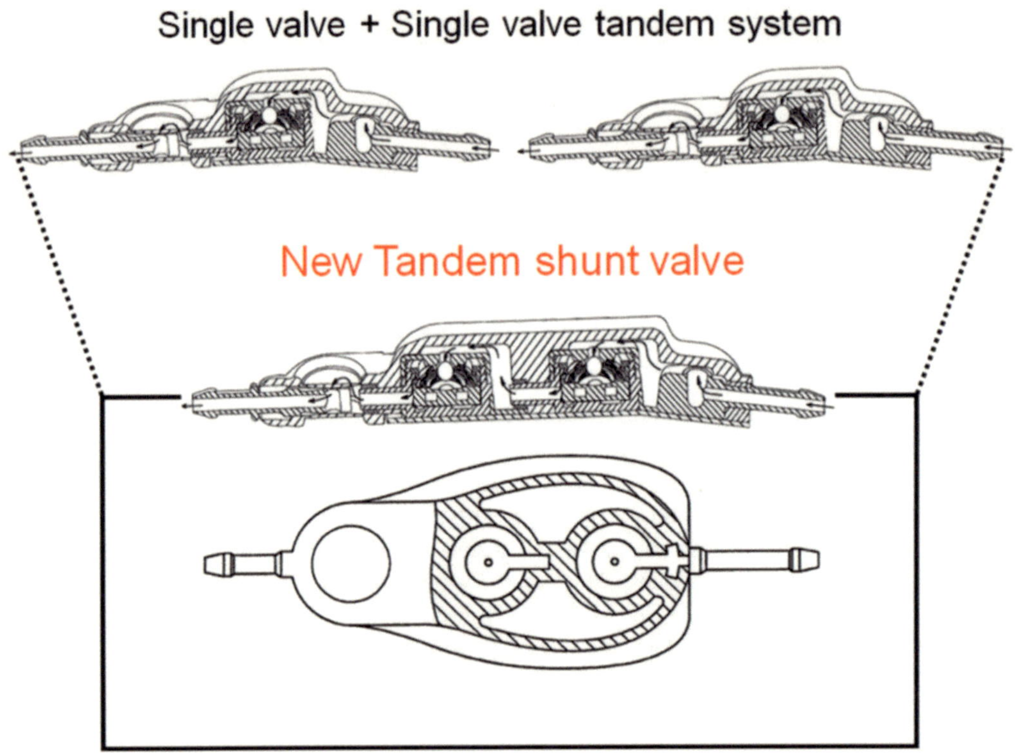

The best combination of the CSF flow and the final ICP condition is through a tandem shunt valve containing two programmable valves. This tandem shunt valve is compact and about the same size as today's single shunt valve.

Fig. 7. The new tandem shunt valve idea model

5. References

[1] Barnett, GH.; Hahn, JF.& Palmer, J. (1987). Normal pressure hydrocephalus in children and young adults. *Neurosurgery,* 20: pp. 904-907.

[2] Black, PM. Hakim, R. & Bailey, NO. (1994). The use of the Codman-Medos programmable Hakim valve in the management of patients with hydrocephalus: illustrative cases. *Neurosurgery,* 34: pp. 1110-1113.

[3] Faulhauer, K. & Schmitz, P. (1978). Overdrainage phenomena in shunt treated hydrocephalus. *Acta Neurochir* 45: pp.89-101.

[4] Hakim, S.(1973). Hydraulic and mechanical mis-matching of valve shunts used in the treatment of hydrocephalus: the need for a servo-valve shunt. *Dev Med Child Neurol,*15: pp.646–653.
[5] Maixner, WJ. et al. (1990). Ventricular volume in infantile hydrocephalus and its relationship to intracranial pressure and cerebrospinal fluid clearance before and after treatment. *Apreliminary study. Pediatr Neurosurg,*16(4–5): pp. 191–196.
[6] Rekate, HL. (1994). The usefulness of mathematical modeling in hydrocephalus research. *Childs Nerv Syst,* 10(1): pp. 13–18.
[7] Boon, AJ. et al. (1998). Dutch Normal-Pressure Hydrocephalus Study: randomized comparison of low- and medium-pressure shunts. *J Neurosurg,* 88(3): pp. 490–4959.
[8] McQuarrie, IG.; Saint-Louis, L. & Scherer, PB. (1984). Treatment of normal pressure hydrocephalus with low versus medium pressure cerebrospinal fluid shunts. *Neurosurgery,* 15(4): pp. 484–488.
[9] Zemack, G. et al. (2003). Clinical experience with the use of a shunt with an adjustable valve in children with hydrocephalus. *J Neurosurg,* 98(3): pp. 471–476.
[10] Zemack, G. & Romner, B. (2000). Seven years of clinical experience with the programmable Codman Hakim valve: a retrospective study of 583 patients. *J Neurosurg,* 92(6): pp. 941–948.
[11] Pollack, IF.; Albright, AL. & Adelson, PD. (1999). A randomized, controlled study of a programmable shunt valve versus a conventional valve for patients with hydrocephalus. Hakim–Medos Investigator Group. *Neurosurgery,* 45(6): pp. 1399–1408; discussion pp. 1408–1411.
[12] Aschoff, A. et al. (1995). Overdrainage and shunt technology. A critical comparison of programmable, hydrostatic and variableresistance valves and flow-reducing devices. *Childs Nerv Syst,* 11 (4): pp. 193–202.
[13] Trost, HA. et al. (1991). Testing the hydrocephalus shunt valve: long-term bench test results of various new and explanted valves. The need for model for testing valves under physiological conditions. *Eur J Pediatr Surg,* 1(Suppl 1): pp. 38–40.
[14] Kestle, J. & Walker, M. (2005). A multicenter prospective cohort study of the Strata valve for the management of hydrocephalus in pediatric patients. *J Neurosurg,* 102 (Suppl 2): pp. 141–145.
[15] Drake, JM.; da Silva, MC. & Rutka, JT. (1993). Functional obstruction of an antisiphon device by raised tissue capsule pressure. *Neurosurgery,* 32(1): pp. 137–139.
[16] Lumenta, CB.; Roosen, N. & Dietrich, U. (1990). Clinical experience with a pressure-adjustable valve SOPHY in the management of hydrocephalus. *Childs Nerv Syst,* 6(5): pp. 270–274.
[17] Piatt, JH Jr. (1995). Cerebrospinal fluid shunt failure: late is different from early. *Pediatr Neurosurg,* 23(3): pp. 129–133.
[18] Matsumae, M. et al. (1989). Quantification of cerebrospinal fluid shunt flow rates. Assessment of the programmable pressure valve. *Childs Nerv Systx,* 5(6): pp. 356–360.
[19] Faulhauer, K. Schmitz, P. (1978). Overdrainage phenomena in shunt treated hydrocephalus. *Acta Neurochir,* 45: pp. 89–101.

[20] Pudenz, RH. Foltz, EL. (1991). Hydrocephalus: overdrainage by ventricular shunts. A review and recommendations. *Surg Neurol,* 35(3): pp. 200–212.

[21] Kamiryo, T. et al. (1991). Intracranial pressure monitoring using a programmable pressure valve and a telemetric intracranial pressure sensor in a case of slit ventricle syndrome after multiple shunt revisions. *Childs Nerv Syst,* 7(4): pp. 233–234.

11

Complex Hydrocephalus

Nasser M. F. El-Ghandour
Department of Neurosurgery, Faculty of Medicine
Cairo University
Egypt

1. Introduction

Hydrocephalus arising from intraventricular septations is known as complex or loculated hydrocephalus. Many synonyms for complex hydrocephalus have been used in the literature such as compartmentalized or loculated hydrocephalus. Complex hydrocephalus remains a challenging neurosurgical problem. Definitive treatment is surgical, yet the approach remains controversial. Traditional treatment consisted of shunting, often requiring the placement of multiple shunt systems and multiple revisions (Ross et al., 1994; Schultz & Leeds 1973).

Some neurosurgeons advocated stereotactic aspiration of the cysts and communication of the compartments (Mathiesen et al., 1993; Ross et al., 1994), others recommended microsurgery with lysis of intraventricular cysts. Good results are reported after using the transcortical approach (Sandberg et al., 2005) or the transcallosal approach (Nida & Haines, 1973). Early experience with neuroendoscopic management is promising. Endoscopy offers a simple means of communicating isolated cerebrospinal fluid spaces and ventricles by membrane fenestration. This can be done through the same burr hole as that for the placement of a ventricular catheter. In some cases, neuroendoscopy has led to eliminating or avoiding the need for shunting (EL-Ghandour, 2006, 2008).

2. Historical perspectives

Before the advancement of neuroendoscopy, microsurgery was the primary method for fenestration of intraventricular cysts. In 1972, Rhoton and Gomez reported a case of multiloculated hydrocephalus which was operated by microsurgical fenestration (Rhoton & Gomez, 1972). In their case, multiloculated hydrocephalus was converted to a univentricular system via a small corticectomy using the microsurgical technique. The hydrocephalus was then managed by a single shunt with good short term results.

In 1982, Kleinhaus et al reported the first successful endoscopic fenestration procedure in a child who had a ventricular cyst. In their case, the bronchoscope has been used as the neuroendoscope (Kleinhaus et al., 1982). In 1986, Powers performed endoscopic fenestration of ventricular cyst using a flexible steerable endoscope and argon laser (Powers, 1986). In 1992, Powers used the same technique and performed successful fenestration in five out of seven patients (Powers, 1992).

Saline torch was used for ventricular cyst fenestration by Heilman and Cohen in 1991 (Heilman & Cohen, 1991) and by Manwaring in 1992 (Manwaring 1992). In 1993, Nida and Haines reported their experience in treating 6 patients with multiloculated hydrocephalus by transcallosal fenestration of intraventricular septations with significant decrease in postoperative shunt revision rate (Nida & Haines, 1993). Lewis et al in 1995 published the first report including a group of patients with loculated hydrocephalus (21 uniloculated and 13 multiloculated) operated by endoscopy (Lewis et al., 1995).

In 2008, EL-Ghandour reported the largest group of patients with multiloculated hydrocephalus (24 pediatric patients) operated by endoscopic cyst fenestration resulting in avoiding, eliminating or simplifying the use of shunts, with significant decrease in postoperative shunt revision rate. The results reported in this study is comparable to or even much better than those obtained previously by using the microsurgical technique. However, the endoscopic procedure has the advantage of being minimally invasive (EL-Ghandour 2008).

3. Classification

Complex hydrocephalus is classified as either uniloculated or multiloculated. Uniloculated hydrocephalus means the presence of a single cyst inside the ventricular system, whether supratentorial (isolated lateral ventricle) or infratentorial (isolated fourth ventricle). Multiloculated hydrocephalus means the presence of multiple cysts or locules isolated by multiple intraventricular septations. Uniloculated hydrocephalus is generally congenital with unaffected cerebrospinal fluid pathways, whereas multiloculated hydrocephalus is generally postinfectious or postinflammatory with obliterated subarachnoid spaces.

The distinction between both types is important because their pathogenesis, success of treatment and prognosis markedly differ. Consequently, it has been concluded that the 2 divergent types of complicated hydrocephalus should not be included in a single study (El-Ghandour, 2006, 2008).

4. Etiological factors

4.1 Uniloculated hydrocephalus

Many designations for uniloculated hydrocephalus have been used such as unilateral hydrocephalus or isolated lateral ventricle. Many types of cysts can exist within the ventricular system. Uniloculated hydrocephalus occurs if the lateral ventricle becomes trapped due to obstruction of foramina of Monro by noncolloid neuroepithelial cysts such as ependymal, choroid plexus or arachnoid cysts (Abtin & Walker, 1998). Arachnoid cysts although typically extradural, can present within the ventricles, as well as choroid plexus cysts, neoplastic cysts, and parasitic cysts (hydatid and cysticercotic cysts).

It has also been described in shunted myelodysplastic children who were treated by low pressure shunt inserted in the contralateral ventricle. The ipsilateral ventricle continues to overdrain through the low pressure shunt, whereas the contralateral or the remainder of the ventricular system becomes dilated. Most of these patients remain asymptomatic and require no treatment. However, if the patient shows progressive enlargement of the lateral ventricle contralateral to the shunt and symptoms occur, further treatment is necessary. Upgrading the shunt valve pressure or simply adding shunt to the contralateral side, has been recommended (Berger et al., 1990).

The most common presentation of uniloculated hydrocephalus is found in the shunted patients. Inflammatory and reactive changes related to shunt catheters, bleeding, infection and scar tissue formation can lead to obstruction or occlusion at the foramen of Monro, thus providing an isolated ventricle. Congenital anatomical causes may be present as well. (Abtin & Walker 1998).

The fourth ventricle can also become isolated due to obstruction of cerebrospinal fluid at the level of the aqueduct of Sylvius and the fourth ventricle outlets, in patients in whom a shunt has already been placed for postmeningitic or posthemorrhagic hydrocephalus. The cerebrospinal fluid produced from the choroid plexus gradually accumulates, resulting in progressive dilatation of the fourth ventricle followed by compression of the brain stem and cerebellar parenchyma. A well functioning lateral ventricular shunt not only decreases the supratentorial pressure, but also reduces the pressure needed inorder to keep the aqueduct open, which occasionally leads to aqueductal collapse. Consequently, the lateral and third ventricles become decompressed, thus leaving the fourth ventricle dilated.

Conventionally, isolated fourth ventricles have been managed by insertion of a ventriculoperitoneal shunt into the fourth ventricle or by craniotomy and microsurgical aqueductal canalization or microsurgical fenestration of the outlets of the fourth ventricle. With the advent of endoscopy in neurosurgery, isolated fourth ventricle is more often treated by endoscopic procedures such as endoscopic third ventriculostomy and aqueductal reconstruction by aqueductoplasty with or without aqueductal stenting (Mohanty, 2005).

4.2 Multiloculated hydrocephalus

Multiloculated hydrocephalus has many synonyms such as multilocular hydrocephalus, polycystic hydrocephalus, polycystic brain disease or intraventricular septations. The ventricular system may become trabeculated or encysted following bacterial meningitis or germinal matrix hemorrhage (Eller & Pasternak 1985; Schultz & Leeds 1973). Predisposing factors include a low birth weight, premature birth, perinatal complications and congenital central nervous system malformations (Albanese et al., 1981). In a study including 24 pediatric patients with multiloculated hydrocephalis operated by endoscopic cyst fenestration, neonatal meningitis was the most common cause (9 cases), followed by intraventricular hemorrhage (6 cases), postoperative gliosis due to previous shunt infection (6 cases) and multiple neuroepithelial cysts (3 cases) (EL-Ghandour, 2008).

In another study including 34 cases of complex hydrocephalus operated by endoscopy, among 21 cases of uniloculated hydrocephalus, 15 cases (71%) were caused by noncolloid neuroepithelial cysts, 3 cases (14%) by choroid plexus cysts, 2 cases (10%) by postoperative gliosis, and 1 case (5%) by meningitis. Among the 13 cases of multiloculated hydrocephalus included in the same study, 4 cases (31%) were caused by intraventricular hemorrhage, 4 cases (31%) by multiple neuroepithelial cysts, 3 cases (23%) by meningitis and 2 cases (15%) by postoperative gliosis (Lewis et al., 1995).

5. Incidence

Complex hydrocephalus is mainly detected in children especially neonates, without any significant variable incidence between boys and girls. The incidence of neonatal meningitis ranges from 0.13% to 0.37% in full-term infants, and from 1.36% to 2.24% in preterm infants.

Hydrocephalus as a sequela of neonatal meningitis is well described, with an incidence of up to 31% (Albanese et al., 1981; Kalsbeck et al., 1980).

Only few reports exist on the rarer subgroup that develop multiloculated hydrocephalus. Many patients with bacterial meningitis also develop ventriculitis, reported as many as 92% of cases on autopsy and 100% of cases seen clinically (Albanese et al., 1981). Postmeningitic hydrocephalus is often believed to be communicating in nature due to an insult at the arachnoid granulations. Based on the pathological findings, however, components of both communicating as well as obstructive hydrocephalus may be present.

6. Pathophysiology

The pathogenesis is still unclear, but believed to be secondary to inflammatory changes and gliosis after ventriculitis, especially commom when caused by Gram-negative organisms (Kalsbeck et al., 1980). It seems that the common link between neonatal meningitis, shunt infection and intraventricular hemorrhage is the resultant ventriculitis. It is believed that the septations giving rise to multiple loculations probably represent the organization of intraventricular exudates and debris produced by ventriculitis, regardless of whether it is chemical or infectious in origin. An inflammatory response at the ependymal surface could encourage proliferation of subependymal glial tissue, upon which exudates and debris organize and serve as a nidus for the formation of septations that span the ventricles.

The septations not only alter the ventricular anatomy, but also disrupt the normal flow of cerebrospinal fluid leading to its accumulation within a loculated cavity with progressive dilatation and mass effect (Nida & Haines, 1993). Grossly, the usual findings are ventricular dilatation, and compartmentalization by membranes. The membranes appear translucent and vary in thickness. Microscopically the septations are composed of fibroglial elements with round and polymorphonuclear cells. The characteristic findings of chronic ventriculitis are frequently present, such as subependymal gliosis, small areas of denuded ependyma, and glial tufts extending through the denuded ependyma into the ventricular lumen (Schultz & Leeds, 1973).

7. Clinical features

Presenting symptoms are mainly those related to increased intracranial pressure leading to macrocephaly in infants and headache in older children. Other symptoms include seizures, gait ataxia, and hemiparesis. Developmental delay is reported to be more common in multiloculated than uniloculated cases. It has been mentioned that neurological status in this patient population is extremely poor.

Patients with multiloculated hydrocephalus are notoriously difficult to treat, and are often compromised intellectually. In a study including 33 pediatric patients who underwent craniotomies for fenestration of progressive multiloculated hydrocephalus, 29 patients (87.9%) were severely delayed or vegetative. Many patients were nonverbal or minimally verbal, nonambulatory, had significant motor deficits, had significant spasticity and experienced seizure disorders (Sandberg et al., 2005).

In a study including 10 pediatric patients with multiloculated hydrocephalus caused by neonatal meningitis, ventriculitis or intraventricular hemorrhage, who were treated surgically (6 patients underwent craniotomy and trancallosal fenestration and 4 patients were treated by shunting), most of the patients were found to be seriously affected. The children reported in this study had detectable cognitive deficits, ranging from profound psychomotor retardation to mild learning disability (Nida & Haines, 1993).

In a study including 34 patients with complex hydrocephalus operated by endoscopy (21 uniloculated and 13 multiloculated), the presenting symptoms were headache in 14 cases (41.2%), developmental delay in 11 cases (32.4%), macrocephaly in 6 cases (17.6%), seizures in 5 cases (14.7%), gait ataxia in 2 cases (5.9%), and progressive hemiparesis in 2 cases (5.9%) (Lewis et al., 1995).

In another study including 24 pediatreic patients with multiloculated hydrocephalus (21 cases were infants younger than 2 years of age), operated by endoscopic cyst fenestration, all patients (100%) presented with head enlargement, 18 patients (75%) presented with developmental delay, 4 patients (16.7%) with epilepsy, and 2 patients (8.3%) with hemiparesis (El-Ghandour, 2008).

8. Diagnostic studies

8.1 Ultrasound

The use of ultrasound is a well established diagnostic method for neonates and patients with open fontanel (Machado et al., 1991). It is useful in the evaluation of patients with complex hydrocephalus, often demonstrating the cyst walls and revealing any compartmentalization that has occurred. Its advantages include that it is nonradiating, noninvasive, gives a multiplanar view and patients don't require sedation. Nevertheless, it is operator-dependant and it couldn't be considered a definitive preoperative diagnostic modality.

8.2 Computed tomography scan

Plain CT scan shows disproportionate hydrocephalus, and can be used for screening of patients. However, the cysts usually have a density similar to that of cerebrospinal fluid, and the walls are usually transparent making it usually difficult to visualize the cyst walls accurately. Often CT scan shows transversely oriented septations of varying thickness and nonuniform distribution, changing the ventricular system into one of irregular contour.

Although the septations may not be visible in the early disease process, retrospective temporal review often delineates pattern of progressive compartmentalization and asymmetrical hydrocephalus. The initially documented ventricular pattern gradually becomes unrecognizable, so that ultimately the cerebral mantle encloses a large single multiloculated cavity. In advanced stages, it may be difficult to recognize the ventricles and other anatomical structures of the brain (Nida & Haines, 1993). However, CT scan is unable to identify communication or noncommunication between cavities.

8.3 Magnetic resonance imaging

Magnetic Resonance Imaging with gadolinium is considered to be the diagnostic method of choice for patients with complex hydrocephalus. Its advantages over the CT scan include the multiplanar view providing a detailed picture in three different planes (axial, coronal, sagittal), and it is more sensitive in revealing septations. The difference in protein content of these cysts may delineate them from the cerebrospinal fluid containing ventricular system. It can also occasionally show the etiological factor as well, such as a neuroepithelial cyst. However, MR imaging fails to provide accurate information on communication or noncommunication of the compartments in multiloculated hydrocephalus.

8.4 Contrast CT ventriculography

Contrast material injected into the ventricular system or the cyst verifies noncommunication of the cyst with the ventricular system and defines the margins of the compartments. It can be done by injecting 1-2 ml of metrizamide directly into the proximal catheter of a pre-existing shunt system, by cannulating the cyst with a 22-gauge spinal needle, or by placing an external ventricular drain. The patient's head is then rotated back and forth inorder to allow the contrast matrial to spread inside the cavity, thereby showing any comartmentalization. A second CT scan is usually done 30-60 minutes after the contrast injection.

Contrast CT ventriculography, provides absolute confirmation of noncommunicating loculations, and allows direct visualization of sequestrated ventricular compartments. However, in multiloculated hydrocephalus, it requires multiple punctures for different compartments inorder to delineate the presence or absence of communication among them. Simultaneous sampling of cerebrospinal fluid for analysis of protein content may also indirectly support the presence of noncommunicating cysts (Nida & Haiens, 1993).

9. Surgical management

The definitive treatment of complex hydrocephalus is surgical. However, a high proportion of patients have a history of prematurity and/or central nervous system infection, and require medical treatment not only for intraventricular hemorrhage but also for any associated co-morbidities. The goals of surgery are to control hydrocephalus, simplify complex shunts (that is, replacing multiple shunts with a single shunt comprising only 1 intraventricular catheter, 1 reservoir, and 1 peritoneal catheter), reducing shunt revision rate, avoiding implanting shunts if possible, and decreasing operative morbidity.

9.1 Ventricular shunting

The basic underlying pathophysiological problem is that ventricular compartmentalization interferes with the proper drainage of the dilated ventricular system, making therapeutic shunting difficult. Consequently, placement of multiple shunt systems should be done inorder to drain loculated ventricular compartments that do not communicate with each other (Kaiser, 1986). The disadvantage of additional proximal shunt catheters is that multiple noncommunicating ventricular compartments are often present, and a second or even a third ventricular catheter may not adequately drain cerebrospinal fluid from all the compartments.

The greater the number of operative procedures and hardware placed, the greater will be the risk of infection. Moreover, when a shunt malfunction or infection is suspected in a patient with complex shunt systems, both diagnosis and surgical treatment can become quite complicated. Consequently, such procedure is usually followed by multiple shunt revisions and is associated with high morbidity and mortality rates. In one series a 54%

mortality rate was reported with the remaining patients severely impaired (Kalsbeck et al., 1980). For these reasons it is better to avoid multiple shunt systems if possible (Sandberg et al., 2005). Insertion of multiperforated ventricular catheter together with puncture of the membranes has also been suggested for control of compartmentalization (Kalsbeck et al., 1980), however, this has not proven to be a reliable method.

9.2 Stereotactic procedure

Many reports stress the operative simplicity and low complication rate of the stereotactic procedure in the treatment of intraventricular cysts. However, the initial enthusiasm for stereotactic aspiration has been tempered by its lack of success in treating some patients. In some patients, a mobile cyst with tough outer capsule may be pushed away by the needle and become resistant to stereotactic puncture (Ross et al., 1994).

Moreover, stereotactic aspiration is considered to be a blind technique (i.e. there is lack of intraoperative visual control) (Hellwig et al., 2008). Most importantly, simple aspiration may lead to high recurrence rate (up to 80%), because the stereotactic procedure fails to devascularize the cyst or to create a large window (>1 cm) in the cyst wall (Mathiesen et al., 1993).

9.3 Microsurgical treatment

Reports of complex hydrocephalus treated by craniotomy and lysis of ventricular cysts have been infrequent and include small groups of patients. Good results were reported in a series of 6 patients operated by transcallosal approach (Nida & Haines, 1993), and in a series of 31 patients operated by transcortical approach (Sandberg et al., 2005). Advocates for using the microsurgical procedure say that adequate hemostasis can be confidently achieved because the intraventricular septations are dissected under direct visualization. Bleeding can be more easily controlled during microsurgery, which permits the bimanual use of the standard instrumentation, such as bipolar cautery, regulated suction, with the ability to apply topical hemostatic agents (Levy et al., 2003).

They also claim that the creation of multiple wide fenestrations can be easily performed during the microsurgical procedure because the surgical microscope provides better visualization of the various compartments and membranes under higher magnification (Sandberg et al., 2005). The stereoscopic view provided by the surgical microscope, gives the surgeon a superior depth perception, particularly during deep dissection. The familiarity of traditional microsurgical techniques makes open procedures more accessible to most neurosurgeons, avoiding the potentially hazardous learning curve needed for endoscopy (Levy et al., 2003).

Nevertheless, there are many drawbacks for this procedure. First, the transcallosal surgery is technically demanding and carries the risks of sagittal sinus thrombosis, venous infarction from division of bridging veins, inadvertant damage to the pericallosal arteries, and injury to the fornix with cognitive sequelae (Jeeves et al., 1979). Second, the transcortical approach is sometimes associated with seizures and may lead to subdural collection postoperatively, because the cortical mantle is often thinned out from hydrocephalus (Kalsbeck et al., 1980). Third, the loss of cerebrospinal fluid during cyst decompression leads to collapse of the ventricular walls (Powers, 1992). Finally, a second craniotomy may be required to reach additional cysts within the fourth ventricle, or to place a shunt.

9.4 Endoscopic treatment

The significant potential morbidity of microsurgical technique and the high failure rate of ventriculoperitoneal shunting, prompted neurosurgeons to search for an alternative procedure. The ability of the endoscope to bring into communication isolated loculated compartments within the ventricular system with minimal cortical disruption has been recently advocated as an alternative to the use of complex shunt systems or microsurgery. The endoscope is an ideal instrument for exploration of fluid-filled cavities, and the intraventricular location of these cysts makes them accessible for the endoscopic procedure. Endoscopy is a safe and effective treatment option for complex hydrocephalus, it is less invasive and offers greater operative simplicity than microsurgery. Patients recover on the ward after endoscopic fenestration of ventricular cysts and can be discharged the following day if there are no associated medical problems; in comparison, patients spend at least 1 day in the intensive care unit after the microsurgical procedure (Lewis et al., 1990).

Endoscopic fenestration combines both advantages, the minimal invasiveness of stereotactic fenestration, and the effectiveness of microsurgery. A single burr hole provides rapid access to the entire ventricular system and avoids the pitfalls of transcallosal approach. In cases of uniloculated hydrocephalus, ventriculocystostomy offers the best chance for treating these patients. Septum pellucidotomy or septostomy can be also performed endoscopically to treat isolated lateral ventricles. Fenestration of the septum pellucidum to connect the two lateral ventricles in patients with isolated lateral ventricle will preclude the need for two shunts in the majority of patients. Isolated fourth ventricle can be also treated endoscopically by aqueductoplasty and/or aqueductal stenting (Cinalli et al., 2006). In cases of multiloculated hydrocephalus, endoscopic cyst fenestration provides wide communication between the ventricular compartments and offers the greatest possibility of avoiding the need for additional shunt catheters (El-Ghandour, 2008).

9.4.1 Endoscpic tools

Flexible endoscopes have been preferred by some neurosurgeons (Lewis et al., 1995), due to its flexibility and steerability which provides increased maneuverability. However, it requires a significant amount of expertise and its main role in multiloculated hydrocephalus in the author's view is navigating the ventricular system and performing aqueductoplasty in cases with isolated fourth ventricle. The author prefers rigid endoscopes because they have greater light intensity and superior optics which allow better visualization. The limited maneuverability of the rigid endoscopes is usually offset by careful selection of the burr hole placement site and by widening the outer edge of the burr hole which provides greater freedom in maneuvering the endoscope and selecting different trajectories (El-Ghandour, 2008).

9.4.2 Endoscopic trajectory

The approach is individually designated in each case depending on location of the cysts, entry site of the pre-existing ventricular catheter, and the need for the placement of a new shunt. Cysts located anteriorly are approached through a standard midpupillary coronal burr hole, whereas an occipital or posterior parietal route is used for posterior or temporal loculations. The burr holes are bevelled laterally to allow the endoscope to reach the contralateral ventricle, and the trajectory is planned to fenestrate the maximum number of cysts, this can be achieved by projecting the best angle with the aid of preoperative coronal and sagittal MR imaging. Sometimes it is not possible to fenestrate all intraventricular cysts because of the high risk of damaging important neural structures during septostomies. The ventricular system or the cyst is cannulated with a 14-F peel-away sheath and stylet. Care is taken to prevent the release of cerebrospinal fluid before the endoscope is introduced. After withdrawal of the stylet, a 2 mm-diameter rigid lens (wide-angle, straight-forward, 0 degree) with angled eye piece and working channel diameter of 3 mm is inserted. In severe cases with more areas of hydrocephalus, working through multiple burr holes (multiportal) ensures more successful localization (El-Ghandour, 2008).

9.4.3 Cyst localization

Intraoperative ultrasonography has proven to be extremely useful both in localization, and assisting in directing the endoscope to the desired location providing an ongoing intraoperative orientation. It gives live feedback of the surgical progress. It is also useful in determining depth of the cysts and presence of any solid structures beyond the cyst walls, as well as any shift of internal contents during or after the fenestration. One can make evaluation concerning successful fenestration and communication between various compartments by viewing saline jet bubbles flowing from one cyst to another as seen on ultrasound. However, its disadvantages include its operative dependability, requirement of a window in the cranial vault, and potential crowding of the operating suite (Abtin & Walker, 1998).

Frameless stereotaxy or neuronavigation has increased the accuracy and safety of endoscopy, and it can be used in conjunction with endoscopy inorder to overcome the problem of distorted anatomy. However, the disadvantage of frameless technology is that the patient is often a young child and the head cannot be secured to the operating table by a 3-pin holder. Without rigid fixation, the head cannot remain in a constant position with respect to the stereotactic arc after markers are registered; consequently a high percentage of errors may occur and the patient may need to undergo re-registering. Recently, simultaneous image-guided MR imaging and endoscopic navigation without rigid cranial fixation (pinless frameless stereotactic assembly) has been used in infants. However, errors may still occur as a result of shifting of intracranial structures after ventricular or cystic access. The frameless system, as opposed to intraoperative ultrasound, is not real time. Consequently, both systems can be used during the same procedure inorder to take advantage of the strengths of both (Abtin & Walker, 1998).

There are not many data on the role of neuronavigation in conjunction to neuroendoscopy in the treatment of multiloculated hydrocephalus in the published literature. In a recently published study, 16 children with multiloculated hydrocephalus were operated by endoscopically navigated procedure. In all children, sufficient drainage of the multiloculated ventricular system was reported. In this series, the authors mentioned that they didn't encounter significant problems with the occurrence of intraoperative brain shift. They attributed this observation to 2 reasons: 1) The majority of opened compartments were small, and each by itself constituted only a small portion of the whole compartmented ventricular system. 2) Continuous irrigation has been used throughout the procedure, thereby maintaining the existing anatomy and dimensions of the penetrated cysts and parts of the ventricular system as much as possible (Schulz et al., 2010)

9.4.4 Operative findings

In most cases, it is difficult to recognize the ventricle and other anatomical structures of the brain due to severe anatomical distorsion. Differentiation between the ependyma and cyst wall is crucial, the latter is usually light blue in color, variable in thickness (translucent in early cases), and usually mobile with cerebrospinal fluid pulsations. A yellow discolouration of the ependyma due to previous intraventricular hemorrhage is sometimes noticed, and glial tufts extending into the ventricular lumen are frequently present. All patients with complex hydrocephalus who presented in an advanced stage, had more ventricular distortion and thicker membranes. Consequently long delays before fenestration is usually accompanied by progressive loculation and worse prognosis (El-Ghandour, 2008).

9.4.5 Endoscopic cyst fenestration

Different methods of fenestrating intraventricular cysts have been reported such as steerable fiberscope, argon laser, Nd:YAG (neodymium:yttrium-aluminum-garnet) laser, saline torch, and bipolar cautery. Cyst fenestration is performed in a relatively avascular segment of the cyst wall. The fenestration is widened to more than 1 cm in diameter to prevent early reclosure. This is achieved sharply by widening the initial hole or connecting multiple holes by using the bipolar electrode. A very wide fenestration has been advocated by some authors (EL-Ghandour, 2008), because of the high incidence of reclosure of small openings due to the low pressure differential across cyst walls as well as the inflammatory origin of the disease (Figs. 1A & B). Devascularization of the cyst wall is done by coagulating its vascular supply to prevent or slow its regrowth. Pulsed irrigation with lactated Ringer solution is used to prevent thermal injury and collapse of the ventricles. Any bleeding from the cyst wall usually stops with irrigation or coagulation. After completion of cyst fenestration, real-time ultrasound can be used while injecting saline into the cyst to confirm successful communication with the ventricular system (Lewis et al., 1995).

9.4.6 Septum pellucidotomy

It is a well recognized, minimally invasive technique that is used in the treatment of isolated lateral ventricle, obviating the need for two shunts, and in some cases, the need for any shunting. Finding and fenestrating the septum in a patient with both lateral ventricles dilated is a simple task, but unfortunately, most patients requiring this procedure have one collapsed ventricle and one grossly dilated ventricle. It is extremely difficult to identify the septum pellucidum in these patients, that frameless stereotaxy or neuronavigation is recommended.

The burr hole is placed more lateral to the standard position, approximately 5-6 cm lateral from the midline. A rigid endoscope is then passed into the nondilated lateral ventricle and through the septum pellucidum under direct vision. Reaching the septum by introducing the endoscope through the dilated ventricle is risky, because the opposite ventricle is often

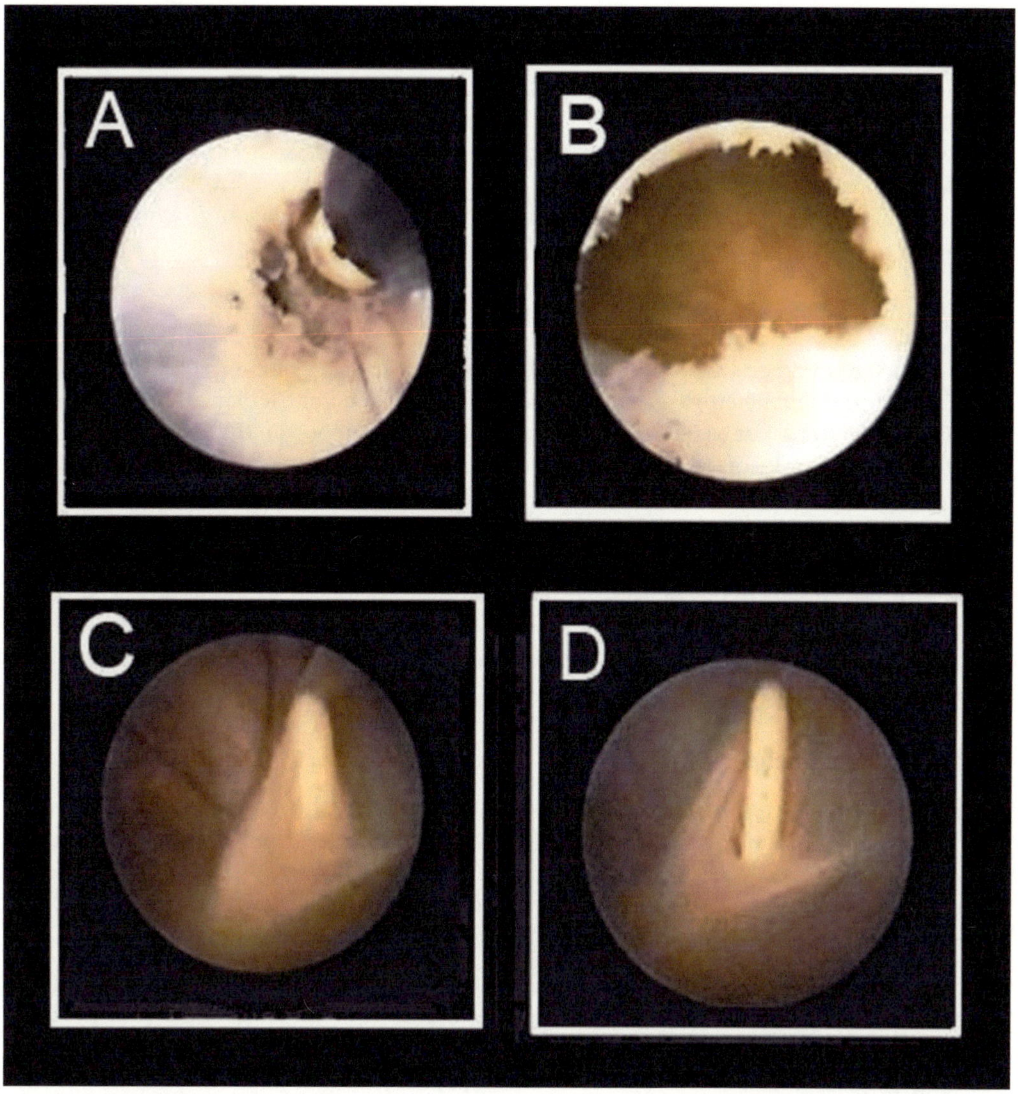

Fig. 1. A, intraoperative photograph showing bipolar electrode coagulating the cyst wall and making initial perforation. B, very wide fenestration is done in order to avoid reclosure. Note yellow discolouration due to previous intraventricular hemorrhage. C, preexisting ventricular catheter is seen obstructed by adherent membranes. D, tip of the catheter after being dissected so that it can be withdrawn safely without risking intraventricular hemorrhage. [Reprinted with permission from El-Ghandour NM (2008). Endoscopic cyst fenestration in the treatment of multiloculated hydrocephalus in children. *J Neurosurg Pediatr,* Vol 1, No. 3, (March 2008), pp:217-222, ISSN 1933-0707].

small and penetrating into the opposite ventricular wall is a potential complication. Significant delay between entering the lateral ventricle and piercing the septum may cause excessive cerebrospinal fluid to escape and this can result in an error due to the theoretical risk of brain shift.

The septum contains relatively avascular tissue, and generous septostomy can be performed safely, taking care to avoid injuring the fornices or corpus callosum. The precise anatomical position of the thinnest part of septum pellucidum is above and infront of the foramen of Monro. The use of lasers or cautery is extremely valuable in performing the septum fenestration, because it allows the surgeon an opportunity to make a larger opening. Large vessels should not be encountered during the procedure. If vessels are seen through the endoscope or if there is significant hemorrhage, this means that the endoscope is passing through or above the corpus callosum (Teo, 1998).

9.4.7 Endoscopic third ventriculostomy

It is a challenge to do endoscopic third ventriculostomy in cases of complex hydrocephalus especially in multiloculated cases, due to the changes in the ventricular architecture to the extent that the third ventricle could not be identified in most of the cases. It has been reported that the role of endoscopy is limited to fenestration, and patients (especially infants) will still need shunts to treat hydrocephalus because of immaturity of the subarachnoid cerebrospional fluid dynamics. Moreover, the pathophysiological mechanism that initially caused the septations are likely responsible for the deficiency of the absorptive capacity of the subarachnoid space due to scarring of arachnoid granulations (Teo, 1998). Nevertheless, performing endoscopic third ventriculostomy and eliminating the need for placing shunts in patients with multiloculated hydrocephalus has been reported recently by some authors (El-Ghandour, 2006, 2008).

9.4.8 Aqueductoplasty

The ideal candidate for this procedure is the premature neonate who has an isolated fourth ventricle. When the fourth ventricle expands through the tentorial incisura, endoscopic fenestration into the trigone or occipital horn of the lateral ventricle is possible. However, when a symptomatic isolated fourth ventricle remains within the posterior fossa, aqueductoplasty with or without a silastic stent becomes the procedure of choice.

The procedure is performed using the flexible endoscope which is introduced through a standard midpupillary coronal burr hole into the lateral ventricle, and hence into the third ventricle. Once the aqueduct is identified, the glial membrane, which invasively covers the orifice, is punctured with a 5-F transluminal angioplasty balloon catheter and dilated to a balloon inflation diameter of 3 mm. Cerebrospinal fluid should be observed flowing through the dilated canal. A small length of silastic tubing may be left in the aqueduct to maintain patency.

However, implanting stents carries the risk of stent dislodgement and migration (Mohanty, 2005). Manipulation of the aqueduct may also traumatize the tegmentum of the midbrain ventrally and the tectal plate dorsally. The clinical manifestation of this traumatization is the development of postoperative dysconjugate eye movements that usually resolve with time (Teo, 1998).

9.4.9 Endoscopic shunt retrieval

Removal of old malfunctioning ventricular catheters under endoscopic guidance is considered to be one of the most important roles of endoscopy in the treatment of complex hydrocephalus. Ventricular catheters embedded in scar tissue or adherent to the choroid plexus, which previously could not be withdrawn safely without risking intraventricular hemorrhage, can now be removed under direct vision with endoscopic assistance. The YAG laser can be used to coagulate the choroid plexus and to cut along the interface of the scar and the silicone tubing in order to dislodge the catheter. Because pulsed irrigation causes movement of the choroid plexus and cyst wall, irrigation is discontinued when firing the laser. The laser is used in a fluid medium to avoid thermal injury to the surrounding structures. When removing an embedded ventricular catheter that has been placed through an occipital approach, a coronal or anterior frontal approach is preferred because the laser can be used at a trajectory perpendicular to the catheter tubing (Lewis et al., 1995).

In another study including 6 patients with pre-existing malfunctioning shunts who had previously undergone shunt drainage through occipital burr holes, another burr hole was done 2-3 cm above the old one through which the endoscope was introduced parallel to the ventricular catheter with slight inclination towards the area of scarred-in catheter tip. Four out of these 6 patients (67%) had complex shunts and simplification was performed in 3 of them (50%). The obstruction was proximal due to the presence of adherent membranes. The author found it very difficult to retrieve a pre-existing ventricular catheter in 2 out of these 6 patients (33%) which necessitated the use of bipolar diathermy probe to dissect and dislodge the tip of the catheter from adherent surrounding membranes (Figs.1C & D), so that it can be withdrawn gently and safely without risking intraventricular hemorrhage. It has been concluded that retained pre-existing malfunctioning ventricular catheters in multiloculated hydrocephalus could not be withdrawn safely without endoscopic assistance (El-Ghandour, 2008).

9.4.10 New shunt placement

Some neurosurgeons prefer placing an external ventricular drain routinely after endoscopic cyst fenestration and postponing shunting procedure to a later date (Abtin & Walker, 1998). The author doesn't put an external drain routinely except if there is intraventricular bleeding, and prefers to place a new shunt during the same session of endoscopic cyst fenestration. It has been reported that external drainage might lead to cyst collapse and initiate or accelerate early closure of the cyst fenestrations due to interference with the already existing cerebrospinal fluid pressure gradients (El-Ghandour 2008).

After removing the old catheter, the surgeon places a new catheter in the optimum position under direct endoscopic visualization. Both shunt retrieval and placement of new shunt can be performed during the same session of endoscopic cyst fenestration, provided there is no intraventricular bleeding. However, if there is bleeding it is better to insert an external ventricular drain and postpone the shunt procedure until a later date, to avoid its malfunctioning by the bloody cerebrospinal fluid (El-Ghandour, 2008).

There are many techniques which can be used for endoscopic shunt placement. The ventricular catheter may be loaded on an endoscope with the tip of the endoscope exposed for visualization. The shunt may then be placed directly into a ventricle through the appropriate trajectory, while looking through the shunt with the endoscope to confirm the shunt catheter position. If the ventricular catheter tip is in an inappropriate position, the shunt is withdrawn and modification of the trajectory may be made.

Another technique, which applies to neurosurgeons using a rod lens endoscope system, involves placing an appropriate-sized peel-away catheter into a ventricle, then placing the endoscope through the peel-away catheter. In this way, the potential shunt position is confirmed and length of the ventricular catheter can be estimated. Once the peel-away catheter is in a satisfactory position, the endoscope is withdrawn and the ventricular catheter is passed into the desired depth. The peel-away catheter is then removed while the ventricular catheter is held gently with a smooth forceps, leaving the ventricular catheter in the appropriate place (Brockmeyer, 1989).

9.4.11 Repeated endoscopic procedure

In a study including 24 pediatric patients with multiloculated hydrocephalus operated by endoscopic cyst fenestration, a repeat endoscopic procedure was necessary in 8 out of 24 patients (33%), among the mean follow-up period (30 months). At the second procedure persistent cysts unrecognized from the first operation were encountered in 5 patients (21%) and reclosure was found in the remaining 3 patients (12.5%). It was also noticed that patients in whom shunts were placed before endoscopic cyst fenestration had a 7.5 risk of having a repeat endoscopic procedure more than patients in whom endoscopic cyst fenestration preceded shunt placement (El-Ghandour, 2008).

While another contributing factor may exist which is the increased severity of multiloculated hydrocephalus in the former group of patients that might increase the incidence of repeat procedure, the difference in incidence between both groups is still highly significant. The incidence of 13% repeat rate detected in patients where endoscopic cyst fenestration was performed prior to shunting is comparable to the 16% incidence reported in a group treated by craniotomy (Nida & Haines, 1993).

The statistically significant difference between the increased incidence of a repeat endoscopic procedure in patients who were shunted before endoscopic cyst fenestration as compared to patients on whom endoscopic cyst fenestration preceded shunt placement ($p<0.001$, highly significant), makes it clear that early diagnosis and fenestration is critical in obtaining the best results in treating these patients. This better prognosis in the latter group can be explained by the thinner ventricular septations with easier fenestration, less vascular cyst wall and less likelihood for postoperative reclosure (El-Ghandour, 2008).

10. Complications

There is no much information about complications connected with the use of neuroendoscopic procedures in the treatment of complex hydrocephalus in the published clinical data. Major complications of cyst fenestration and septostomy include ventricular hemorrhage, ventriculitis, injury to adjacent neural tissue, and cerebrospinal fluid leakage. Hemorrhage and ventriculitis may lead to further loculations. The risk of injury to adjacent neural tissue can be minimized by careful planning of the surgical approach and by having a knowledge of the neural structures beyond the point of fenestration. Consequently, orientation is critical and the intraoperative use of ultrasound and stereotaxis in conjunction with endoscopy are so helpful (Abtin & Walker, 1998).

It has been mentioned that the surgeon's ability to control unexpected hemorrhage during endoscopic fenestration of ventricular cysts is suboptimal and could lead to catastrophic complications (Nida & Haines, 1993). However, recent studies didn't report any significant bleeding during endoscopic treatment of complex hydrocephalus. In a study including 24 pediatric patients with multiloculated hydrocephalus operated by endoscopic cyst fenestration, minor intraoperative arterial bleeding was encountered in 2 patients (8%), but terminating the procedure was not necessary, and the bleeding stopped within few minutes with irrigation. None of the patients required craniotomy nor suffered a postoperative neurological deficit or seizures. There was no deaths (0%) and morbidity was minimal. It included cerebrospinal fluid leakage in 2 patients (8%) which stopped spontaneously within 3 days (El-Ghandour, 2008). Among 34 cases of complex hydrocephalus (21 uniloculated and 13 multiloculated) operated by endoscopic procedure, cerebrospinal fluid leakage occurred in 1 case (3%) and central nervous system infection occurred in 1 case (3%) (Lewis et al., 1995).

11. Outcome and prognosis

The outcome depends on the surgical procedure adopted, as well as the type of complex hydrocephalus. The outcome is evaluated by the incidence of improvement of hydrocephalus in postoperative MR imaging, avoiding or eliminating the need for shunting, simplifying complex shunt systems, and reducing shunt revision rate. Uniloculated hydrocephalus is easier to treat endoscopically than multiloculated hydrocephalus and consequently, it carries a better prognosis. It has been reported that 84% of patients undergoing endoscopic cyst fenestration for unilateral hydrocephalus have either remained shunt free or not required additional shunt placement (Abtin & Walker, 1998).

In a series of 6 patients with multiloculated hydrocephalus operated by transcallosal fenestration of intraventricular septations, a significant decrease in the rate of shunt revision per year was reported from a mean of 2.75 shunt revision per year (over an observation period of 44.5 months) to 0.25 per year (over a median follow-up period of 27 months) (Nida & Haines, 1993).

Successful communication between the isolated cavities can be confirmed postoperatively by contrast-enhanced CT ventriculography (Fig. 2). In a series of 24 pediatric patients with multiloculated hydrocephalus operated by endoscopic cyst fenestration, improvement of hydrocephalus was detected in postoperative imaging in 18 patients (75%), where there was an apparent decrease in the cyst size or ventricular size and restoration of normal ventricular architecture (Figs. 3-5). The need for shunt was avoided in 3 patients (12.5%) who were treated by endoscopic cyst fenestration and endoscopic third ventriculostomy (El-Ghandour, 2008).

In a group of 6 patients with malfunctioning pre-existing shunts included in the same study, endoscopy reduced the shunt revision rate from 2.9 per year before fenestration (among a mean observation period of 12.3 months) to 0.2 per year after fenestration (among a mean follow-up period of 27.3 months) ($P<0.01$, highly significant) (Table 1). Four of these 6 patients had complex shunt systems, and simplification was performed in 3 of them (75%).

However, all the 6 patients required a single repeated endoscopic procedure, endoscopic cyst fenestration was repeated in all of them (100%), and shunt revision was done in 3 patients (50%). Patients in whom shunts were placed before endoscopic cyst fenestration, more frequently needed a repeat endoscopic cyst fenestration (6 out of 6) than patients in whom endoscopic cyst fenestration preceded shunt placement (2 out of 15) with a relative risk ratio 7.5:1 ($p<0.001$, highly significant). In these 2 patients, endoscopic cyst fenestration was repeated without shunt revision. In other words, none of the 15 patients (mean age 9.1 months) in which endoscopic cyst fenestration preceded shunting, required shunt revision among the mean follow-up period of 30.7 months.

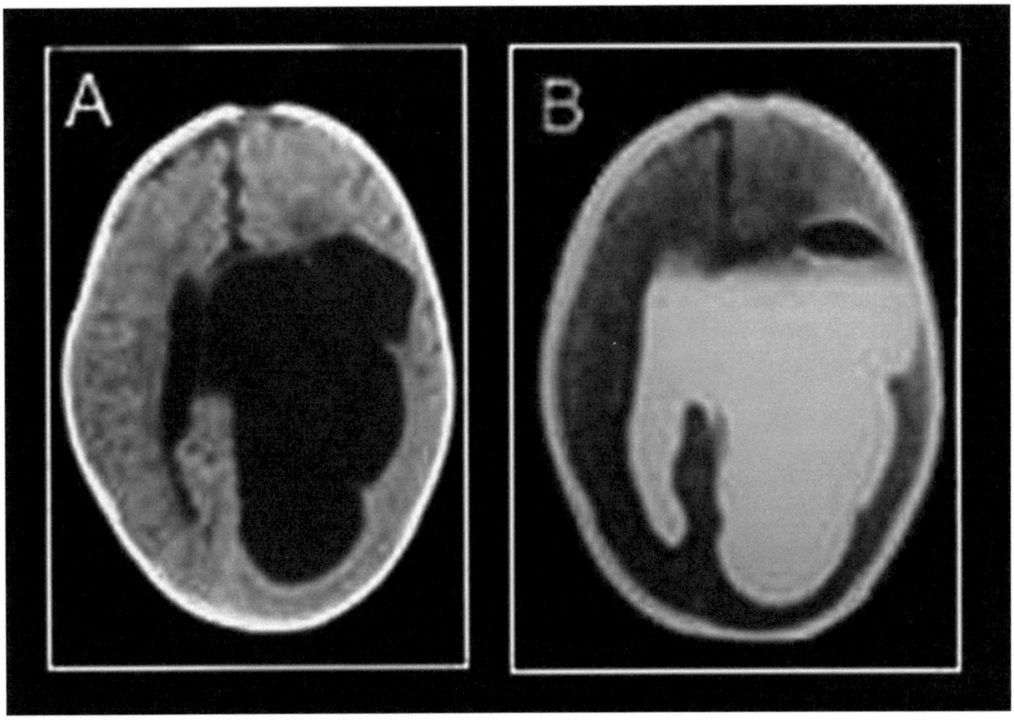

Fig. 2. A, Preoperative CT scan axial view of a 5 months old male patient with multiloculated hydrocephalus. B, postoperative CT ventriculography performed 1 week after surgery showing the contrast material evenly filling the entire ventricular system confirming communication among all cavities. The presence of air within the cyst is an indication of successful fenestration [Reprinted with permission from El-Ghandour NM (2008). Endoscopic cyst fenestration in the treatment of multiloculated hydrocephalus in children. *J Neurosurg Pediatr,* Vol.1, No. 3, (March 2008), pp:217-222, ISSN 1933-0707].

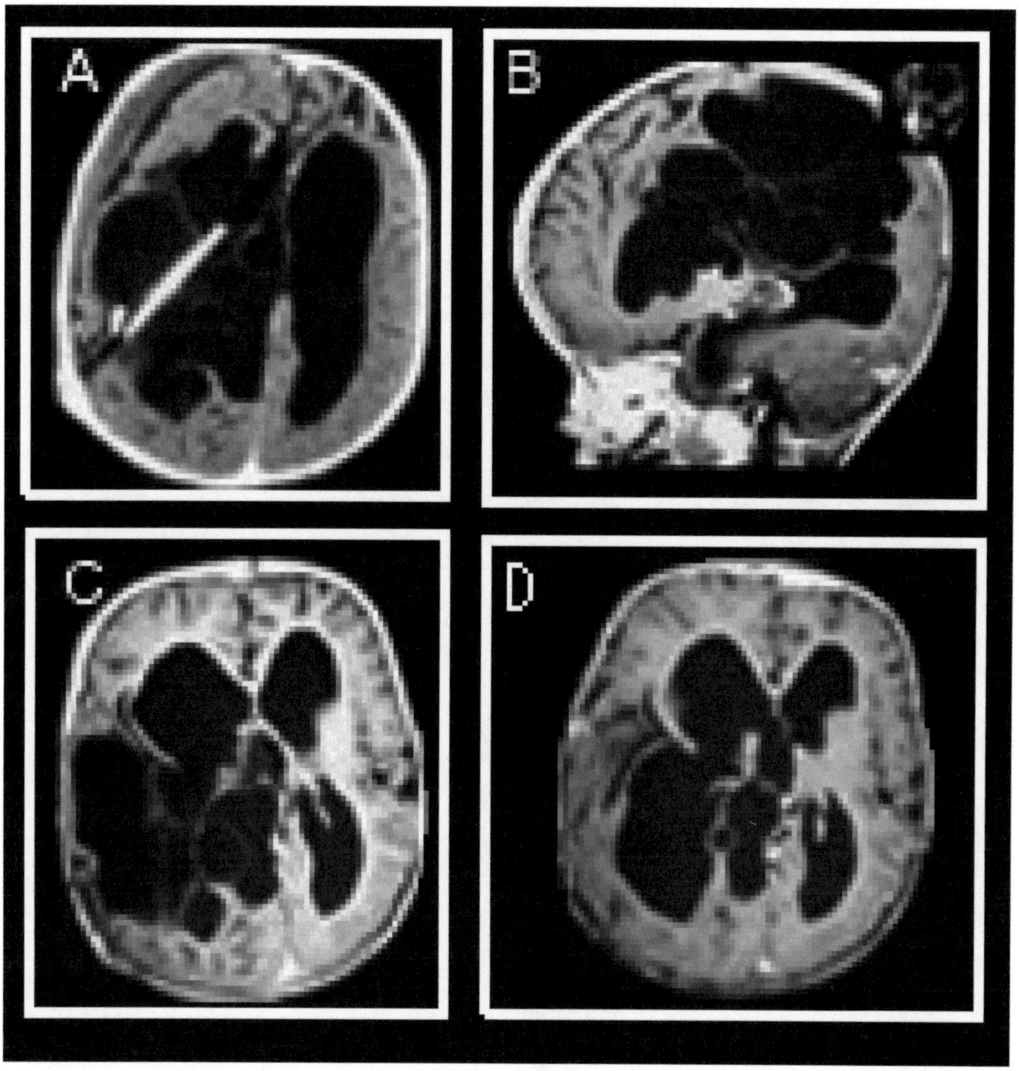

Fig. 3. A, preoperative CT scan of a 1 year old male patient with severe multiloculated hydrocephalus due to gliosis secondary to shunt infection. Note complex malfunctioning shunts. B, preoperative sagittal MR imaging of the same case. C, axial MR imaging performed 3 months after surgery. D, axial MR imaging performed 1 year after surgery showing improvement of hydrocephalus, increase in cerebral mantle, and restoration of ventricular architecture [Reprinted with permission from El-Ghandour NM (2008). Endoscopic cyst fenestration in the treatment of multiloculated hydrocephalus in children. *J Neurosurg Pediatr*, Vol.1, No. 3, (March 2008), pp:217-222, ISSN 1933-0707].

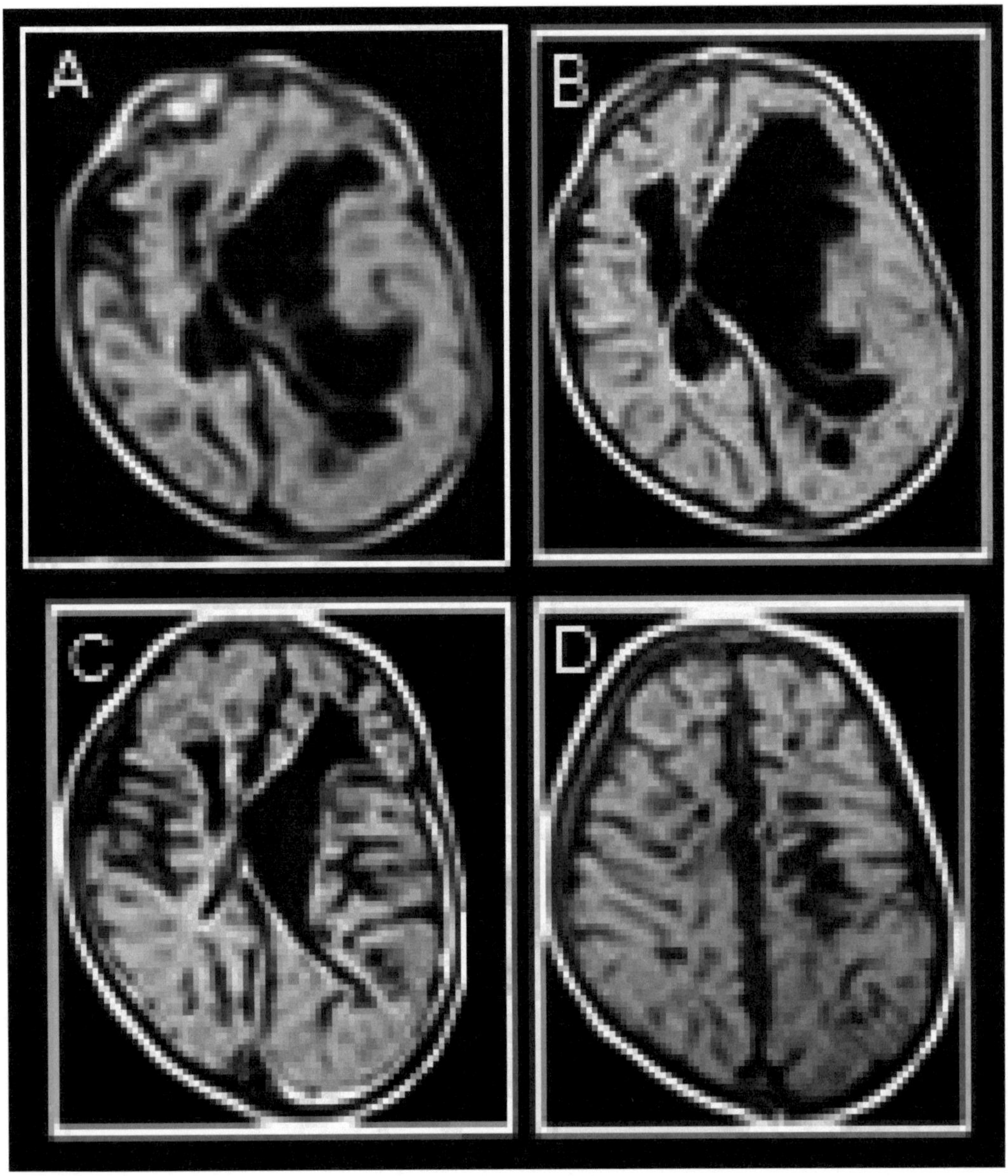

Fig. 4. A, B, preoperative axial MR imaging of a 7 months old male patient with multiloculated hydrocephalus due to intrauterine toxoplasmosis infection. C, axial MR imaging performed 3 months after surgery showing improvement of hydrocephalus. D, axial MR imaging performed 1 year after surgery showing complete resolution of hydrocephalus [Reprinted with permission from El-Ghandour NM (2008). Endoscopic cyst fenestration in the treatment of multiloculated hydrocephalus in children. *J Neurosurg Pediatr,* Vol.1, No. 3, (March 2008), pp:217-222, ISSN 1933-0707].

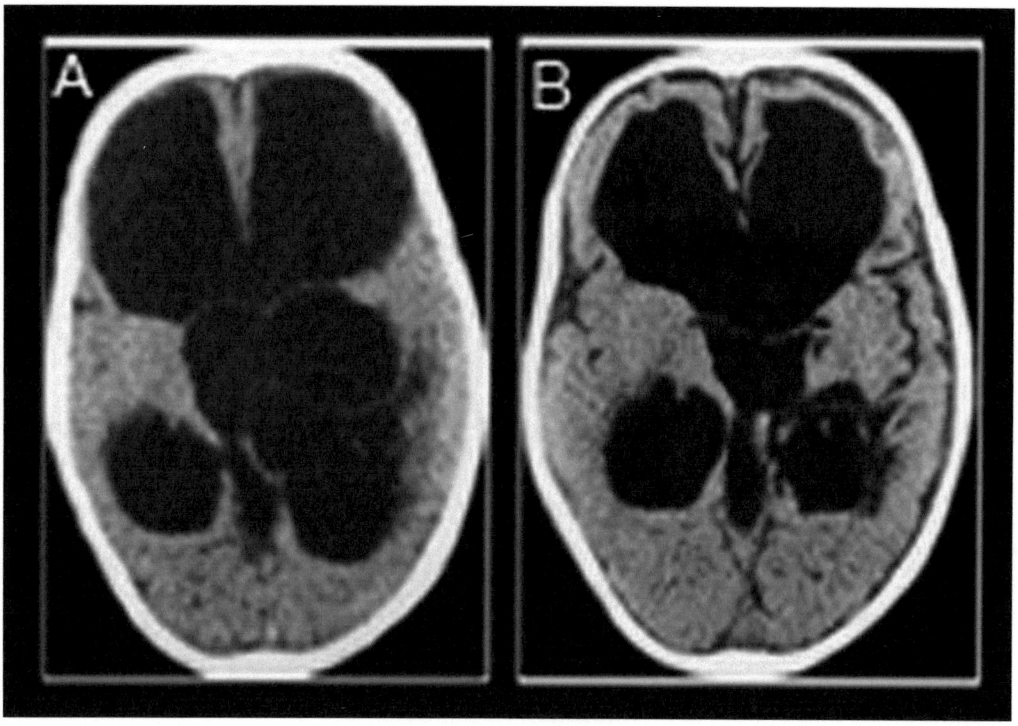

Fig. 5. A, preoperative CT scan axial view of a 1.5 years old female patient with multiloculated hydrocephalus. B, postoperative CT scan performed 3 months after surgery showing improvement of hydrocephalus, increase in cerebral mantle, opening of subarachnoid space, and restoration of ventricular architecture. This patient has been operated through a biportal technique (left coronal + left occipital burr holes) [Reprinted with permission from El-Ghandour NM (2008). Endoscopic cyst fenestration in the treatment of multiloculated hydrocephalus in children. *J Neurosurg Pediatr,* Vol.1, No. 3, (March 2008), pp:217-222, ISSN 1933-0707].

Case No.	Age at ECF (mos)	Observation Period (mos)		No of Revisions		No of Revisions / year	
		Pre ECF	Post ECF	Pre ECF	Post ECF	Pre ECF	Post ECF
1	12	9	36	4	0	5.33	0
2	24	18	21	4	1	2.66	0.57
3	16	9	9	1	0	1.33	0
4	36	15	42	3	1	2.40	0.28
5	8	5	26	1	0	2.40	0
6	36	18	30	5	1	3.33	0.39
Mean	22.0	12.3	27.3	3	0.5	2.91	0.21
S.D.	12.1	5.4	11.6	1.7	0.55	1.34	0.24
Median	20.0	12.0	28.0	3.5	0.5	2.54	0.14

Table 1. Age, observation period in months (mos), and shunt revision rates before and after endoscopic cyst fenestration (ECF), in 6 patients with multiloculated hydrocephalus presented with preexisting shunts. [Reprinted with permission from El-Ghandour NM (2008). Endoscopic cyst fenestration in the treatment of multiloculated hydrocephalus in children. *J Neurosurg Pediatr,* Vol.1, No. 3, (March 2008), pp:217-222, ISSN 1933-0707].

12. Conclusions

Complex hydrocephalus is a challenging problem in pediatric neurosurgery. Early diagnosis and treatment is the key for a better prognosis, therefore a high threshold of alertness is needed among pediatricians in dealing with patients having meningitis or intraventricular hemorrhage or premature infants. Multiplanar MR imaging is the preferred diagnostic modality. The definitive treatment is surgical, yet the approach remains controversial. Cyst fenestration is the main strategy of treatment, and it can be done either microsurgically or endoscopically, aiming at improving hydrocephalus, reducing number of shunts and shunt revision rate. However, the endoscopic treatment has the advantage of being minimally invasive. It is worthy to mention, that multiloculated hydrocephalus carries a worse prognosis than uniloculated hydrocephalus.

13. References

Abtin K & Walker ML (1998). Endoscopic management of complex hydrocephalus. In: *Intracranial Endoscopic Neurosurgery,* Jimenez DF, pp. 135-145, AANS publication committee, ISBN 0-9624246-6-8, Illinois.

Albanese V, Tomasello F & Sampaolo S (1981). Multiloculated hydrocephalus in infants. *Neurosurgery,* Vol 8, No 6, (June 1981), pp. 641-646, ISSN 0148-396x

Berger MS, Sundsten J, Lemire RJ, Silbergeld D, Newell D & Shurtleff D (1990). Pathophysiology of isolated lateral ventriculomegaly in shunted myelodysplastic children. *Pediatr Neurosurg,* Vol 16, No 6, (1990), pp. 301-304, ISSN 1016-2291

Brockmeyer DL (1998). The use of endoscopes for shunt placement. In *Endoscopy of the central and peripheral nervous system,* King W, Frazee J & De Salles A, pp. 91-99, Thieme, ISBN 0- 86577-690-3, New York

Cinalli G, Spennato P, Savarese L, Ruggiero C, Aliberti F, Cuomo L, Cianciulli E & Maggi G (2006). Endoscopic aqueductoplasty and placement of a stent in the cerebral aqueduct in the management of isolated fourth ventricle in children. *J Neurosurg* Vol. 104 (1 Suppl), No. 1, (January 2006), pp. 21- 27, ISSN 0022-3085

El-Ghandour NM (2006). Multiloculated hydrocephalus: A study of 24 patients operated by endoscopic cyst fenestration. *Neurosurgery,* Vol. 59, No. 2, (August 2006), p 477, ISSN 0148-396x (Abstr).

El-Ghandour NM (2008). Endoscopic cyst fenestration in the treatment of multiloculated hydrocephalus in children. *J Neurosurg Pediatr,* Vol.1, No. 3, (March 2008), pp. 217-222, ISSN 1933-0707

Eller TW & Pasternak JF (1985). Isolated ventricles following intraventricular hemorrhage. J *Neurosurg,* Vol. 62, No. 3, (March 1985), pp. 357-362, ISSN 0022-3085

Heilman CB & Cohen AR (1991). Endoscopic ventricular fenestration using a " saline torch". *J Neurosurg,* Vol. 74, No. 2, (February 1991), pp. 224-229, ISSN 0022-3085

Hellwig D, Bauer BL, Schulte M, Gatscher S, Riegel T & Bertalanffy H (2008). Neuroendoscopic treatment for colloid cysts of the third ventricle : the experience of a decade. *Neurosurgery,* Vol. 62, No. 6 (Suppl 3), (June 2008), pp. 1101 -1109, ISSN 0148-396x

Jeeves MA, Simpson DA & Geffen G (1979). Functional consequences of the transcallosal removal of intraventricular tumors. *J Neurol Neurosurg Psychiatry.* Vol. 42, No. 2, (February 1979), pp.134-142, ISSN 0022-3050

Kaiser G (1986). The value of multiple shunt systems in the treatment of nontumoral infantile hydrocephalus. Childs Nerv Syst, Vol. 2, No. 4, (April 1986), pp. 200-205, ISSN 0939-0146

Kalsbeck EJ, DeSousa AL, Kleiman MB, Goodman JM & Franke EA (1980). Compartmentalization of the cerebral ventricles as a sequela of neonatal meningitis. *J Neurosurg, Vol.* 52, No. 4, (April 1980), pp. 547-552, ISSN 0022-3085

Levy ML, Wang M, Aryan HE, Yoo K & Meltzer H (2003). Microsurgical keyhole approach for middle fossa arachnoid cyst fenestration. *Neurosurgery,*Vol. 53, No. 5 (November 2003), pp. 1138-1145, ISSN 0148-396x

Lewis AI, Keiper GL & Crone KR. (1995). Endoscopic treatment of loculated hydrocephalus. *J Neurosurg,* Vol.82, No.5, (May 1995), pp. 780-785, ISSN 0022- 3085

Machado HR, Martelli N, Assirati JA Jr & Colli BO (1991). Infantile hydrocephalus: brain sonography as an effective tool for diagnosis and follow-up. *Childs Nerv Syst,* Vol. 7, No. 4, (April 1991), pp. 205-210, ISSN 0939-0146

Manwaring K (1992). Endoscopic ventricular fenestration. In: *Neuroendoscopy,* Manwaring K & Crone K, pp 79-89, Mary Ann Liebert , ISBN 0913113573, New York

Mathiesen T, Grane P, Lindquist C & von Holst H (1993). High recurrence rate following aspiration of colloid cysts in the third ventricle. J *Neurosurg, Vol.* 78, No. 5, (May 1993), pp. 748-752,. ISSN 0022- 3085

Mohanty A (2005). Endoscopic options in the management of isolated fourth ventricles. Case report. *J Neurosurg: Pediatrics,* Vol. 103, No. 1, (July 2005), pp. 73-78, ISSN 0022-3085

Nida TY & Haines SJ (1993). Multiloculated hydrocephalus: Craniotomy and fenestration of intraventricular septations. *J Neurosurgery,* Vol. 78, No.1, (January 1993), pp. 70-76, ISSN 0022-3085

Powers SK (1986) Fenestration of intraventricular cysts using a flexible, steerable endoscope and the argon laser. *Neurosurgery,* Vol. 18, No. 5, (May 1986), pp.637-641, ISSN 0148-396x

Powers SK (1992). Fenestration of intraventricular cysts using a flexible, steerable endoscope. *Acta Neurochir (Wien)*. Vol. 54, (1992), pp. 42-46, ISSN 0065-1419

Rhoton AL Jr & Gomez MR (1972). Conversion of multilocular hydrocephalus to unilocular. Case report. *J Neurosurg*. Vol. 36, No. 3, (March 1972), pp. 348-350, ISSN 0022-3085

Ross DA, Muraszko K & Dauser R (1994). A special cyst puncture catheter for use in thick-walled or mobile intracranial cysts. *Neurosurgery*, Vol. 34, No. 1, (January 1994), pp. 191-192, 0148-396x

Sandberg DI, McComb G & Kreiger MD (2005). Craniotomy for fenestration of multiloculated hydrocephalus in pediatric patients. *Neurosurgery*, Vol. 57 (1 Suppl), No. 1, (July 2005), pp. 100-106, 0148-396x

Schultz P & Leeds NE (1973). Intraventricular septations complicating neonatal meningitis. *J Neurosurg, Vol.* 38, No. 5, (May 1973), pp. 620-626, ISSN 0022-3085

Schulz M, Bohner G, Knaus H, Haberl H & Thomale UW. (2010). Navigated endoscopic surgery for multiloculated hydrocephalus in children. *J Neurosurg: Pediatr*, Vol. 5, No. 5 (May 2010), pp. 434-442, ISSN 1933-0707

Teo C (1998). Endoscopy for the treatment of hydrocephalus. In *Endoscopy of the central and peripheral nervous system*, King W, Frazee J & De Salles A, pp. 59-67, Thieme, ISBN 0- 86577-690-3, New York

12

Recognition of Posture and Gait Disturbances in Patients with Normal Pressure Hydrocephalus Using a Posturography and Computer Dynography Systems

L. Czerwosz[1], E. Szczepek[1,2], B. Sokołowska[1],
J. Jurkiewicz[1,2] and Z. Czernicki[1,2]
[1]*Mossakowski Medical Research Centre, Polish Academy of Sciences, Warsaw,*
[2]*Warsaw Medical University, Warsaw,*
Poland

1. Introduction

There are great difficulties in clinical practice to differentiate between normal pressure hydrocephalus (NPH) and brain atrophy (Tans 1979, Galia at al. 2005). The consequences of inaccurate diagnosis are serious therefore we observe steady searching of new non-invasive or minimal-invasive diagnostic methods.

The purpose of this study is to quantify the characteristics of the postural sway and locomotion in NPH patients in two states: before and after shunt implantation and to compare posture and gait features among: NPH, brain atrophy patients and healthy persons.

Assessment of stability and balance system consist in quantitatively measuring and analysing movements of the centre of foot pressure (COP). Position of COP steadily changes due to the so called postural sways, and of course due to voluntary moves. Enlarged sways, observed in normal pressure hydrocephalus, are not however specific and cannot give simple diagnosis. Postural balance can be impaired due to pathology in various organs including vestibular and cerebellar disorders and various forms of ataxia (Mohan at al. 2009), Parkinsonism (Bloem at al. 1995, Stolze at al. 2001, Jagielski at al. 2006), multiple sclerosis (Kessler at al. 2011) and even alcohol dependence (Wöber at al. 1998) and muscle fatigue or aging (Błaszczyk and Michalski 2006).

Evaluation of gait relates to postural stability in standing upright position. The gait disturbance is probably the most prominent clinical feature of NPH and it is often the first NPH symptom to develop (Radvin 2008). Gait disturbances are part of so called Hakim triad (Hakim & Adams 1965). NPH gait disturbances are very characteristic and rely on shuffling manner of walking, without raising the feet as if they were glued to the floor. This kind of gait is called also magnetic. Gait disturbances are still not fully described quantitatively due to lack of reliable, specific parameters measuring most typical features of gait in NPH.

Some papers related to postural stability and gait evaluation in NPH have already been published by Szczepek and Czerwosz (Szczepek at al. 2008, Czerwosz at al. 2008, 2009). The current study is trying to summarize some of our results.

2. Methods

Recently rapid development of precise methods of quantitative measurements of body position while standing or walking has been observed. Two techniques used by us in our investigations should be discussed here:

1. static posturography - measurement of body sways while standing on a force plate,
2. dynography - measurement of gait.

In both systems the resultant force - feet pressure acting on the horizontal surface (XY) is calculated on the basis of some number of pressure sensors. The most important is the point of application of this force. This point is called Centre of foot/feet Pressure (COP). In static conditions the COP point is a projection of the Centre of Gravity (COG) position - on the XY horizontal plane. COM and COG signals are highly correlated (Błaszczyk 2008). It has been documented that COG signal can be extracted from COP by low-pass filtering (Benda et al. 1994). The high frequency component comes in dynamic and realistic conditions from inertia forces that influence COP instantaneous location. Inertia forces arise from accelerations of the body while it is swaying or moving - losing and recovering balance (Newton's second law of motion).

2.1 Posturography

The instantaneous COP xy position can be calculated on the basis of instantaneous values of $p_1(t)$, $p_2(t)$, $p_3(t)$, $p_4(t)$ forces measured on four corners of the square plate; d is a length of it's side. In case of our device: d= 40 cm.

$$\begin{cases} x(t) = \frac{d}{2}(-p_1(t) + p_2(t) + p_3(t) - p_4(t)) / (p_1(t) + p_2(t) + p_3(t) + p_4(t)) \\ y(t) = \frac{d}{2}(+p_1(t) + p_2(t) - p_3(t) - p_4(t)) / (p_1(t) + p_2(t) + p_3(t) + p_4(t)) \end{cases} \quad (1)$$

To obtain the exact position of COP, the p_n forces must be reduced by tare weights measured independently on each corner. The real force plate is shown on **Figure 1**; p_n forces are pointed and orientation of xy plane is given by X and Y axes. All $p_n(t)$ values, and therefore x(t) and y(t) change in time. In practice we collect them in 0.01 seconds intervals (sampling frequency 100 Hz) in digital form with 12 bit accuracy. Data were low-pass filtered (15 Hz cut-off frequency). Trajectory can be observed on-line and off-line in an analogue way on a chart called posturogram or stabilogram.

A single measurement on a force plate takes usually 30-60 seconds. The resultant time had to be reduced due to some artefacts related to unsolicited activity of the patient such as his movement or speaking influencing the outcomes. Removing artefacts is still an unresolved problem in posturography due to questionable difference between unsolicited movement and essential balance restoration, especially in case of large sways.

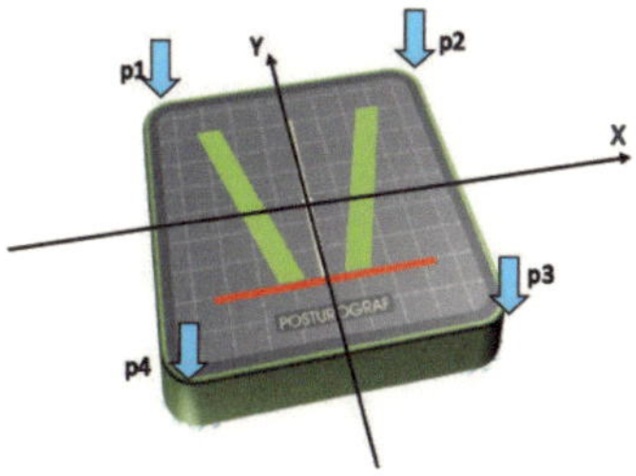

Fig. 1. Force plate.
There are four sensors measuring forces on each corner: p1, p2, p3, p4.
Y represents forward-backward, anterior-posterior sways, in sagittal plane,
X represents left-right, mediolateral sways, in frontal plane.

2.2 Examples of posturographic measurements

Figure 2 shows six examples of posturographic measurements with eyes open (EO) or closed (EC). The two first trajectories belong to NPH patient in acute state, before shunt

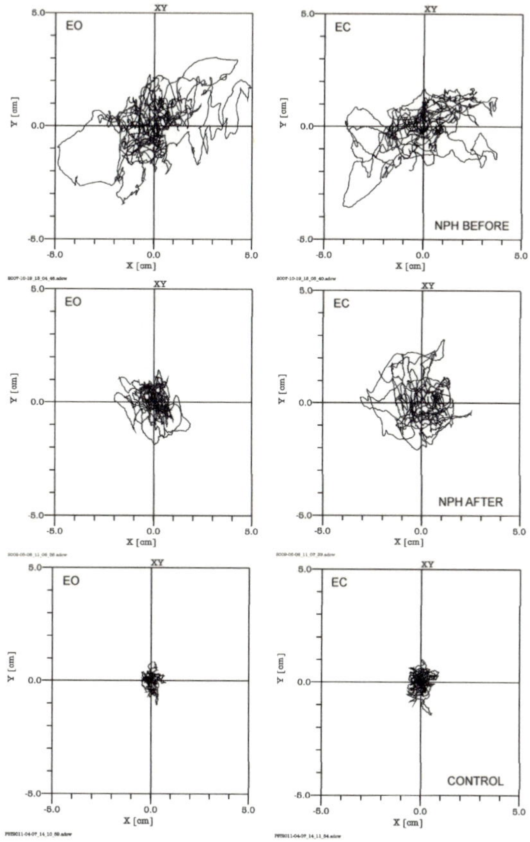

Fig. 2. Examples of measurements - from top: NPH BEFORE - NPH patient before shunt implantation measured with eyes open (EO - left) and closed (EC- right), NPH AFTER - NPH patient after surgery. CONTROL - healthy person.

implantation. The next two were measured after surgery; the last two belong to a healthy person. As one can see, there are big differences in the shapes of the trajectories, especially NPH patient before surgery demonstrates very large sways - both, with eyes open and closed. Sways of the NPH patient are very large both for EO and EC. After surgery sways are reduced but they are still larger than in a healthy person.

2.3 Posturography parameters

COP trajectory represents sways of an object standing in upright position for some time. There is some number of various metrics developed that evaluate average or typical "behaviour" of the curve in many aspects (Baratto at al. 2002, Raymakers at al. 2005).

The starting point of our analysis was to define the global parameters expressing the "size" of sways. We have taken into consideration:

- R - average COP sway Radius,
- A - Area of developed surface of COP trajectory, AS - Area Speed
- L - Length of COP trajectory, V - Velocity.

An average Radius of sway is a simple average of distances between curve samples and (0,0) point on XY plane - coordinate origin. Actually all points of the curve have been shifted by $(\bar{x},\bar{y})$ vector beforehand and thus (0,0) turns into the "centre of gravity" of all samples ($\bar{x}$ denotes average value of all x_i). This simple way of calculating R has been applied by Czerwosz and Szczepek in their papers (Czerwosz at al. 2008, 2009, Szczepek at al. 2008) and also Mraz at al. 2007, Bosek at al. 2005, Kubisz at al. 2011.

Calculation of developed area bases on all available samples. The developed surface consists of triangles created from every two consecutives COP positions sampled every 0.01 second and the coordinate origin (0,0). Let's compare this surface to wooden pencil shavings when sharpening a pencil. **Figure 3** shows the idea of the calculation on a piece of COP curve. The area depends on the number of samples - thus it depends on measurement duration. It is easy to normalize it dividing the area by measurement duration. In this way we are obtaining Area Speed (AS) in mm^2/sec.

The length of COP trajectory is calculated as a simple sum of consecutives segments between COP positions sampled every 0.01 second. Length after division by measurement duration becomes a Velocity (V) in mm/sec.

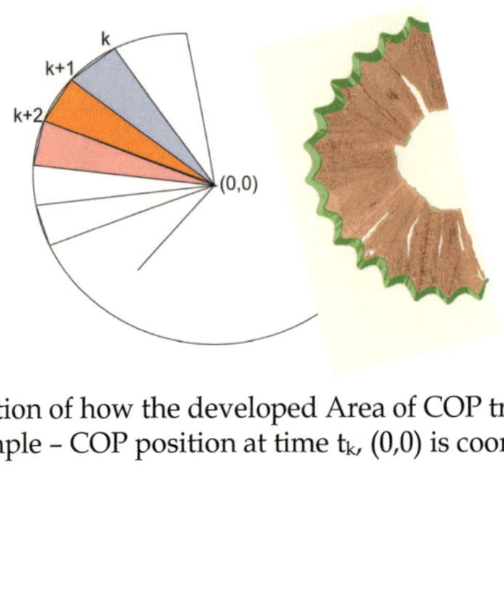

Fig. 3. Graphical explanation of how the developed Area of COP trajectory is calculated. k is a serial number of xy sample - COP position at time t_k, (0,0) is coordinate origin.

Each parameter can relate to two measurement conditions: eyes either open (EO) or closed (EC). In order to express change in value of some parameters due to different conditions one can use simple difference (2). For computational reasons in advanced statistical analysis sum of the same parameters (3) has been introduced.

$$D_x = X_{EC} - X_{EO} \quad (2)$$

$$S_x = X_{EC} + X_{EO} \quad (3)$$

where X can be R, A, AS, L, or V.

A derived parameter - the vision index (4) has been developed on the basis of Radius, Area, Area speed, Length or Speed to express difference of chosen parameter in relation to its mean value. Index is an absolute, dimensionless number with theoretical range [-100%, 100%]. Zero means no difference. One should notice that I_x is bigger for bigger D_x and smaller S_x and vice versa: I_x gets smaller for smaller D_x and bigger S_x. A similar index related to the parameters measured in two different conditions have been introduced by Mraz as ICOP (Mraz at al. 2007).

$$I_x = (X_{EC} - X_{EO})/(X_{EC} + X_{EO}) * 100\% \quad (4)$$

where X can be R, A, AS, L, or V. EC means „eyes closed", EO - „eyes open ", while measurement has been performed. We have made use of vision indices related to radius, area and length. Notice that the index related to area is equal to the index related to area speed ($I_{AS} = I_A$) and the index related to length is equal to the index related to velocity ($I_V = I_L$).

Let's take sight index of radius as an example. Exact way of calculation I_R is given below:

$$I_R = (R_{EC} - R_{EO})/(R_{EC} + R_{EO}) * 100\% \quad (5)$$

2.4 Dynography

Computerized dynography (Infotronic 2007) is a gait analysis system which consists of two soles containing sensors sensible to a foot pressure acting on the ground. These sensors measure the vertical ground reaction forces and their distribution during walking. It's a good alternative to much less quantitative gait scale - for measuring gait impairment of NPH patients (Boon at al. 2007). Another alternative is camera based system but then the only information that is provided are body parts positions and angles without any data related to forces. Walking on a treadmill gives just the speed of gait; to measure more gait features some extra instrumentation should be added. In this study we don't take advantage of forces explicitly, but our system (see below) uses them internally to determine gait phases. Other alternative method of gait evaluation can be performed on two or more joined force plates. This method limits gait to only few steps because of size. It can easily be used for gait analysis in small animals (Voss at al. 2007).

Special boot for dynography is presented in **Figure 4** (on the left side). There are eight sensors inside each sole located as shown in the middle picture. Actually eight histograms are shown here on the sole, not sensors, but they are distributed just as sensors. Histogram height expresses instantaneous or average force acting on a sensor. The picture on the right shows how the point of application of the resultant ground reaction force is being displaced while stance phase of gait cycle. This point is the Centre of foot/feet Pressure (COP) and its position changes during each step. The overall load, the value of resultant ground reaction changes due to inertia forces as well.

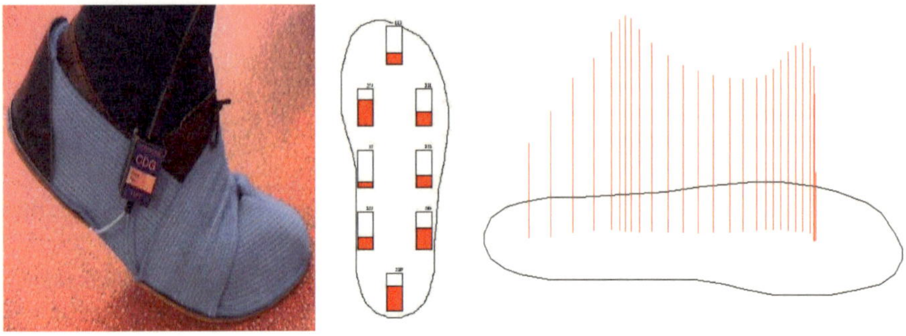

Fig. 4. Left: A boot for dynography with eight sensors inside its sole. Middle: Histograms express instantaneous or average force acting on each sensor. Right: displacement of resultant ground reaction force along a foot. (Pictures from Ultraflex system - Infotronic Company 2007).

The displacement of COP presented in **Figure 4** relates to single foot only. In this case COP position is calculated on the basis of eight sensors. **Figure 5** presents so called gait-lines where successive COP positions of each step are drawn overlapped. Gait-lines of each foot are calculated independently. Pictures on the right side are averaged over all gait cycles of 20 seconds walking. Gait-line represents stance phase of gait from initial contact, while a heel touches the ground till toe off moment (Perry & Burnfield 2010). COP can also be calculated on the basis of 16 sensors enclosed in two soles - from both feet. Cyclogram arises if connecting successive COP positions of each step and drawing the lines overlapped. They are presented in **Figure 6**. Pictures on the right side are averaged over all gait cycles. During double support the COP position lies somewhere between the feet depending on the load ratio and its position changes from one side to another. During single support COP is located within single foot boundary.

Let there be N sensors. N = 8 or N = 16. Let i be the number of a sensor: $1 \leq i \leq N$. Let the position of sensor i be (x_i, y_i). Let $F_i(t)$ be the force at moment t acting on sensor i.

Coordinates of the COP at moment t can be calculated from equations (6) - see Jeleń at al. 2008.

$$\begin{cases} x(t) = \sum_{i}^{N} F_i(t) * x_i \, / \sum_{i}^{N} F_i(t) \\ y(t) = \sum_{i}^{N} F_i(t) * y_i \, / \sum_{i}^{N} F_i(t) \end{cases} \tag{6}$$

Equations (6) are very similar to (1) related to force plate, only the number of sensors (N = 4) and its positions are different. The gait-lines and cyclograms are normalised and related to dimensionless foot length, therefore all distances and speed can be calculated only if the total distance that the person has walked has been entered. Data is sampled with the frequency equal to 100 Hz.

2.5 Examples of dynography measurements

Pictures in **Figure 5** show examples of gait-lines; pictures in **Figure 6** - cyclograms obtained for NPH patient before and after shunt implantation and for healthy person. Gait-lines and cyclograms show gait in compact way. The symmetry of gait and regularity of cycles can

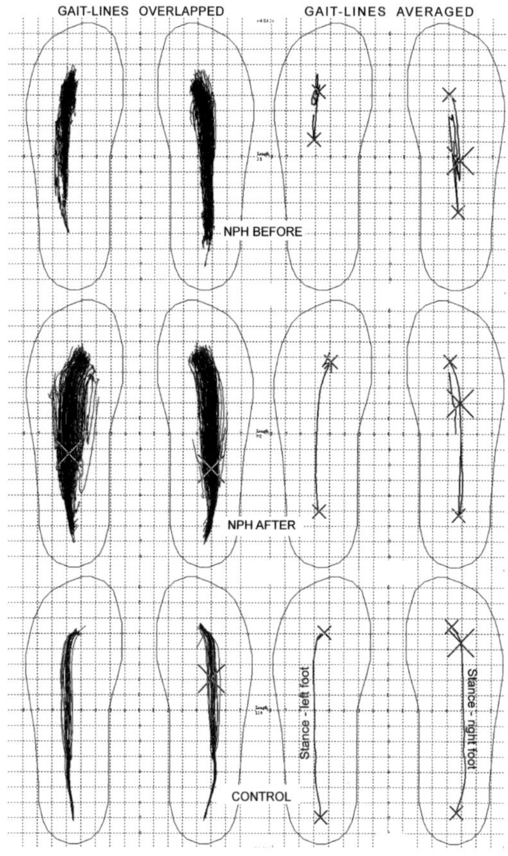

Fig. 5. Examples of gait-lines. The left pictures show overlapping gait cycles measured by 8 sensors in each foot. Pictures on the right side are averaged. The upper gait-lines represent NPH patient before shunt implantation (NPH BEFORE). Gait-lines in the middle belong to NPH patient after surgery (NPH AFTER). Lower gait-lines have been measured in healthy person (CONTROL). Lines representing the Stance gait phase are annotated in the bottom picture.

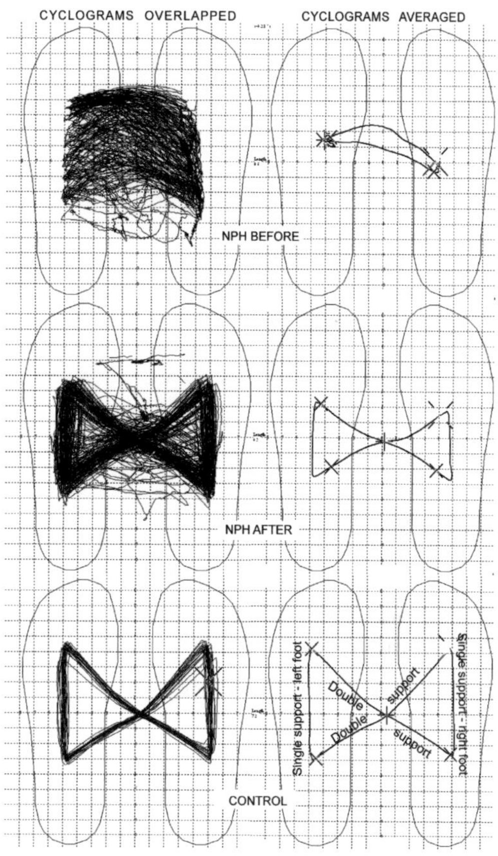

Fig. 6. Examples of cyclograms. The left pictures show overlapping gait cycles measured by 16 sensors in both feet. Pictures on the right side are averaged. Successive panels are: NPH patient before shunt implantation (NPH BEFORE), NPH patient after surgery (NPH AFTER), healthy person (CONTROL). Lines representing the Single and Double Support gait phases are annotated in the bottom picture.

easily be observed. One can notice shuffling gait of NPH patient (before surgery) - there is almost no single support phase - the patient only slightly rises his feet. The whole stance phase is consisting of double support.

2.6 Dynography parameters

After data collection CDG software recognizes gait phases and calculates gait parameters. Gait was described in our research as a duration of a single (SSUP) and double support (DSUP) and duration of a stance phase (STANCE). These measures relate to the left and right leg independently. The phases are shown in **Figure 7**.

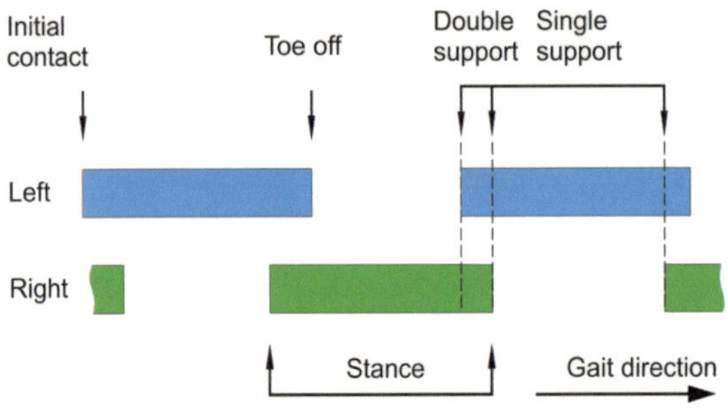

Fig. 7. Phases of gait cycle.

2.7 Hardware and software usage

For posturographic measurements Pro-Med (Poland) force plate (Olton & Czerwosz 2006) was used by us. The software for data collection and analysis has been written by the author (Leszek Czerwosz).

For measurement of ground reaction forces in walking we used the Ultraflex Computer DynoGraphy system from Infotronic Company (Netherlands). Applications of CDG system in NPH are not aware. Explanations of usefulness of this system are provided by Bhargava at al. 2007, Majumdar at al. 2008, Jeleń at al. 2008.

2.8 Statistical methods

Wilcoxon matched pairs test for intragroup and Mann-Whitney U test for between-group comparisons were performed in our studies (Czerwosz at al. 2008, 2009, Szczepek at al. 2008). Non-parametric ANOVA Kruskal-Wallis test (Kruskal & Wallis 1952) was used while comparing more cohorts and then Bonferroni correction (Dunn 1961) for post-hoc comparisons.

There is much confusion related to the application of corrections if performing post-hoc comparisons, especially if testing schema is a priori established. It is hard to accept the fact that the result of one statistical test, i.e. while comparing statistically the NPH and CONTROL groups, can be influenced by other tests, while collecting some extra data, for example ataxia group and by performing other comparisons. We will of course change the level of significance required for rejection the null hypothesis to $p<0.016$ in case of three group analysis that we perform in this study. And we are introducing pattern recognition methods for differentiation of groups to avoid purely academic arguments.

All the nonparametric analyses were conducted using Origin software (OriginLab Corporation) and PASW Statistics (IBM-SPSS Statistics).

We applied pattern recognition algorithms - two advanced statistical methods: Dicriminant Analysis (DA) and k-Nearest Neighbour method (K-NN) (Devijver and Kittler 1982, Duda at al. 2001). DA calculations were performed by means of PASW Statistics. For K-NN calculations (Jóźwik at al. 2011, Sokołowska at al. 2009) a computer programme developed by Adam Jóźwik was used.

The K-NN classifier is a pattern recognition algorithm for recognizing classes of objects. Objects are just vectors of features which values can be measured in patients. Thus an object represent a patient in n-dimensional space, where n is a number of features - measured parameters for each patient. The k-NN algorithm requires a reference set of objects with known class membership. Class means the same as patient group. Any new object, from outside the reference set, is assigned to the class most frequently represented among its k nearest neighbours, searched in the reference set. The leave-one-out method is used to experimentally establish the best value of k giving minimal misclassification rate.

The DA and K-NN methods differ absolutely because DA is a strictly parametric method related closely to the analysis of variance (ANOVA) and produces, among other, linear combination of features (parameters or variables). There is a fundamental assumption that all independent variables have to be normally distributed. In our case - there is no proof for normal distributions, therefore DA outcomes may not be reliable. For the K-NN method it is not important whether distributions are normal.

Pattern recognition methods have already been used in relation to some gait parameters (Bertrani at al. 1999). They should not be mixed with the pattern recognition of gait (Maduko). Discriminant analysis and neural networks were used for gait classification (Kaczmarczyk at al. 2009).

3. Material

After ethical approval by a local Ethics Committee, posturographic and dynographic recordings were taken from NPH patients and from healthy volunteers. Patients with brain atrophy were also recorded to obtain a comparison group to test the power of calculated parameters and statistical methods in differentiation NPG and atrophy (Tans 1979, Galia at al. 2005).

NPH diagnosis was based on the following criteria

1. Enlargement of brain ventricles seen on CT or MR - Evans' ratio above 0.3 (Evans 1942),
2. Neurological symptoms (Hakim triad - minimum two of three symptoms),
3. Mean intracranial pressure ≥ 10 cmH_2O,
4. Resorption resistance $R \geq 11mmHg/ml/min$.

Infusion test (Śliwka at al. 1984, Czernicki at al. 1984, Czosnyka at al. 1988) is performed on the basis of cerebrospinal intracranial fluid pressure measurement with simultaneous infusion of physiological saline in L4, L5, and S1 regions. Infusion test seems to be the most important and limitative qualification for shunt implantation.

In all cases balance disturbances and impairment of gait was observed.

The ATROPHY group has been formed according to the following inclusion criteria:

1. Enlargement of brain ventricles seen on CT or MR (Evans' ratio above 0.3),
2. Both subcortical and cortical atrophy,
3. No characteristic neurological symptoms,
4. Mean intracranial pressure < 10 cmH_2O,
5. Resorption resistance R < 11 mmHg/ml/min.

Balance disturbances and some impairment of gait were observed in atrophy patients.

Posturography and dynography evaluations were performed in NPH cases before shunt implantation and shortly after the surgery (within seven days).

3.1 Subjects for posturography study

There were 18 NPH diagnosed patients with spontaneous postural sways measured (9 males and 9 females, range: 32-82 y. o., mean: 64.1 ± 13.2 y. o.). The same group was evaluated twice: before and after shunt implantation forming two cohorts: NPH BEFORE and NPH AFTER.

CONTROL group consisted of 47 healthy subjects, aged 60-69, mean: 59.9 ± 7.0 y. o. The data have been collected by Katarzyna Dmitruk (doctor thesis 2005, partially published in Czerwosz at al. 2009).

ATROPHY group was composed from 36 patients (32-75 y. o., mean: 57.0 ± 14.1 y. o.)

3.2 Subjects for dynography study

CDG measurement was performed in 15 patients with the NPH (8 males and 7 females, age range: 32-82 y. o., mean: 63.1 ± 14.3 y. o.) The same group was evaluated twice: before and after shunt implantation forming two cohorts: NPH BEFORE and NPH AFTER but they are not identical with posturography groups, only 11 patients were examined by two methods.

CONTROL group consisted of 24 healthy subjects (5 males, 19 females).

ATROPHY group was composed from 35 patients (21 males, 14 females, range: 32-79 y. o., mean: 64.1 ± 12.3 y. o.).

4. Results

A number of results have been obtained in the posture and gait study. Posturography and dynography results will be reported separately because so far no joined analysis has been made.

4.1 Simultaneous comparison of three groups – posturography

To compare three groups: NPH BEFORE, ATROPHY, and CONTROL non-parametric ANOVA Kruskal-Wallis test was used. The results are in **Table 1**. The groups differ significantly for all parameters. This allows post-hoc comparisons in pairs of groups, applying Bonferroni correction.

NPH AFTER group was not taken into account in above comparison because it is the same group as NPH BEFERE but evaluated in different condition and it should be compared to NPH BEFERE group by means of paired test.

Parameter		χ^2 K-W	p
Radius	Radius - eyes open R_{EO}	55.9	< 0.001
	Radius - eyes closed R_{EC}	45.2	< 0.001
	Sum of radiuses S_R	55.0	< 0.001
	Difference of radiuses D_R	9.8	< 0.007
	Vision index related to radius I_R	10.5	< 0.005
Area speed	Area speed - eyes open AS_{EO}	59.9	< 0.001
	Area speed - eyes closed AS_{EC}	48.0	< 0.001
	Sum of area speeds S_{AS}	56.8	< 0.001
	Difference of area speeds D_{AS}	7.7	< 0.021
	Vision index related to area I_A	10.2	< 0.006
Velocity	Velocity - eyes open V_{EO}	57.5	< 0.001
	Velocity - eyes closed V_{EC}	41.3	< 0.001
	Sum of velocities V_L	50.6	< 0.001
	Difference of velocities D_V	8.6	< 0.014
	Vision index related to velocity I_V	11.6	< 0.003

Table 1. Results of non-parametric ANOVA Kruskal-Wallis test for three groups: NPH BEFORE, ATROPHY, and CONTROL. The significance p was reported as <0.000 in the original SPSS results meaning that only subsequent, not displayed decimal digits can differ from zero; to avoid confusion the true outcome has been approximated to 0.001.

Similar three-group analysis was done for NPH AFTER, ATROPHY, and CONTROL. These groups differ significantly for parameters provided in **Table 2**. There are no significant differences for D_R, D_A, and D_L differences as well as for the vision indices: I_R, I_A, I_L. This is quite obvious if you compare left and right columns in each pair of columns in CONTROL, ATROPHY, and NPH AFTER groups in **Figure 8** - in the upper column chart. Only one chart - the radius chart is presented here. The lower column chart shows vision indices. Indeed CONTROL, ATROPHY, and NPH AFTER columns are very similar.

Parameter		χ^2 K-W	p
Radius	Radius - eyes open R_{EO}	38.0	< 0.001
	Radius - eyes closed R_{EC}	26.9	< 0.001
	Sum of radiuses S_R	32.8	< 0.001
Area speed	Area speed - eyes open AS_{EO}	42.5	< 0.001
	Area speed - eyes closed AS_{EC}	32.2	< 0.001
	Sum of area speeds S_{AS}	38.1	< 0.001
Velocity	Velocity - eyes open V_{EO}	42.8	< 0.001
	Velocity - eyes closed V_{EC}	33.2	< 0.001
	Sum of velocities V_L	38.0	< 0.001

Table 2. Results of non-parametric ANOVA Kruskal-Wallis test for three groups: NPH AFTER, ATROPHY, and CONTROL. Other parameters differentiate not significantly.

4.2 Comparison of groups in pairs – posturography

All collected posturographic data related to the Radius are exhibited in **Figure 8**. There are four groups here; each one consists of EO and EC measurements. Individual values of the Radius in EO and EC measurements are shown overlapped to respective columns.

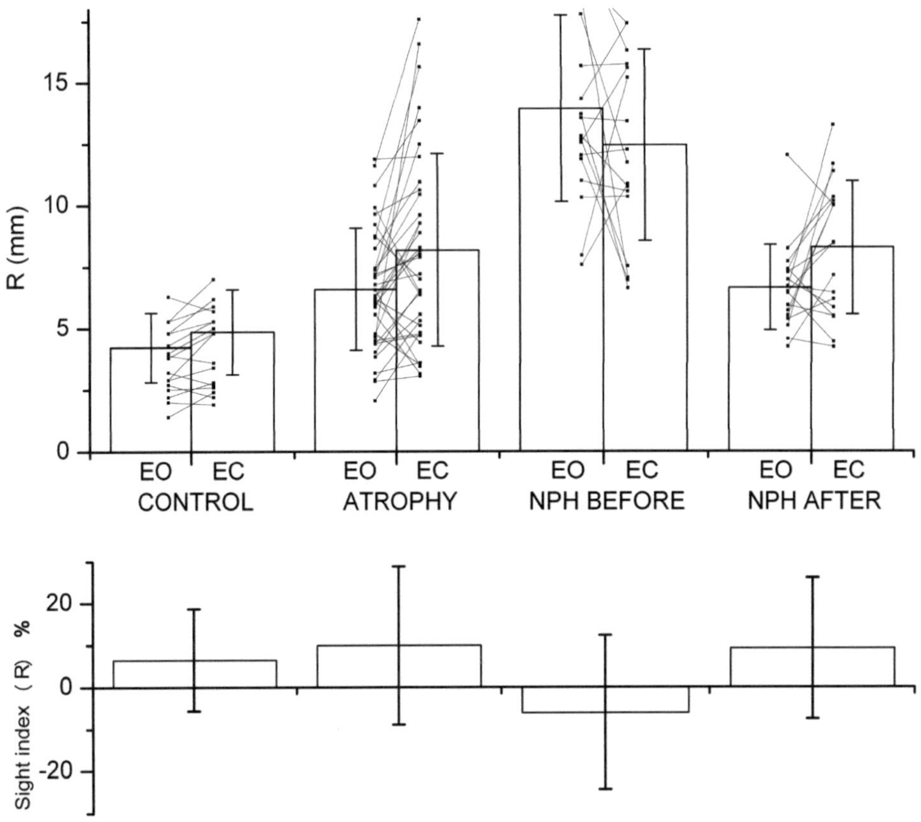

Fig. 8. Upper column chart: Sway Radius - R in CONTROL, ATROPHY, and NPH groups - in patients before and after shunting. Individual values of the Radius are also shown - the lines connect measurements performed with eyes open (EO) or closed (EC). The lower chart expresses vision indices related to radius. Columns represent mean values. Standard deviations are shown as vertical lines.

For comparisons among three groups in pairs see **Tables 3**, **4**, **5**, **7**, and **8**. Nonparametric Mann-Whitney U test with Bonferroni correction was used.

One can notice that NPH BEFORE patients reach largest sways, both with EO and EC (see **Table 3** and **4** respectively). CONTROL group exhibits the smallest sways, both with EO and EC. The same effect can be observed on sums of corresponding parameters (S_X, where X can be R, AS, or V, see **Table 5**). All tested differences of X_{EO}, X_{EC}, and S_X parameters are significant but only V_{EC} and S_V parameters do not differentiate NPH BEFORE and ATROHY pair of groups (**Tables 4** and **5**).

EO		CONTROL	ATROPHY	NPH BEFORE
Radius R_{EO}	AV ± SD mm	4.2 ±1.4	6.6 ± 2.5	13.9 ± 3.8
	CONTROL		p < 0.001	p < 0.001
	ATROPHY			p < 0.001
Area speed AS_{EO}	AV ± SD mm²/sec	13.3 ± 10.2	56.1 ± 84.5	159.5 ± 104.65
	CONTROL		p < 0.001	p < 0.001
	ATROPHY			p < 0.001
Velocity V_{EO}	AV ± SD mm/sec	9.2 ± 4.4	23.2 ± 23.4	35.5 ± 17.7
	CONTROL		p < 0.001	p < 0.001
	ATROPHY			p < 0.001

Table 3. Comparisons among three groups in pairs; measurements were performed with eyes open. Average values(AV) with standard deviations (SD) and significances p of Mann-Whitney U test are given in appropriate table cells. All groups differ in respective pairs of groups.

EC		CONTROL	ATROPHY	NPH BEFORE
Radius R_{EC}	AV ± SD mm	4.9 ± 1.7	8.2 ± 3.9	12.4 ± 3.9
	CONTROL		p < 0.001	p < 0.001
	ATROPHY			p < 0.008
Area speed AS_{EC}	AV ± SD mm²/sec	22.7 ± 22.6	107.8 ± 175.6	140.8 ± 92.2
	CONTROL		p < 0.001	p < 0.001
	ATROPHY			p < 0.011
Velocity V_{EC}	AV ± SD mm/sec	13.5 ± 8.7	33.5 ± 32.0	35.2 ± 17.4
	CONTROL		p < 0.001	p < 0.001
	ATROPHY			n.s.

Table 4. Comparisons among three groups in pairs of groups; measurements were performed in eyes closed condition. All EC parameters but one differentiate these groups. Only average velocity V_{EC} is similar in NPH BEFORE and ATROHY groups.

Sums		CONTROL	ATROPHY	NPH BEFORE
Radius S_R	AV ± SD mm	9.1 ± 2.9	14.7 ± 5.7	26.4 ± 6.3
	CONTROL		p < 0.001	p < 0.001
	ATROPHY			p < 0.001
Area speed S_{AS}	AV ± SD mm²/sec	36.1 ± 30.3	163.8 ± 255.1	300.3 ± 152.9
	CONTROL		p < 0.001	p < 0.001
	ATROPHY			p < 0.001
Velocity S_V	AV ± SD mm/sec	22.8± 12.6	56.8 ± 54.1	70.7± 31.8
	CONTROL		p < 0.001	p < 0.001
	ATROPHY			p < 0.020 =n.s.

Table 5. Comparisons among three groups in pairs of groups. All sums of parameters but one differentiate the groups. Only the sum of average velocities S_V is similar in NPH BEFORE and ATROHY groups.

4.3 Effect of shunt implantation on posturography parameters

One can see in **Figure 9** that radius of sways measured in both conditions: EO and EC in a NPH group before shunt implantation treatment exceeded corresponding values measured in the same patients after surgery.

There is a full set of parameters included in **Table 6** - average values, standard deviation and significance level of nonparametric Wilcoxon paired test. The NPH BEFORE and NPH AFTER groups differ in relation to almost all parameters. The most powerful is radius with EO (R_{EO}) - see also **Figure 9**.

Sways with eyes opened before shunting is much bigger than after surgery.

Parameter			NPH BEFORE	NPH AFTER	p
Radius	R_{EO}	mm	13.9 ± 3.8	6.7 ± 1.7	<0.001
	R_{EC}	mm	12.4 ± 3.9	8.3 ± 2.7	<0.002
	S_R	mm	26.4 ± 6.3	14.9 ± 3.6	<0.001
	D_R	mm	-1.49 ± 4.48	1.62 ± 2.78	<0.007
	I_R	%	-6.09 ±18.9	9.26 ± 7.3	<0.008
Area speed	AS_{EO}	mm^2/sec	159.5 ± 104.6	37.9 ± 17.1	<0.001
	AS_{EC}	mm^2/sec	140.8 ± 92.2	79.4 ± 77.9	n.s.
	S_{AS}	mm^2/sec	300.3 ± 152.9	117.2 ± 88.4	<0.001
	D_{AS}	mm^2/sec	-18.7 ± 124.6	41.5 ± 70.1	<0.043
	I_{AS}	%	-5.2 ± 34.7	15.6 ± 37.7	<0.025
Velocity	V_{EO}	mm/sec	35.5 ± 17.7	18.3 ± 7.4	<0.002
	V_{EC}	mm/sec	35.2 ± 17.4	26.3 ± 17.1	n.s.
	S_V	mm/sec	70.7± 31.8	44.6 ± 23.1	<0.011
	D_V	mm/sec	-0.3 ± 16.2	8.0 ± 12.5	<0.035
	I_V	%	0.7 ± 21.1	13.3 ± 16.1	<0.035

Table 6. Comparisons between NPH BEFORE and NPH AFTER – all parameters are included. Average values with standard deviations and significances p of nonparametric Wilcoxon paired test are given in appropriate table cells.

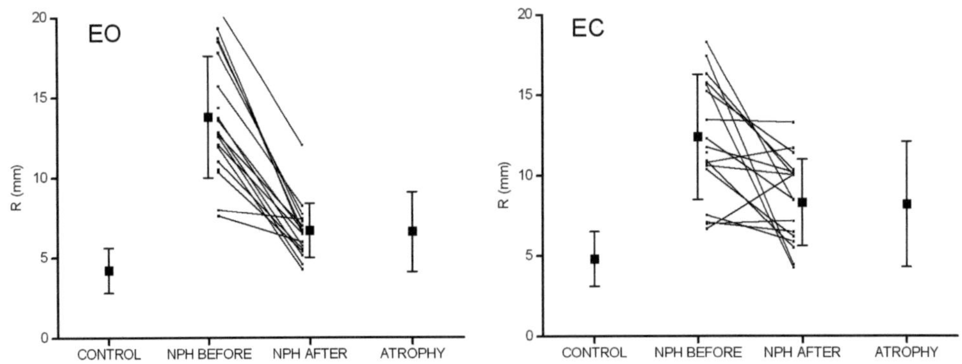

Fig. 9. Mean values of the sway Radius measured with eyes open (EO - left) and closed (EC - right) in NPH patients before and after surgery. Individual R values are given, they are connected with lines. CONTROL and ATROPHY groups are also shown to illustrate effect of shunting against wider background.

4.4 Impact of vision on postural sway characteristics

We introduced EC-EO differences and vision index for explaining in various groups the effect of eye opening or closure on sways. **Table 7** shows D_X and **Table 8** - I_X (where X can be R, AS, or V). The interpretation of differences D_X can be skipped here.

Most interesting features are the vision indices. They differentiate NPH BEFORE group from NPH AFTER and from any other group. **Table 8** shows three comparisons in pairs of groups. The groups NPH BEFORE - ATROPHY significantly differ as well as the NPH BEFORE - CONTROL groups do.

A direct comparison of EO and EC parameters in four groups independently is provided in **Table 9**. Sways with EO and EC seem to be equal in NPH BEFORE group only. In any other group there are significant changes of sways related to the eyes closure. Enlargement of sways is a normal phenomenon after closing eyes, but not in NPH patients in acute state.

Sways of NPH patients do not depend on the sight, they seem to be the same in EO and EC conditions. This observation is the most important result of this study.

4.5 Two dimension analysis – posturography

Much more insight into the data collected is provided in the two dimensional graph. There is four-group scattergram in **Figure 10**. One can see a separation of NPH BEFORE cases and the centroid from all other groups. A separation is statistically significant - see **tables 5** and **8** for NPH BEFORE - CONTROL and NPH BEFORE - ATROPHY data.

Differences		CONTROL	ATROPHY	NPH BEFORE
Radius D_R	AV ± SD mm	0.63 ± 1.19	1.67 ± 3.15	-1.49 ± 4.48
	CONTROL		n.s.	p < 0.013
	ATROPHY			p < 0.008
Area speed D_{AS}	AV ± SD mm²/sec	9.4 ± 17.7	51.7 ± 104.4	-18.7 ± 124.6
	CONTROL		p < 0.031 = n.s.	n.s.
	ATROPHY			p < 0.013
Velocity D_V	AV ± SD mm/sec	4.3 ± 5.7	10.3 ± 14.7	-0.3 ± 16.2
	CONTROL		p < 0.035 = n.s.	n.s.
	ATROPHY			p < 0.007

Table 7. Comparisons of differences D_R, D_{AS}, D_V among three groups in pairs of groups.

Indexes		CONTROL	ATROPHY	NPH BEFORE
Radius I_R	AV ± SD %	6.5 ± 12.1	9.3 ± 19.4	-6.09 ±18.9
	CONTROL		n.s.	p < 0.004
	ATROPHY			p < 0.005
Area speed I_{AS}	AV ± SD %	19.8 ± 23.5	22.1 ± 28.2	-5.2 ± 34.7
	CONTROL		n.s.	p < 0.004
	ATROPHY			p < 0.003
Velocity I_V	AV ± SD %	15.3 ± 13.4	16.3 ± 15.3	0.7 ± 21.1
	CONTROL		n.s.	p < 0.001
	ATROPHY			p < 0.002

Table 8. Comparisons of vision indices I_R, I_{AS}, I_V among three groups in pairs of groups.

Group	parameter		EO	EC	p
CONTROL	R	mm	4.2 ±1.4	4.9 ± 1.7	< 0.001
	AS	mm²/sec	13.3 ± 10.2	22.7 ± 22.6	< 0.001
	V	mm/sec	9.2 ± 4.4	13.5 ± 8.7	< 0.001
ATROPHY	R	mm	6.6 ± 2.5	8.2 ± 3.9	< 0.004
	AS	mm²/sec	56.1 ± 84.5	107.8 ± 175.6	< 0.001
	V	mm/sec	23.2 ± 23.4	33.5 ± 32.0	< 0.001
NPH BEFORE	R	mm	13.9 ± 3.8	12.4 ± 3.9	n.s.
	AS	mm²/sec	159.5 ± 104.6	140.8 ± 92.2	n.s.
	V	mm/sec	35.5 ± 17.7	35.2 ± 17.4	n.s.
NPH AFTER	R	mm	6.7 ± 1.7	8.3 ± 2.7	< 0.035
	AS	mm²/sec	37.9 ± 17.1	79.4 ± 77.9	< 0.014
	V	mm/sec	18.3 ± 7.4	26.3 ± 17.1	< 0.004

Table 9. Comparison of R, AS, and V parameters measured with EO and EC in CONTROL, ATROPHY, NPH BEFORE and NPH AFTER groups separately.

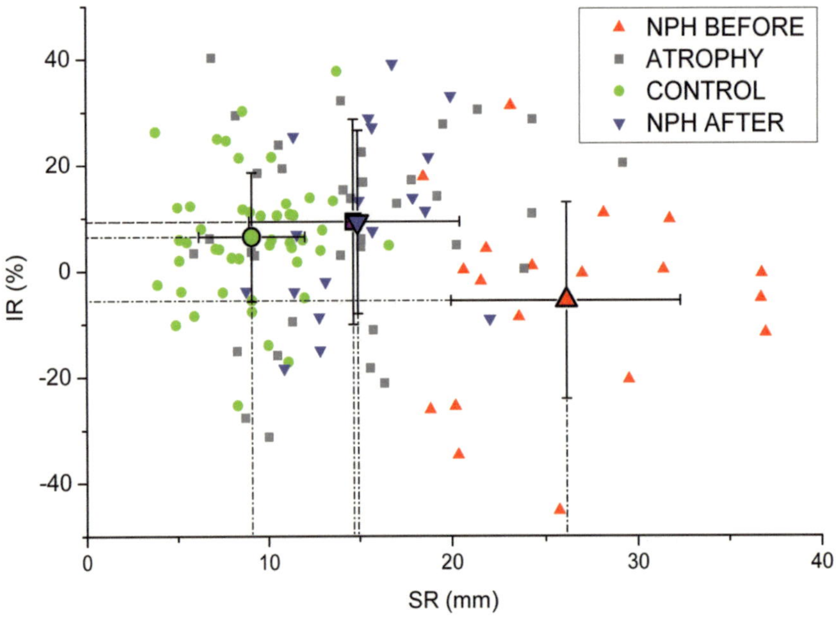

Fig. 10. Scattergram presents all cases in four groups: NPH BEFORE, ATROPHY, CONTROL, and NPH AFTER in I_R (vision index related to radius) versus S_R (sum of R_{EO} and R_{EC}) coordination system. Centroids of the groups are shown with standard deviations. Notice that ATROPHY and NPH AFTER group centroids do overlap.

Two dimensional statistical analysis was performed by means of methods described in the following section.

4.6 k-NN classification of posturografic parameters

All data was analysed by means of two methods: Discrimination Analysis (DA) and k nearest neighbours (K-NN) method. Both methods give similar results for most of classifications.

Feature is a single value of multidimensional vector assigned to any object/case/patient. Groups of patients are called classes within the "classification world". There are 15 features used here as follows: R_{EC}, R_{EO}, AS_{EC}, AS_{EO}, V_{EC}, V_{EO}, S_R, S_{AS}, S_V, D_R, D_{AS}, D_V, I_R, I_{AS}, and I_V, exactly as parameters.

The analysis was performed in several sections. At the beginning every feature was used, one at a time. Then features were grouped into pairs according to the templates: (X_{EO} and X_{EC}), (sums S_X and differences D_X), (sums S_X and vision indices I_X), where X can be R, AS, or V. Features related to R, AS and V were paired separately. Then clusters consisting of six features were applied.

We classified groups/classes in two following schemas – like in traditional analysis: 1) NPH BEFORE, ATROPHY and CONTROL 2) NPH BEFORE and NPH AFTER. Briefing of the classification results is presented below.

Single feature applied individually, classes: NPH BEFORE and NPH AFTER:

There were 15 DA classifications of NPH BEFORE and NPH AFTER classes and 15 K-NN classifications performed. R_{EO} demonstrated the best classification - both methods classified correctly 91.9%/91.9% cases (the first number relates to DA, the second to K-NN). Below there is a list of some best features with outcome better than 75%:

R_{EO}	91.9%/91.9%
S_R	86.5%/89.2%
A_{EO}	86.5%/83.8%
R_{EC}	78.4%/78.4%
S_{AS}	75.7%/78.4%
S_V	75.7%/75.7%

Classification power of vision indices was rather poor; the best was I_R: 67.6%/67.6%.

Two-feature pairs, classes: NPH BEFORE and NPH AFTER:

There were nine DA/K-NN classifications here, the best are:

(R_{EO},R_{EC})	91.9%/94.6%
(S_R,D_R)	91.9%/91.9%
(S_R,I_R)	91.9%/91.9%
(AS_{EO},AS_{EC})	83.8%/83.8%
(S_{AS},D_{AS})	83.8%/78.4%
(S_{AS},I_{AS})	86.5%/83.8%

It is interesting that there are three pairs of features with equal classification power. They relate to the analysis in two dimensions. Notice that (S_{AS},I_{AS}) and (S_{AS},D_{AS}) can be calculated from (AS_{EO},AS_{EC}) using formulas (2),(3), and (4). These dimensions are not completely independent because, for example in the CONTROL group the features R_{EO} and R_{EC} are correlated (R = 0.73); in other groups the correlation is not as high. An example of two-dimensional approach is shown in **Figure 10**.

Six-feature cluster without and with feature selection, classes: NPH BEFORE and NPH AFTER:

Multi-feature classification by K-NN method was also performed with the following features: S_R, S_{AS}, S_V, I_R, I_{AS}, and I_V. Classification without feature selection (all features forced to enter the analysis) resulted in 89.2% of correctly classified cases. Classification with automatic selection of "best" features resulted in 94.6%. The selected features: S_R and I_{AS}.

Single feature applied individually, classes: NPH BEFORE, ATROPHY, and CONTROL:

Three-group classification (NPH BEFORE, ATROPHY and CONTROL) using single features cannot be good both in DA and K-NN methods. The best results reached AS_{EO} - 77.4% of correct classified cases.

Two-feature pairs, classes: NPH BEFORE, ATROPHY, and CONTROL:

There were nine DA/K-NN classifications here, the best are:

(R_{EO},R_{EC})	75.5%/75.5%
(S_R,D_R)	75.5%/76.5%
(S_R,I_R)	73.5%/74.5%

Other pairs of features are worse. Again there is no difference between classification level among pairs (R_{EC}, R_{EO}), (S_R, D_R) and (S_R, I_R).

Six-feature cluster without and with feature selection, classes: NPH BEFORE, ATROPHY, and CONTROL:

DA/K-NN classifications without feature selection (all features forced to enter the analysis):

R_{EO}, R_{EC}, AS_{EO}, AS_{EC}, V_{EO}, V_{EC}	78.4%/73.5%
S_R, D_R, S_{AS}, D_{AS}, S_V, D_V	78.4%/74.5%
S_R, I_R, S_{AS}, I_{AS}, S_V, I_V	79.4%/73.5%

Classifications with feature selection - DA only:

R_{EO}, V_{EC}	80.4%
S_R, D_R	75.5%
S_R, I_R	73.5%

Features selected automatically during analysis were exactly the same as those selected manually during previous stages.

Classifications with feature selection - K-NN only:

R_{EO}, R_{EC}, AS_{EO}, AS_{EC}, V_{EO}	82.3%
S_R, D_R, D_{AS}, S_V	81.4%
S_R, I_{AS}, S_V	79.4%

Here better results were obtained.

Three-class K-NN classifier consist of three two-class sub-classifiers. The results of sub-classification are also interesting. Single feature: S_R demonstrates 100% correctly classified cases in NPH BEFORE - CONTROL sub- classifier. Selection of three features: R_{EO}, D_{AS} and DV classified correctly 94.6% cases in NPH BEFORE - ATROPHY sub- classifier what proofs the existence of **important difference between NPH and atrophy imbalance.** This observation is also an important result of the present study.

4.7 Analysis of gait parameters

Evaluation of gait is performed by means of five gait parameters: time of single supper (T_{SSUP}), time of double support (T_{DSUP}), time of stance (T_{STANCE}), length of single support (D_{SSUP}), and length of double support (D_{DSUP}). Initially ten parameters were involved; they were related to the left and right leg. Average values with standard deviations were plotted in **Figure 11**. Values of the parameters related to the left and right leg were compared statistically by means of nonparametric Wilcoxon paired test in each group separately. There was no difference found between legs. Therefore the outcomes from the left and right leg were combined - cases are not patients now but legs.

Parameter	χ^2 K-W	p
Time of single support (T_{SSUP}) sec	53.3	< 0.001
Time of double support (T_{DSUP}) sec	84.2	< 0.001
Time of stance (T_{STANCE}) sec	83.2	< 0.001
Length of single support(D_{SSUP})	107.3	< 0.001
Length of double support(D_{DSUP})	80.9	< 0.001

Table 10. Non-parametric ANOVA Kruskal-Wallis test for three groups: NPH BEFORE, ATROPHY, and CONTROL. n = 148.

Non-parametric ANOVA Kruskal-Wallis test was used again to compare three groups: NPH BEFORE, ATROPHY, and CONTROL. The results are in **Table 10**. The groups differ significantly for all parameters. This allows making post-hoc comparisons in pairs of groups, applying Bonferroni correction.

One can notice in **Table 11** that the T_{STANCE} is the biggest in NPH BEFORE group. This means slower gait of patients in acute state; time of stance phase T_{STANCE} is more than 130% longer than in CONTROL group (ratio: 1.61/0.68 = 2.36 of values in NPH BEFORE and CONTROL groups). ATROPHY patients show decreased walking pace compared with healthy people, however they have higher gait velocity than NPH BEFORE.

Duration of single support T_{SSUP} in NPH BEFORE group is 70% longer than in CONTROL group (ratio: 0.65/0.38 = 1.71). Duration of double support in NPH BEFORE group is 180% longer than in CONTROL group (ratio: 0.46/0.16 = 2.87). One can see differences in single and double support distributions. In NPH BEFORE group ratio: T_{SSUP} / T_{DSUP} = 0.65/0.46 = 1.41, in CONTROL group: T_{SSUP} / T_{DSUP} = 0.38/0.16 = 2.37. Double support is much longer not only if measured in seconds, but in relation to single support length. If comparing D_{SSUP} and D_{DSUP}, between NPH and CONTROL groups, one can observe strong reduction of single support length. For single support length D_{SSUP} there is a proportion: 1.64/7.13 = 0.23, for double support length D_{DSUP}: 6.28/11.54 = 0.54. ATROPHY group is always in the middle between NPH BEFORE and ATROPHY.

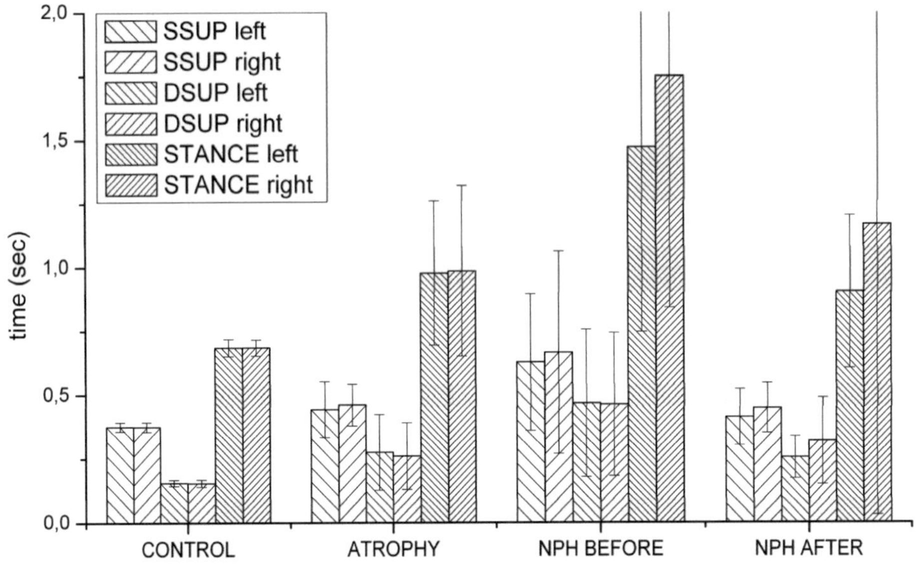

Fig. 11. Average values with standard deviations of times: T_{SSUP}, T_{DSUP}, T_{STANCE} in four groups.

Parameter			CONTROL	ATROPHY	NPH BEFORE
T_{SSUP}	AV ± SD	sec	0.38 ± 0.02	0.45 ± 0.10	0.65 ± 0.33
	CONTROL			< 0.001	< 0.001
	ATROPHY				< 0.001
T_{DSUP}	AV ± SD	sec	0.16 ± 0.01	0.27 ± 0.14	0.46 ± 0.28
	CONTROL			< 0.001	< 0.001
	ATROPHY				< 0.001
T_{STANCE}	AV ± SD	sec	0.68 ± 0.03	0.98 ± 0.31	1.61 ± 0.82
	CONTROL			< 0.001	< 0.001
	ATROPHY				< 0.001
D_{SSUP}	AV ± SD	cm	7.13 ± 0.53	3.29 ± 1.49	1.64 ± 1.17
	CONTROL			< 0.001	< 0.001
	ATROPHY				< 0.001
D_{DSUP}	AV ± SD	cm	11.54 ± 1.85	9.54 ± 1.77	6.28 ± 2.88
	CONTROL			< 0.001	< 0.001
	ATROPHY				< 0.001

Table 11. Comparisons of T_{SSUP}, T_{DSUP}, T_{STANCE}, D_{SSUP}, D_{DSUP} parameters in pairs of groups. Average values with standard deviations and significances p of Mann-Whitney U test are given in appropriate table cells. All differences are significant.

Group	parameter		BEFORE	AFTER	P
NPH n= 15	T_{SSUP}	sec	0.65 ± 0.33	0.42 ± 0.10	< 0.001
	T_{DSUP}	sec	0.46 ± 0.29	0.28 ± 0.14	< 0.001
	T_{STANCE}	sec	1.61 ± 0.82	1.03 ± 0.83	< 0.001
	D_{SSUP}	cm	1.64 ± 1.17	3.55 ± 1.31	< 0.001
	D_{SSUP}	cm	6.28 ± 2.88	8.54 ± 2.96	< 0.001

Table 12. Comparison between NPH BEFORE and NPH AFTER. Average values with standard deviations and significances p of nonparametric Wilcoxon paired test are given in appropriate table cells. All parameters: T_{SSUP}, T_{DSUP}, T_{STANCE}, D_{SSUP}, and D_{DSUP} differentiate significantly NPH stages. All differences are significant.

Parameter			CONTROL n=48	ATROPHY n=35	NPH AFTER n=34
T_{SSUP}	AV ± SD	sec	0.38 ± 0.02	0.45 ± 0.10	0.42 ± 0.10
	CONTROL				< 0.001
	ATROPHY				n.s.
T_{DSUP}	AV ± SD	sec	0.16 ± 0.01	0.27 ± 0.14	0.28 ± 0.13
	CONTROL				< 0.001
	ATROPHY				n.s.
T_{STANCE}	AV ± SD	sec	0.68 ± 0.03	0.98 ± 0.31	1.00 ± 0.78
	CONTROL				< 0.002
	ATROPHY				n.s.
D_{SSUP}	AV ± SD	cm	7.13 ± 0.53	3.29 ± 1.49	3.56 ± 1.28
	CONTROL				< 0.001
	ATROPHY				n.s.
D_{DSUP}	AV ± SD	cm	11.54 ± 1.85	9.54 ± 1.77	8.46 ± 2.79
	CONTROL				< 0.001
	ATROPHY				n.s.

Table 13. Comparisons of T_{SSUP}, T_{DSUP}, T_{STANCE}, D_{SSUP}, D_{DSUP} parameters in group-pairs. Average values with standard deviations and significances p of Mann-Whitney U test are given in appropriate table cells.

Direct comparison of gait parameters between BEFORE and AFTER states in NPH are given in **Table 12**. Because NPH BEFORE and NPH AFTER are paired groups, the Wilcoxon test was used to compare the gait. Differences of all parameters are statistically significant. **Figure 12** shows average values with standard deviations as well as individual values of T_{SSUP}, T_{DSUP}, T_{STANCE} in NPH patients before and after surgery.

After surgery gait of NPH patients resembles gait of patients with atrophy. **Table 13** shows that there is no statistical significant difference between NPH AFTER and ATROPHY groups.

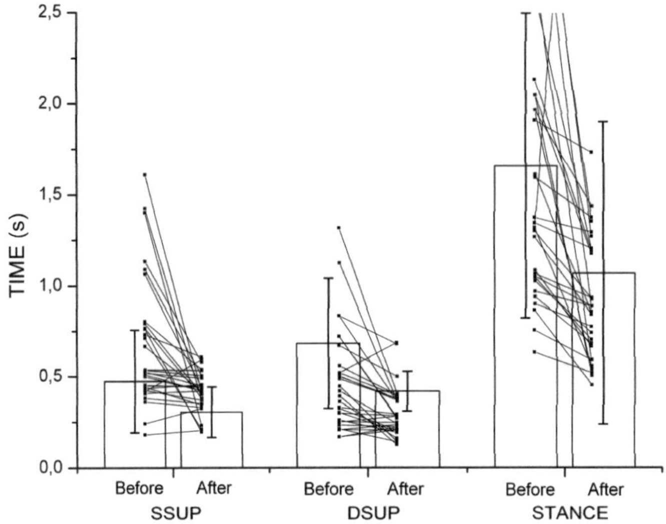

Fig. 12. Mean values of T_{SSUP}, T_{DSUP}, T_{STANCE} in NPH BEFORE and NPH AFTER groups. Individual values of these parameters are given, they are connected with lines. Values for both legs are combined.

4.8 k-NN classification of dynografic parameters

Dynographic parameters were analysed by means of k-NN method in 2008 (Czerwosz at al. 2008). Now the calculations should be repeated with larger number of subjects. Usage of pattern recognition methods can give chance for better evaluation of multi-parameter data.

5. Discussion and conclusions

There are three main theses that come out from this study:

1. Sways in NPH patients before shunting is much bigger than after surgery. This relates mostly to eyes open (EO) condition.
2. Sways of NPH patients do not depends on the sight, they seem to be the same in EO and EC conditions.
3. NPH and atrophy imbalances differ when evaluate by means of more than one parameter (feature). Pattern recognition methods should be used.

There are many proofs of strong relationship between vision and postural control. Vision has a greater influence on standing postural control, resulting in greater sway when individuals are presented with erroneous or conflicting visual cues (Redfern at al. 2001). In impairment of the vestibular system and possibly other sensing systems and probably in cerebellar ataxias, vision can help in balance recovery. In NPH we do not observe any improvement, there is some probability that vision can disturb maintenance of the balance. Interestingly the vision index was slightly negative in NPH BEFORE group, meaning that with eyes closed sways are smaller. Blomsterwall (Blomsterwall at al. 2000) found that healthy individual had a 29% better postural function with open eyes while NPH patients only improved their balance score by 18% with open eye. The impact of vision should be studied farther due to this discrepancy.

6. Acknowledgment

We would like to thank Adam Jóźwik for releasing his K-NN software.

This study was partially supported by grant from the Polish Ministry of Education and Science (Grant No. R13 041 02).

Research support was partially provided by the Biocentrum-Ochota project [POIG.02.03.00-00-003/09 - European Regional Development Fund, the Operational Programme "Innovative Economy" 2007-2013].

7. References

Baratto L, Morasso PG, Re C, Spada G. (2002) *A new look at posturographic analysis in the clinical context: sway-density versus other parameterization techniques.* Motor Control 6(3): 246-70.

Benda, B. J., Riley, P. O., & Krebs, D. E. (1994) *Biomechanical relationship between center of gravity and center of pressure during standing.* IEEE Transactions on Rehabilitation Engineering 2(1): 3-10.

Bertrani A, Cappello A, Benedetti MG, Simoncini L, Catani F. (1999) *Flat foot functional evaluation using pattern recognition of ground reaction data.* Clin Biomech (Bristol, Avon) 14(7): 484-93.

Bhargava P., Shrivastava P., & Nagariya S.P. (2007) *Assessment of changes in gait parameters and vertical ground reaction forces after total hip arthroplasty.* Indian J Orthop 41(2): 158–162.

Bloem B.R., Beckley D.J., Remler M.P. (1995). *Postural reflexes in Parkinson's disease during "resist" and "yield" tasks.* J. Neurol Sci 129: 109-119.

Blomsterwall E., Svantesson U., Carlsson U., Tullberg M., Wikkelsö C. (2000) *Postural disturbance in patients with normal pressure hydrocephalus.* Acta Neurol Scand 102: 284-291.

Błaszczyk J.W. (2008) *Sway ratio - a new measure for quantifying postural stability.* Acta neurobiologiae experimentalis 68 (1): 51-57.

Błaszczyk J.W., Michalski A. (2006). *Aging and postural stability.* Studies in Physical Culture and Tourism 13: 11-14.

Boon AJ, Tans JT, Delwel EJ, Egeler-Peerdeman SM, Hanlo PW, Wurzer HA et al. (1999) *Dutch Normal-Pressure Hydrocephalus Study: the role of cerebrovascular disease.* J Neurosurg 90(2):221-226.

Bosek, M., Grzegorzewski, B., Kowalczyk, A., Lubiński, I. (2005) *Degradation of postural control system as a consequence of Parkinson's disease and ageing.* Neuroscience letters 376(3), 215-20.

Czernicki Z., Szewczykowski J., Kunicki A., Śliwka S., Korsak-Śliwka J., Pawłowski G., Dziduszko J., Mempel E., Jurkiewicz J., Augustyniak B. (1984) *Computerized infusion test II. Clinical use.* Neurol. Neurochir Pol 18 (6): 561-565.

Czerwosz L., Szczepek E., Błaszczyk J.W., Sokołowska B., Dmitruk K., Dudziński K., Jurkiewicz J., Czernicki Z. (2009) *Analysis of postural sway in patients with normal pressure hydrocephalus: effects of shunt implantation.* European Journal of Medical Research 14 Supl 4: 53-58

Czerwosz L., Szczepek E., Sokołowska B., Jóźwik A., Dudziński K., Jurkiewicz J., Czernicki Z. (2008) *Recognition of gait disturbances in patients with normal pressure hydrocephalus using the Computer Dynography system.* Journal of Physiology and Pharmacology 59, Supl 6: 201-207.

Czosnyka M., Wollk-Laniewski P., Batorski L., Zaworski W. (1988) *Analysis of intracranial pressure waveform during infusion test.* Acta Neurochirurgica (Wien) 93, 3-4: 140-145.

Devijver P.A., Kittler J. (1982) *Pattern recognition: A statistical approach.* Prentice Hall, London.

Dmitruk K. (2005) *Analiza wybranych parametrów posturograficznych u ludzi w różnych grupach wiekowych.* Doctor distertation. Nicolaus Copernicus University, Collegium Medicum. Bydgoszcz (in Polish).

Duda R.O., Hart P.E., Stork D.G. (2001) *Pattern classification.* John Wiley & Sons, New York.

Dunn, O.J. (1961) *Multiple Comparisons Among Means.* Journal of the American Statistical Association 56, 52-64.

Evans W.A. (1942) *An Encephalographic Ratio for Estimating Ventricular Enlargement and Cerebral Atrophy.* Arch. Neurol. and Psych 47 (6): 931-937.

Galia G.L., Rigamonti D., Williams M.A. (2005) *The diagnosis and treatment of idiopathic normal pressure hydrocephalus.* Nature Clinical Practice Neurology 2: 375-381.

Hakim S., Adams R.D. (1965). *The Special Clinical Problem of Symptomatic Hydrocephalus with Normal Cerebrospinal Fluid Pressure.* J. Neurol. Sci. 2: 307-327.

IBM-SPSS Statistics. (n.d.) *PASW Statistics v. 18.(previously SPSS – Statistical Package for the Social Sciences).* http://www-01.ibm.com/software/analytics/spss/products/statistics.

Infotronic Company (2007) *Ultraflex system.* Available from: http://www.infotronic.nl/Brochures/English/Model-English-CEGV2-2007.pdf.

Jagielski J., Kubiczek-Jagielska M., Sobstyl M., Koziara H., Błaszczyk J., Ząbek M., Zaleski M. (2006). *Posturography as objective evaluation of the balance system in Parkinson's disease patients after neurosurgical treatment. A preliminary report.* Neurol Neurochir Pol. 40(2): 127-33. In Polish.

Jeleń P., Wit P., Dudziński K., Nolan L. (2008) *Expressing gait-line symmetry in able-bodied gait.* Dynamic Medicine 7:17.

Jóźwik A., Sokołowska B., Nieboj-Dobosz I., Janik P., Kwieciński H. (2011) *Extraction of biomedical traits for patients with amyotrophic lateral sclerosis using parallel and hierarchical classifiers.* International Journal of Biometrics 3, 1: 85-94.

Kaczmarczyk K., Wit A., Krawczyk M., Zaborski J. (2009) *Gait classification in post-stroke patients using artificial neural networks.* Gait & Posture 30: 207–210.

Kessler N., Ganança M.M., Ganança C.F. Ganança F.F., Lopes S.C., Serra A.P., Caovilla H.H. (2011). *Balance Rehabilitation Unit (BRUTM) posturography in relapsing-remitting multiple sclerosis.* Arq. Neuro-Psiquiatr. 69, 3: 485-490.

Kruskal and Wallis (1952) *Use of ranks in one-criterion variance analysis.* Journal of the American Statistical Association 47 (260): 583–621.

Kubisz L., Werner H., Bosek M., Weiss W. (2011) *Posture Stability Evaluation Using Static Posturography in Patients after Cruciate Ligament Reconstruction.* Acta Physica Polonica 119: 957-960.

Maduko E. *Pattern recognition of human gait signatures.* (n.d.) University of Texas at El Paso. Available from: http://faculty.utep.edu/Portals/1255/Elizabeth.pdf.

Majumdar K., Lenka P.K., Kumar R. (2008) *Variability of Gait Parameters of Unilateral Trans-tibial Amputees in Different Walking Speeds.* Indian Journal of Physical Medicine and Rehabilitation 19 (2): 37-42.

Mohan G., Pal P.K., Sendhil K.R., Thennarasu K., Usha B.R. (2009). *Quantitative evaluation of balance in patients with spinocerebellar ataxia type 1: A case control study.* Parkinsonism and Related Disorders 15 (6): 435-439.

Mraz M., Curzytek M., Mraz M.A., Gawron W., Czerwosz L., Skolimowski T., (2007) *Body balance in patients with systemic vertigo after rehabilitation exercises.* J.Physiol Pharmacol 58 (5): 427-436.

Olton J., Czerwosz L. (2006) *Posturograf firmy Pro-Med,* Acta Bio-Optica et Informatica Medica. Inżynieria Biomedyczna 12: 143. (Article in Polish)

Origin Corporation. (n.d.) *Origin-pro software v. 8.* Available from: http://www.originlab.com/index.aspx?go=PRODUCTS/OriginPro.

Perry J., Burnfield J.M. (2010) *Gait Analysis. Normal and Pathological Function.* Slack Inc., Thorofare, New Jersey Second Edition.

Raymakers J.A., Samson M.M., Verhaar H.J.J. (2005) *The assessment of body sway and the choice of the stability parameter(s).* Gait and Posture 21 48–58.

Ravdin L.D., Heather L. Katzen Anna E. Jackson, Diamanto Tsakanikas, Stephanie Assuras, and Norman R. Relkin (2008) *Features of gait most responsive to tap test in normal pressure hydrocephalus.* Clin Neurol Neurosurg. 110(5): 455–461.

Redfern M.S., Yardley L., Bronstein A.M. (2001) *Visual influences on balance.* Anxiety Disorders 15: 81- 94.

Sokołowska B., Jóźwik A., Nieboj-Dobosz I., Janik P., Kwieciński H. (2009) *Evaluation of matrix metalloproteinases in serum of patients with amyotrophic lateral sclerosis with pattern recognition methods.* Journal of Physiology and Pharmacology 60 (suppl 5): 117-120.

Stolze H., Kuhtz-Buschbeck J.P., Drücke H., Jöhnk K., Illert M., Deuschl G. (2001) *Comparative analysis of the gait disorder of normal pressure hydrocephalus and Parkinson's disease.* J Neurol Neurosurg Psychiatry 70:289–297.

Szczepek E., Czerwosz L., Dąbrowski P., Dudziński K., Jurkiewicz J., Czernicki Z. (2008) *Posturography and computerized gait analysis in the Computer Dyno Graphy system as non-invasive methods for evaluation of normal pressure hydrocephalus progression.* Neurologia i Neurochirurgia Polska 42, 2: 139–152. (Article in polish)

Śliwka S., Pawłowski G., Korsak-Śliwka J., Szewczykowski J., Czernicki Z. (1984) *Computerized infusion test I. The method.* Neurol Neurochir Pol, 18 (6): 553-560.

Tans J.T.J. (1979) *Differentiation of normal pressure hydrocephalus and cerebral atrophy by computed tomography and spinal infusion test.* Journal of Neurology 222, 2: 109-118.

Voss K., Imhof J., Kaestner S., Montavon P.M. (2007) *Force plate gait analysis at the walk and trot in dogs with low-grade hindlimb lameness.* Vet Comp Orthop Traumatol, 20: 229-304.

Wöber C., Wöber-Bingo C., Karwautz A., Nimmerrichter A, Walter H. and Deecke L. (1998). *Aataxia of stance in different types of alcohol dependence – a posturographic study.* Alcohol & Alcoholism 33, 4: 393-402.